Mastering LEPTIN

THIRD EDITION

Byron J. Richards, CCN

with **Mary Guignon Richards**

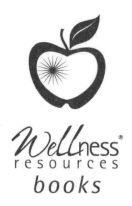

Wellness®
resources
books

NOTE TO READERS

The information presented in this book is for educational and informational purposes. It is not intended as a diagnoses or treatment of any medical condition. The information given is not medical advice nor is it presented as a course of personalized treatment. Before changing any medical treatment or before discontinuing any course of medical treatment you may now be undergoing, you should consult your physician. The reader should not stop prescription medications without the advice and guidance of his or her personal physician. Any application of the material set forth in the following pages is at the reader's discretion and sole responsibility.

MASTERING LEPTIN
Third Edition

Published by Wellness Resources Books
A division of Wellness Resources, Inc.
www.wellnessresources.com, www.masteringleptin.com
Minneapolis, Minnesota 55439 U.S.A.

Printed in the United States of America

International Standard Book Number: 978-1-933927-25-1
Previous Edition International Standard Book Number: 0-9727121-2-9
Library of Congress Control Number: 2002117389

This book is dedicated to
those who wish to take charge
of their health and help their friends
and family to do the same.

For leptin news, weight loss tips, and natural health options,
visit www.wellnessresources.com/leptin or call 800-717-9355

CONTENTS

INTRODUCTION

THE INFORMATION IN THIS BOOK represents one of the most significant advancements in our understanding of health in recent times.

As a clinician and a health educator on the leading edge of applied clinical nutrition, we have had the opportunity to help many thousands of people achieve a better level of health. We have been a place of last resort for many individuals over the years, those unable to be helped by the traditional Western medical approach.

We solve tough problems. This makes it much easier for us to help people who are not having difficult issues. Certainly, the consumer demand to understand natural options for health has never been higher.

The information in this book is truly groundbreaking. We can say this because we work day in and day out on the front lines. We know what is going on in our field. We know what is being told to the public and what is being taught to our peers.

The significant undertaking of reading, understanding, compiling, and coordinating thousands of current studies, including the most recent and up-to-date ones, makes this work truly unique. Its usefulness will be broadly realized because so many people in search of answers to their health issues will find solutions here. This has been our mission, our purpose for tackling this tremendous undertaking: to help as many people as possible to live healthier, thus happier lives.

The general public has no workable way to figure out what to eat, let alone how to lose weight and keep it off. America is getting fatter and sliding down a path of poor health. There exists an ever-growing epidemic of obesity and diabetes in our society, never before seen. Overall health problems are getting worse. Disease is more rampant than ever. Real solutions are lacking.

This problem is about to change with the information in this book. The discovery of leptin in 1994 marked a major change in traditional theories of health. Leptin is a powerful hormone: it controls and permits other hormones to function – or not function.

The discovery of leptin and what it means, now backed by undeniable science, puts to rest some of the oldest arguments about the nature of disease itself. We now know that malfunctioning genes and leptin, overburdened by a variety of stressors, are the actual cause of disease.

Restoring these genes and related hormonal rhythms to a condition of healthy function will dramatically improve the quality of health of any person who chooses to follow this path. If enough individuals in society follow this path, then health care costs will plummet and the so-called diseases of aging will greatly decrease.

There is no longer a need to look for the cause of these diseases. There is only a need to work out the best approach to solving them.

Mary and I have been working with people to help them solve health issues for over twenty years. We have wanted to write a book for many years, but have not had the time. Between developing and running a busy practice, raising children, and everything else that goes on in life, it just was not practical. Several years ago, we finally decided we would make the time to write our book; we knew it was the right time.

I am very proud of how Mary has taken care of herself over the years. It is not that she has had a stress-free life; far from it. She runs our busy business, has raised four children, and has helped me more than anyone could imagine.

Our cover picture was taken four months after Mary's fiftieth birthday, yet she looks much younger. She is full of energetic vitality, has no hormonal issues at menopause, is at her optimum body weight and maintaining it, and has never had a significant illness or disease.

This is a true testament to the workability of what we are teaching. The principles in this book work in the real world; they help solve real problems. Even healthy people will benefit by applying the information in this book, by slowing down the rate of aging and preventing disease.

Our initial idea for a book was to write on the subject of how to age without wear and tear. A big part of this was going to be about getting to a proper body weight and staying there. We have a tremendous amount of knowledge and experience in these areas.

As we began to put this book together and document how our program works in terms of the scientific rationale, it became clear we would need to tackle the monumental task of explaining leptin to the general public, a task that has not been done before.

There are over five thousand published scientific articles on the subject of leptin. Many of these studies seem conflicting and are rather confusing. One minute leptin was good, the next minute it was bad.

Leptin was a big problem for a fat mouse, yet it was not really a problem for overweight people, or was it? Was it causing diabetes or preventing diabetes? Was it causing cancer or preventing cancer? Was it causing heart disease or preventing heart disease? Was it causing hormonal problems or was it the problem itself? Was it fostering pregnancy or causing infertility? Or did it not matter one way or the other?

The contradictions were overwhelmingly interesting and intriguing. Thus began a journey that will forever change the way we view health.

In a sense, it felt as if we had struck gold. Everything began to come together, like a complex puzzle falling into place. As we figured out the complexity of leptin, we could apply it to everything we had learned in the past twenty years. We now understood even more clearly the specific nature of weight problems, hormonal problems, fibromyalgia, thyroid problems, metabolic syndrome X, heart disease, and cancer. We saw the true significance of this information we had uncovered.

Mary and I have been an inseparable team. We are an example of the whole being greater than the sum of its parts. In this book, I have done the highly technical research, study, and compilations. Mary has helped to turn it into plain English, ensuring its clarity, applicability, and usefulness. Her unique skills and experience, her compassion and intelligence, enable her to teach people to become more empowered with information that can improve their lives.

Writing this book was a difficult and sometimes grueling task, as the information regarding leptin is highly technical and complex and does not follow simplistic cause-and-effect thinking. While we may wish our bodies worked in simplistic ways, they do not.

Health is a reflection of an elegant and harmonic symphony of well-coordinated rhythm and timing. A healthy body is reflected in the efficiency and quality of millions of simultaneous and synchronized events. Leptin is the guiding energetic regulator that permits this to happen properly.

We have gone to great lengths to provide the appropriate scientific references to document this information and these discoveries, with over seven hundred scientific studies referenced. Enjoy and learn from an amazing array of up-to-date scientific findings at the cutting edge of modern science.

With the evaluation and interpretation of this breakthrough science, and placing it in its applicable context, this book will become a useful tool for every reader.

Our main goal for undertaking this project is to help the general public to make constructive changes in a wide variety of ways that directly affect health, to become more educated about their health, and to be better able to take charge of it.

With the introduction of the term Health Asset Manager™ as an essential concept in health self-care, we teach the importance of taking charge of one's health, thus making possible an improved quality of life.

This information directly relates to overcoming our societal issue of obesity. However, it is a great deal more than that. It is the essence of quality health in all areas.

Our extensive documentation makes this book an excellent reference tool for any student or health professional who wants to get up to speed on the subject of leptin, to understand its importance and role in overall health and how to master it.

It is our hope that our readers will pass a copy of this book along to their physicians. This information is not yet known – not known by the general public and not known by doctors and other health-care practitioners. No doctor can do an ongoing good job without understanding the many ramifications of leptin for health and disease and for the numerous medications they prescribe on a daily basis. The information on leptin is of primary importance to every aspect of medicine and quality of medical care.

The time we have put into this book causes us to remember why we never had time to write a book in the first place. Nevertheless, we managed to finish our project.

We are very proud to be the first to explain the diverse nature of leptin and how important *Mastering Leptin* is to the health and well being of everyone.

It is our wish that this book brings you more knowledge and useable health information, so that you and your loved ones may live a healthier and happier life, now, and into the future.

Byron Richards
December 2002

TWO YEARS LATER

It has been a little over two years since our first edition of *Mastering Leptin* was released to the public. During that time the number of leptin studies in scientific literature has jumped from 5,000 to over 8,800. Brilliant scientific research is unraveling the complexity of leptin and pinpointing its precise mechanisms of operation. There is a worldwide scientific push to gain a much better understanding of obesity and related disease.

Our government has announced that 365,000 people are now dying each year of obesity-related preventable disease. Heart disease, diabetes, and cancer are directly caused by leptin-induced obesity. Obesity may soon overtake smoking as the number-one cause of preventable death in America.

In addition to mortality, quality of life is seriously affected even in people who are simply overweight and not obese: fatigue, stress, depression, sleep apnea, snoring, and arthritis are just a few of the inflammatory problems directly caused by obesity.

The health of the mother before conception, during pregnancy, and following birth are now moving to the forefront of medical concern. Mastering Leptin is the first writing to explain the dramatic nature of these pregnancy-related discoveries and how they can help countless women have healthy pregnancies and give birth to children who are much less likely to become obese.

A frequent comment from many readers of our book is, "I asked my doctor about leptin and he had never heard of it before." In reality, this is a rather sad commentary on the current state of Western medicine in our society. It shows very clearly that science is far ahead of the type of medical care a person receives when walking into a doctor's office.

Leptin's role in health is not passive or secondary. Drugs given to "manage the symptoms" of a problem frequently adversely interact with leptin, making underlying health problems worse. Yet, the very individuals responsible for delivering medical care do not understand the current science about what they are doing.

It is not that there is one poorly done leptin study hidden away in the scientific literature. There are thousands of studies, many conducted by the finest scientists in the world, with the most sophisticated genetic research tools available.

The sobering truth is that doctors do not know about leptin because they have not been given a leptin drug to prescribe. And if they did have a leptin drug, it would be administered based on a lab-test number on paper, with a limited understanding of what is going on inside the body. Current medical care is based on drug-dispensing guidelines, not on an understanding of how the body works and how its problems can be fixed so that they actually go away.

State governments pass medical licensing laws that pass as officially sanctioned care. The American public is currently stuck with a care system based on unsafe drug dispensing; this is the legal standard for health management. This system is driven by the marketing and profits of drug companies. It is in the best interest of these companies to sell drugs and to convince as many people as possible to take drugs. It is in their best interest to suppress any competition. Out-of-control health care costs, unhealthy people, and a monopoly on the primary-care options given to the majority are a dream come true for these companies and their bottom line. Is this in the best health interests of individuals?

The discoveries relating to leptin show the glaring weakness of the American health system. Leptin science, which is relevant to virtually anything a doctor does, is widely unknown by the practicing medical profession.

Our idea of individuals empowering themselves to become better informed about their own health and thus make better decisions for themselves, is more vital than ever.

We have been flooded with stories of personal health improvement by those following *The Leptin Diet* guidelines in our book. This has been very gratifying.

The explosion in leptin science since our first printing has served to validate the principles we outlined. Confirmation of leptin's involvement in thyroid issues is now firmly documented.

A wealth of new information is uncovering the precise communication strategies leptin employs to carry out its diverse regulation of the energy systems in the human body. Of particular interest is the explosion of information regarding uncoupling proteins. These are a primary tool leptin uses to enhance metabolism and prevent obesity and heart disease.

Serious dangers regarding the ingestion of MSG and its contribution to the obesity epidemic can now be understood. All pregnant and lactating women should make it a priority to avoid MSG. The reality is that MSG should be removed from the food supply. It is an unsafe neurotoxin that dysregulates leptin and contributes to obesity and therefore disease. Since 2004 this problem has become crystal clear in the scientific literature. It took American health officials ten years to admit that folic acid should be given to prevent fifty thousand neural tube defects a year. Considering we are facing an obesity epidemic, how long will the public warnings take this time?

Many of the new studies on leptin focus on cardiovascular health. It is now recognized in the scientific literature that leptin problems are a primary cause of cardiovascular disease. Leptin problems are directly involved with high cholesterol, high blood pressure, and risk for stroke and heart attack. Doctors are complacently handing out cardiovascular medication without understanding of the most current underlying scientific principles actually causing the problems. While they are asleep on their watch, heart disease continues to be the number-one killer in America.

Individuals have many options for improving health. These options are grounded in new science. It is science based on restoring health by fixing problems in natural balance. Drugs will always have a relevant place, but not as a prime force in solving the emerging obesity epidemic and preventing the hundreds of thousands of deaths each year that are the direct consequence of preventable and reversible obesity. Constructive and consistent individual actions are the only remedy. Either we either take effective personal action, or collectively as a society we will drain our nation's energetic vibrancy, quality of health, and financial resources by paying for the care of all those who did not take responsibility for themselves. There is no quick fix for obesity.

Mastering Leptin is more important than ever. In our second edition, we have integrated many of the key recent studies as well as expanded diet-related tips to help individuals stay on track. We have added 90 pages and cited over 130 of the newest and most relevant scientific findings.

It is vital that individuals stand up for health freedom and free access to nutritional options. Nutritional science offers tremendous potential to help solve the obesity epidemic and break out of a rut of inefficient metabolism and yo-yo dieting. Readers of our book are consistently asking for more supplement guidelines and information, which we have provided at Wellness Resources for over twenty years.

Leptin is incredibly complex: thus, living in harmony with it involves at least a basic understanding of how it works and how it relates to stress eating, disease risk, thyroid function, food cravings, weight loss, and preventing the yo-yo diet problem.

If you have read various health books while trying to solve a variety of problems, you will find *Mastering Leptin* quite refreshing. Truly understanding this book takes some focus and energy. Our book goes far deeper than the typical diet book, which merely introduce basic ideas. *Mastering Leptin* links diet directly to disease and actually explains it in plain English.

If this is your first health book, many of the terms will be new. The chapters are written in a sequence that builds understanding. Many people who truly want to understand *Mastering Leptin* read it several times, as it is packed with information. If you just want a quick way to get started on a healthy diet, read chapters 14 and 27. Then start at the beginning and work your way through.

Mastering Leptin offers true hope for individuals who have struggled with body weight. Finally there are answers that do not rely on some type of fad diet. *The Leptin Diet* is a common-sense way to eat that enables metabolism to run faster on less food. It improves energy, mood, vitality, and the feeling of good health, and significantly reduces the risk for the primary diseases of aging.

Byron Richards
February 2005

SIX YEARS LATER

Mastering Leptin has taken on a life of its own, and continues to be widely read. When we first wrote the book it was hastily sent to press as we were so excited to be the first to explain leptin and the Leptin Diet® to the general lay public. The Third Edition of *Mastering Leptin* has been freshly edited from cover to cover, making it much easier for you to read.

The information in this book remains accurate and timely, a testament to the validity of our interpretation of emerging research. While many in today's world continue to struggle with metabolism and obesity, many thousands of others have found *Mastering Leptin* – opening the door to a whole new world of weight-loss solutions that really work.

There are now over 15,000 studies relating to leptin in the scientific literature. For the latest information on leptin please visit my website at www.WellnessResources.com. Here you will find the latest studies and news on leptin, thyroid, weight loss, and many other health topics of importance.

Be in the know! Take charge of your health and learn to master leptin – you health depends on it.

Byron Richards
January 2009

PART ONE

The Scope of Leptin

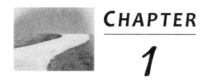

CHAPTER

1

The Most Powerful
Hormone in the Human Body

THE TWENTIETH CENTURY saw Americans transformed from fit to fat. Scientific advancements have enabled many Americans to live longer but not necessarily healthier. Heart disease, cancer, obesity, diabetes, osteoporosis, and serious age-related mental decline, including Alzheimer's, are problems that plague our society and show no signs of improvement.

The cost to treat these problems is staggering in terms of the money spent on care, the burden placed on caretakers, rising health-care costs, lost productivity, and the personal loss of quality of life.[1]

Surgeon General David Satcher calls obesity in America an epidemic. Two out of three American adults are classified as overweight or obese, compared with one in four in the early 1960s. A person is obese who weighs twenty percent more than the maximum healthy body weight.

Our nation's health-care costs jumped to $1.424 trillion in 2001, up from $1.310 trillion in 2000. Health-care spending averages about $5,000 per person. Prescription-drug spending comprises $140 billion of total health spending: obesity, which is a preventable disease, accounts for $117 billion per year. The prescription-drug and obesity costs are directly related to individuals not keeping themselves in a healthy condition of natural balance.

When individuals fail to make good personal health choices during the course of their life, it affects more than just themselves and their families. There is a significant economic burden to society as well.

A recent study published in the *Journal of the American Medical Association* shows that the consequences of being overweight are worse than previously known, causing significantly reduced lifespan. If a person is overweight at age forty, life is shortened by three years. If a person is obese at age forty, it shortens life by six-seven years. If an overweight person also smokes, it shortens life by thirteen years. If obesity starts at a younger age, the problem is even worse. The life of a twenty-year-old obese male is shortened by thirteen years.

Health officials plead with the public to eat better and exercise more, a plea falling on deaf ears. The need for a real solution to these problems has never been more important.

THE SCIENTIFIC BREAKTHROUGH SOLUTION

Somewhat quietly, at the end of the twentieth century, a hormone called leptin was discovered. The immense importance of this hormone was not immediately recognized. In fact, all that it does is not yet fully understood.

One thing is very clear: mastering leptin transforms the subjects of weight management and disease prevention in an astounding way, opening the door for solving many major health issues that afflict the majority of Americans.

THE POWER OF LEPTIN

Leptin is the hormone secreted by fat cells contained in white adipose tissue. It is the most significant hormone that exists, in terms of understanding the function of the human body.

Leptin is essential for survival. It has a regulating effect on other hormones, not in a passive way but as a prime controlling signal. Leptin tells thyroid hormones, adrenal hormones, pancreatic hormones, and sex hormones how to perform. Leptin can function without any help from these other hormones, but these other hormones cannot function properly without leptin.

This new information reveals that leptin is the single most important hormone known to humankind. Interestingly, it was not discovered until 1994, and its comprehensive role has not been written about for broad public knowledge.

Leptin is secreted by white adipose tissue, the undesirable fat that accumulates on the abdomen, buttocks, and thighs. What was once considered something to liposuction out of the body is now seen as a most important endocrine organ. This is a rather amazing turn of events.

LEPTIN PROBLEMS

Leptin is responsible for bizarre and erratic behavior and cravings related to food, including the inability to attain and maintain a healthy body weight. Leptin is essential for survival; without it, the human race would have perished from starvation long ago. However, in the land of food on every corner, it is also the hormone that fuels addictive and compulsive behavior. It is the reason why individuals will "start their diet tomorrow".

The food pyramid, even though its creators may have been well intentioned, is an eating method that induces serious health issues. There is one healthy way to eat. It is a way that maximizes the efficient function of leptin. All this information is new. Low-fat diets are incredibly destructive, as are high-fat diets. Understanding leptin finally puts to rest the conflicting diet information that is currently running rampant in society.

Problems with leptin set the stage for serious health issues. In addition to obesity, this includes anorexia, immune problems, bone loss, gastrointestinal problems, liver problems, cognitive problems, nerve problems, heart disease, and cancer.

Leptin is a hormone; it carries on communication within your body. Leptin-related problems occur as a result of a breakdown in communication. In some cases, this means not enough leptin; in other cases, it means too much leptin.

When leptin problems are magnified, there is a serious risk for disease. Leptin problems cause excess internal friction, meaning that cells in general begin to "overheat" or become overly stressed. This sets the stage for serious disease.

SUMMARY

Anyone who wishes to be healthy while growing older would be wise to learn what leptin is all about. We are entering a new era of health and wellness, wherein the understanding of genes and molecules can be translated into tangible and realistic ways to improve health.

There is no need to wait for some startling drug discovery to improve life. The information is already available, and the tools for improvement already exist.

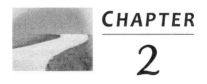

CHAPTER
2

Be a Health Asset Manager™

QUALITY OF HEALTH is our most important asset. Everyone should know enough about health to stay on a good track and have appropriate solutions in the event that health problems arise. We need to be able to think for ourselves, make correct decisions, and take effective action.

In terms of health, this requires an ability to understand one's own body and to have enough knowledge to implement solutions to keep on a healthy track. This is the bare minimum expertise required to stay in charge of one's own health.

Understanding leptin will help improve health IQ. There is no simplistic and false leptin premise like there is with "good" and "bad" cholesterol. Too many Americans are illiterate on the subject of health, a sad state of affairs directly contributing to out-of-control health-care costs and burdens. Many Americans have poor ability to implement even rudimentary health data and to translate it into correct action.

There is only one solution to these problems, on both an individual and a society-wide basis: that is for individuals to learn to become much more responsible for their own health. This means having the knowledge and skills to manage the most important personal asset, health. We call this becoming a *Health Asset Manager*.

DO NOT BECOME PART OF THE PROBLEM
People are continuing to get fatter and unhealthier. Four hundred

thousand Americans a year die from obesity-related issues.[2,3] It does not matter how much public-health officials warn us about the need to exercise and eat better; the majority of people in America cannot seem to get on track and stay there.

In order to improve personal health we must be able to think with health data. This requires a whole set of correct ideas relating to health and the ability to implement those ideas. Without intelligent health decision-making our country's health-care woes and costs will continue to spiral out of control.

Empowering yourself with useful knowledge is the first step to becoming a competent *Health Asset Manager*.

ON THE CUTTING EDGE OF SCIENCE

Much of the information in this book is new, even to health professionals. A new health paradigm will evolve from this information, one focusing on solutions that are in the best health interests of the individual.

There must also be a framework in one's mind for evaluating health information. If, every time there is a health problem, all one does is "follow the advice of my doctor," then that is the individual's personal health paradigm. Such advice may be good or bad, but that person's thinking ends there.

In the new health paradigm, individuals will need to take charge of their own health. This is a much greater level of personal responsibility, especially in non-emergency situations. This means understanding options, doing personal research on the pros and cons of any important decision, fitting the information discovered into a workable way of thinking about optimum health, and initiating life skills adequate to implement knowledge in order to get health-producing results.

Scientific health discoveries are happening at a breakneck pace. It is sometimes years before essential discoveries are implemented in day-to-day health care. Many traditional ways of looking at health information are quickly becoming obsolete, even though drugs continue to be prescribed that are not in harmony with current science.

For example, there is a tremendous amount of new and astounding scientific information about what is happening at the cellular level in terms of molecules, genes, and disease processes. Virtually all drugs on the market today have been approved for safe use without ample or any consideration given to this important science. It already costs drug companies millions of dollars to bring a drug to the market. Now that there is new science which gives new meaning to "safe," what should be done to verify safe use of current drugs?

These are political and financial questions, and the powers that be will not wish to revisit the safety of already approved medications. In many cases, it is not difficult to figure out which medications should be on the dangerous list. At the conclusion of this book, it will be clear why any medication that causes weight gain as a side effect or makes insulin resistance worse, and there are many, is a contributing causative factor to major diseases, when a person uses them over time. For the consumer, it places new emphasis on actually needing a medication before simply taking it on an ongoing basis.

THE FUNDAMENTALS OF BEING A COMPETENT *HEALTH ASSET MANAGER*

Here are the key points about thinking with health data and making good personal health decisions. These are useful ideas to guide decisions and integrate information in a productive way. These tools for thinking with health data will enable you to process health information more effectively, so that your most important personal asset, your own health, can be properly cared for.

Individual responsibility for health decisions.

Gone are the days of relying on anyone else but ourselves, at least in the final analysis. Information and education are the keys to personal empowerment. Asking intelligent questions and not robotically following instructions will be a hallmark of this approach.

There usually is one individual in the family, frequently the mother, who will learn this way of thinking and act as a valuable resource for other family members. The advantage here is that this individual has only the best health interest of the other family members in mind.

The quick-fix mentality is replaced with proactive health behavior. Society is currently conditioned to believe that there is a drug for everything. But, there will never be a single drug that stops bone loss. An individual is not going to arrive at age fifty-five, discover there is a bone-loss issue, take a drug, and solve the problem.

The handwriting has been on the wall for over twenty years. Stress, lack of fitness, not enough sleep, overeating, undereating, and lifestyle abuse are among the many factors that contribute to the problem. Problems with leptin are a major cause of bone loss.

The solution involves learning to master leptin. Following a healthy lifestyle is the underlying foundation in this new way of looking at health. This is a lifelong commitment to a healthy lifestyle.

Relational thinking will dominate over cause-and-effect thinking. Virtually all of Western medicine is based on cause-and-effect thinking. Name the illness or disease, and name the drug. Medicate the problem, or operate on the problem. Apply as many such treatments as possible to increase the statistical chance of improvement. This has resulted in the evolution of a long list of specialists, who scrutinize cause and effect in narrow areas of health, frequently ignoring consequences or relevant information in other aspects of health.

This way of thinking is important for specific problems that have defined causes (a small percentage of actual health issues). Our lawsuit-happy culture leads medical practitioners to use progressively invasive methods attempting to find a cause that frequently does not exist. It also leads to excessive and harsh treatments for problems, just to be on the "safe side."

It is evident that the human body functions in a complex and inter-related way, wherein multiple mechanisms are at work at the same time. In many situations, the "cause" is an inability of the body to tolerate the effects of multiple stressors. This results in symptoms that defy cause-and-effect thinking.

The ability to figure out what these interrelationships mean is an important part of "health intelligence." Leptin is the key hormonal signal that crosses virtually all areas of body function. It is the key that unravels the great mysteries of health.

Healthy function and efficiency are far more important than number management.

Currently, a great deal of emphasis is placed on using drugs to force certain numbers on lab tests into normal range. This includes blood pressure, cholesterol, and clotting times, to name a few. In the new way of looking at health, numbers that are out of range will be viewed as symptoms of an imbalance in the body, not the cause of a problem. Improving numbers by improving healthy function will be a sign of a skilled health practitioner.

Drugs will be used primarily as temporary solutions, as needed, until healthy function can be restored. By asking the doctor how long you must take a medication, or what else can be done so the medication is not needed, or how willing the doctor is to work on employing other solutions, you can quickly tell if this is the type of doctor wanted on your health team.

When a doctor can helpfully and intelligently answer such questions, you can have confidence that their training and areas of expertise include a more synergistic and functional understanding of health. This gives you more options for integrating a variety of strategies to improve issues and get on a healthy course of action.

It will be decades before the general medical profession has this level of knowledge and expertise, even though it is fundamental in order for them to do a good job. In the meantime, this places an even higher priority on point number one, individual responsibility for health decisions.

Function will also have greater meaning than lab test numbers in general. For example, the clear symptoms of a poor metabolism will take on more importance than "normal-range thyroid scores." The solution will not be giving out thyroid hormone; the solution will be resolving the stressors on metabolism that cause the hypothyroid symptoms. Leptin issues will be recognized as the prime cause of the great majority of slow metabolic conditions.

It will also be imperative to determine how efficiently your body is working. For example, the number of immune cells that exist is not as important as how well the immune cells work. The properly trained and well-armed immune cell will take considerable priority over an immune cell that cannot get the job done. Understanding leptin provides key working knowledge as to the cause of immune deficiency, cancer, and autoimmune problems.

There is no reason for any doctor in the United States not to become an expert in this subject. Leptin affects all aspects of medicine and every medical specialty as a primary causative issue.

There are many shades of gray.
The difference between optimum health and a disease can be found in progressively less efficient function on many levels. Traditional medicine is based on the belief that a person is either healthy or diseased. This form of logic has little to do with current scientific discoveries relating to disease. It is an old way of thinking about health, one whose time has passed.

Take, for example, the issue of calorie burning: on one end is optimum function; on the other end is the diabetic. In between are a thousand shades of gray that represent various levels of less efficient calorie metabolism. Leptin is the key to understanding how a person becomes diabetic. This is true for both type I diabetes and especially type II diabetes.

Individuals need to learn what symptoms go with what problems. Part of health intelligence is the ability to see a small problem developing and to take effective action to return it to a more optimal function. This is a life skill, not a paper-and-pencil test. Only when a large number of individuals personally have this skill will current obesity-driven disease trends improve. It is important to catch problems at an early stage rather than letting them evolve into more complex issues.

A greater importance on saving for older age.
The quick-fix mentality and excessive-stress lifestyles will be replaced by a more prudent understanding of the long-term consequences of current actions on future health. Everyone knows they need to save money for retirement; this is called financial reserves. Some people do it better than others. It takes some restraint not to spend everything on a current "want," so as to have stability in the future.

The same concept applies to being a competent *Health Asset Manager*. An important aspect of health is that every part of your body has different types of reserves which provide stability to health. When reserves run low, then health problems are prevalent and risk factors skyrocket. There are many types of reserves that relate to health: antioxidant reserves, mineral reserves, alkaline reserves, and energy reserves, to name a few. The demands of stress tend to drain health reserves, just as financial problems drain savings.

Any person who needs caffeine or antidepressants to function has a clear warning that energetic reserves are lacking. Building up reserves that have been drained takes time, minimally three-six months. It is also a lifelong commitment to doing things correctly, similar to managing a regular savings plan.

The skill with which a person builds and maintains important health reserves determines the quality of health that is established for a lifetime.

Even decisions made early in life affect one's overall reserves in the long run. It is never too late, and seldom too early, to begin being a good *Health Asset Manager*.

Timing is everything.
Timing is a powerful principle for health-related decisions. When you eat is oftentimes more important than what you eat.

Getting your body into rhythm is fundamental health principle that will solve many problems that you may not have thought were related. Leptin responds to specific rhythmic patterns and is a fundamental hormone in regulating your body rhythms.

These principles can be applied by forward-thinking physicians. The emerging field of chronotherapy shows that the timing of medication administration is of profound importance to cardiovascular health,[4,5] cancer treatment,[6] mental health,[7,8] sleep disorders,[9] and asthma,[10,11] and will eventually relate to many aspects of medicine.[12,13]

When your body is working in harmony, it has much less internal friction and much less wear and tear. Leptin is doing what it is supposed to be doing instead of causing problems to your health. There is little reason why most Americans cannot maintain vibrant health until the age of one hundred.

SUMMARY

Every individual faces numerous health decisions on a day-to-day basis: the food that is eaten or not eaten, the exercise completed or not, the procrastination on starting a healthy lifestyle pattern, the list continues. At the end of the day and the end of the week, look back and see what you have actually done. Only in this way can you have an objective view of what your entire mind, subconscious plus conscious, has set as priorities.

True health intelligence is based on the ability to translate useful information into constructive behavior. This means having a clear understanding of health information. This means having the skills to take charge of life and the subconscious mind. This means learning to master leptin.

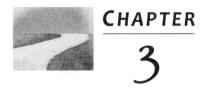

CHAPTER

3

What is Natural Balance?

HOMEOSTASIS is a key principle of health. It is defined as the ability of your body to establish stability, regardless of the stress it is under, by regulating internal physiologic responses. Homeostasis is the key to being able to bounce back, to recover, and to tolerate stress of any type. It is the essence of natural balance.

Problems with the hormone leptin involve the loss of natural balance in regulating food intake, fat storage, and metabolic rate throughout the body. In essence, leptin either allows or restricts energy production, making this hormone of prime importance. Proper functioning of leptin also prevents fat from being deposited in places that should not have fat, such as your liver, kidneys, arteries, and heart. Correct leptin function is crucial for the healthy operation of any system or cell in your body.

For people who fail to understand what this means, proper health-related decisions will be difficult to make. When individuals or health practitioners do not understand natural balance, they focus on symptom suppression and number management, rather than on true health.

THE WESTERN MEDICAL VIEW

Historically in Western medicine, homeostasis was considered to be a divine principle, something that was always there. This was an essential belief underpinning the entire paradigm of Western medicine. A great majority of the protocols used today in Western medicine are still based on this assumption.

These beliefs support the idea that almost anything can be done to the body to eradicate a disease or germ and it will automatically bounce back to normal. Unfortunately, modern molecular science proves that this is not the case.

During the evolution of Western-medical thinking, the "cause" of disease was considered to come from outside the individual. The classic example is the germ theory of disease. This led to treatments involving antibiotics to eradicate the cause, immunizations to bolster defense against the cause, and surgery to remove the cause.

The thought is that diseased cells, like cancer cells, must be eradicated at all costs. A "successful" treatment is the complete removal of the offending, diseased cells. Then, once these cells are removed, natural balance will simply reappear in a healthy state.

Cancer treatment involves drugs, surgery, radiation, chemotherapy, and anything else that aids the complete eradication of the cancer. Since modern medicine is unable to determine if complete eradication of all cancer cells has occurred, the approach calls for as many therapies as possible, for as long as possible, in order to increase the statistical chance that all cancer cells are killed. Drugs are frequently used as a follow-up to treatment in an effort to prevent a recurrence of the problem.

Little or no attention is given to why cancer occurred in the first place, what is fueling it in the present, or how to restore natural balance to prevent it from coming back. It is much easier to give the treatments and drugs, hoping that the physical body can tolerate them long enough to kill the cancer. It is common knowledge that many forms of cancer are resistant to current medical therapies.

This type of medical thinking evolved with the creation of immunizations and was reinforced with the discovery of antibiotics. A whole economy and numerous vested interests have grown around this thinking, facilitating the use of drugs and/or surgeries. It has a degree of workability and enough of a track record to pass as standard medical care. This does not mean it is the best care or best option; it is simply an agreed-upon level of care.

KEEP ALL BODY PARTS IF POSSIBLE!

In 2001, over 600,000 gall bladders were removed. Many times these surgeries were performed even though the individual did not experience a significant problem. The rationale is that because the gall bladder has stones in it, it is diseased. The gall bladder is seen as the cause of a problem or as a potential cause of a problem.

Insurance pays for this operation, and it is considered safe because humans can live without a gall bladder. Little attention is given to why a person forms stones, how to clean up a gall bladder that makes stones, what happens to the overall natural balance of a person with a poorly functioning gall bladder, or what happens to natural balance in a person without a gall bladder.

It is easier and more cost effective to take out the gall bladder and send the person on his way, with little advice about what to do next. While it is true the person may need such an operation, it is also common that there are other options.

Surgery should only be performed when truly needed. Unless the person takes charge, he or she is caught up in the automatic gall-bladder-removal production line. Since estrogen imbalance fuels gall bladder problems, ninety percent of gall bladder operations are performed on women. The female reproductive system is another favorite surgical target. A basic rule of natural health is to try, as much as possible, to keep all body parts.

MALFUNCTIONING NATURAL BALANCE

Currently, it is inconvenient for Western medicine to think of homeostasis in any other terms than as a system which is always operational and healthy. However, what if a malfunction of the homeostatic system is the cause of a health problem? What if the inability to bounce back or self-regulate causes problems?

In reality, new discoveries show that homeostasis malfunction is the prime cause of virtually all serious diseases. What we formerly considered to be "causes" are stressful irritants that strain homeostasis until the body breaks down. Science now shows that various stressful irritants change the natural defense systems so that they begin to work against the body and cause disease.

Leptin is the essential hormone that controls energy balance and metabolism in the human body. Problems with leptin disrupt the natural balance of homeostasis and are, therefore, the cause of a great majority of health problems. Leptin is the prime controller of natural balance, as will be clear by the end of this book.

The homeostatic system cannot be surgically removed. Leptin cannot be removed from the human body. A malfunction in the homeostatic system cannot be corrected with a drug. When an imbalance causes anxiety, the nervous system can be drugged to a point where it cannot generate anxiety; however, drugs only suppress symptoms while the underlying problems worsen.

Blood pressure can be forced down with medication, but then what has been done to general circulation? Cholesterol can be lowered with drugs, but what has been done to the liver, overall steroid synthesis in the human body, and normal muscle function? Hot flashes can be stopped with estrogen, but will excess estrogen cause cancer?

Current Western medical dogma, in the drug-dispensing trenches, does not want to have to evaluate these complexities. It wants to employ a system of standard medical protocols, focusing on drugs and surgeries, relying on test scores to indicate correct response to a particular therapy. It wants to believe that homeostatic systems in the human body will be unharmed no matter what is done to them. The new science shows this method of practicing medicine has significant shortcomings.

HOW THE WESTERN MEDICAL VIEW TOOK POWER

The debate over the cause of disease is not new. In the nineteenth century, it played out in the French Academy of Science with the classic battle between Antoine Bechamp and Louis Pasteur. Bechamp believed that the cause of disease was deterioration in the internal health of the person, a breakdown of homeostasis or natural balance. Pasteur believed the sole cause of disease was germs from the outside.

Pasteur's research led to the first marketable drugs for immunizations and the birth of the pharmaceutical industry. His ideas were backed by considerable money: that is why today his name is known and Bechamp's is not recognized.

The discovery of penicillin in the 1930s ushered in the era of antibiotics. Penicillin is a poison derived from fungus, a poison that kills bacteria. The seemingly instantaneous results of this antibiotic sealed the fate of other natural medical ideas of that time.

Western medical ideas became the dominant theme in health care, with huge money and legal forces placed behind their implementation and competitive survival. At the time of their evolution, the science supporting them seemed to provide an acceptable level of workability.

The discovery of penicillin led to massive pharmaceutical research, looking for more antibiotics. Research quickly showed that most of the new antibiotics being developed kept killing the tested animals, as the drugs were too toxic. Most of this research has never been made public.

Today, germs have built resistance to most antibiotics. A major health crisis has resulted because stronger antibiotics are simply too toxic for humans to consume. Even if an individual is very healthy and never uses antibiotics, there is still a chance of being infected with one of these superbugs that has been created from the overuse of antibiotics. These new superbugs are very hard to eradicate once they settle into a person's system. Just when the illness seems to be over, the bug flares up again and there is a recurrence.

One drug that evolved in the early antibiotic research was cyclosporine, allowed for use as an anti-rejection drug for transplant surgery. The drug was originally intended as an antibiotic but was too toxic to give to the general public. It found a market niche because it poisons the immune system to a point that the immune system will not reject a donor organ. This drug currently has a needed role in transplant surgery; if not for that role, it would not be on the market at all.

Unfortunately, long-term use of this drug invariably results in a significantly increased risk for heart disease[14] and cancer.[15] When doctors employ drugs for unapproved use, a common practice, major problems can occur. For example, when cyclosporine is used to treat autoimmune skin problems, the result can be a fatal cancerous fungal infection.[16,17]

This book makes it clear that when leptin is mastered, many autoimmune problems will simply go away. Older therapies that rely on toxic immunosuppressive drugs are no longer the primary approach. There is a huge difference between poisoning the immune system and returning the immune system to natural function.

THE MEDICATION TRADE-OFF

There is a price to pay for almost any medication. That price is based on the toxicity of the drug as well as how that drug may dysregulate natural function in the process of trying to produce a "desirable" result. Some undesirable side effects may be noticed in a matter of days or weeks; others are more insidious and may slowly emerge over a period of years.

What constitutes a desirable result depends on the situation. Medical emergencies require drugs to facilitate care. A heart recovering from a heart attack requires medications to ensure that it does not have to work too hard while it regains strength. There are numerous appropriate uses of medication. Most of them involve short-term use for a definable amount of time. They are used to help get the body back on track so that it can function on its own. It is like using a cast to allow a broken bone to heal. Once the bone is healed, the cast is discarded. Few would argue against the use of any medication in this context. Even antibiotics have an appropriate use to combat acute infections.

In the case of drugs and ongoing use, negative effects are cumulative and progressive over time. For example, let us say that a doctor wants to lower cholesterol with medication. A statin drug is given to lower the cholesterol to an acceptable number. Since this medication interrupts natural signals to synthesize steroidal hormones in the body, and since steroidal hormones help regulate homeostasis, especially the ability to adapt to stress, what will be the effect? It will vary dramatically from person to person. Some will feel miserable right away. Others will lose five to fifteen percent efficiency in their natural-balance system. They will not feel the same, but they accept it.

After a number of years on a cholesterol-lowering medication, this lack of efficiency has a domino effect on many other systems in the body that are not directly related to steroid synthesis, they are only indirectly related because the body is not working as well, and so a new symptom or problem crops up somewhere else. This requires a new medication to address that symptom, and the cycle goes on and on. This type of medical-symptom and number-management approach is definitely in the interest of drug companies and not in the long-term health interest of individuals.

The human body is not composed of drugs. It is made up of proteins, carbohydrates, fats, water, vitamins, minerals, and numerous other substances that facilitate healthy function and structure. These substances work together in an effort to maintain natural balance. The human body performs millions of self-regulatory steps every minute in an attempt to deal with stress and maintain natural balance.

Drugs are powerful. They force self-regulation to take a back seat and thereby force natural balance to take a back seat as well. It is impossible to predict all consequences of any drug taken for a long period of time. Furthermore, the current guidelines for safe use of drugs need major re-evaluation in light of new scientific discoveries about the causes of disease. Consumers must be warned of the potential life-threatening risks of long-term use of numerous medications.

SCIENCE FORGES NEW GROUND

Molecular medicine has opened a new Pandora's Box. The very scientists looking for the causes of diseases and seeking to improve treatments are proving the unthinkable! They are showing that the causes of cancer, heart disease, and age-related diseases are changes in the body's own regulatory communication systems. The same gene and hormonal signals that are essential for survival are turned upside down and used against the person to cause cancer and heart disease. This is an amazing discovery; one that fundamentally alters the way health care should be viewed.

This is great news for individuals who are truly interested in their own quality of health. These discoveries translate to realistic and practical steps that can be taken by anyone to dramatically improve their quality of health and reduce their risk for serious disease, regardless of their genetic risk factors.

SUMMARY

This book is written for those who want to better understand their own health options and who are interested in truly improving and maintaining their quality of health. It teaches the key principles of self-care, the essence of being a *Health Asset Manager*. It is about empowering individuals to be in charge of their own health and to be responsible for the final decisions on their health.

The stressors inherent in modern society are enough to throw any person's health out of balance. It is easy to get off track to the point where symptoms are bad enough that doctors recommend a drug. This is especially true in the baby-boom generation that is growing older. Ask questions and learn to take charge. Knowledge is power; there are options.

The goal is managing health in a way that keeps the quality of health intact. The bottom line is improved quality of health.

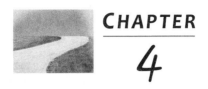

CHAPTER

4

Fat and Leptin – The New Reality

THE OLD VIEW OF FAT was that it primarily acted as a place for the body to store extra calories. No higher-level thinking or more prestigious purpose was given to fat; it simply became the undesirable extra weight that many people carried around.

That view of fat changed dramatically and forever in 1994 with the discovery of leptin.[18] And with this discovery, the basis of Western medicine theory of the last hundred years will need to change.

Leptin is a hormone that is secreted by fat cells in white adipose tissue *(figure 1)*. Leptin was found to be a signal to the brain, having a primary influence on body weight. It was also discovered to be involved with insulin, cardiovascular health, reproductive function, sex hormones, immune function, adrenal function, stress, thyroid function, bone health, cancer, and inflammation. Indeed, it has a major determining role in many aspects of healthy function.

When leptin falls out of natural balance and loses its ability to communicate efficiently, health problems follow. Thus, the concept of fat as a storage place has been transformed to fat as a major endocrine organ, like the thyroid gland, adrenal glands, and sex glands.[19]

THE SUBCONSCIOUS ANTI-STARVATION PRINCIPLE

While there is an optimum body weight for health as well as for our own concept of ourselves, your subconscious brain has its own ideas about how much you should weigh.

Your subconscious brain does not care about body weight from the point of view of how you look. Your subconscious brain has no idea if you think you are fat or at the right body weight. Your subconscious brain cannot see your body in the mirror. In fact, your subconscious brain does not even know how much fat is actually stored. Yet, your subconscious brain is in primary control of your eating behaviors.

Your brain is concerned with surviving, especially on a subconscious basis. It is concerned about replenishing body fat back to a proper amount for survival. If your body is in a state of natural balance, it has the ability to normalize itself at a reasonable weight.

Your brain senses how much fat is on hand by a system of communication with fat cells. The primary hormone secreted by fat cells is called leptin. When your brain senses that leptin levels are normal, then there is no need to store extra calories as fat. These are core survival mechanisms programmed into human survival genetics, and they are more powerful than a person's willpower.

Leptin is how the human race has survived in response to times when there was little food. However, in today's society there is a new problem called "food is everywhere." From a genetic and evolutionary point of view, we do not have a lot of experience with chronic overeating, and your subconscious brain gets very confused by this behavior. Your brain no longer properly senses the leptin message and becomes leptin resistant. Once this problem sets in, a person keeps eating and gets fatter, and the confused metabolism responds as if it were starving.

Worse yet, excess leptin reinforces the problems that set the stage for cardiovascular disease, cancer, and the diseases of aging.

The bottom line is that a fundamental principle of survival is turned against the individual and ends up causing major health problems, one of which is being overweight. This is a breakdown of natural balance.

THE DISCOVERY OF LEPTIN

There is a type of mouse called an *ob/ob* mouse. It is always hungry and cannot stop eating. It gets to be three times the weight of a regular

What is Leptin?

Figure 1

 Leptin is a hormone secreted by fat cells in white adipose tissue, which is sent to the brain to let it know how much fat is stored.

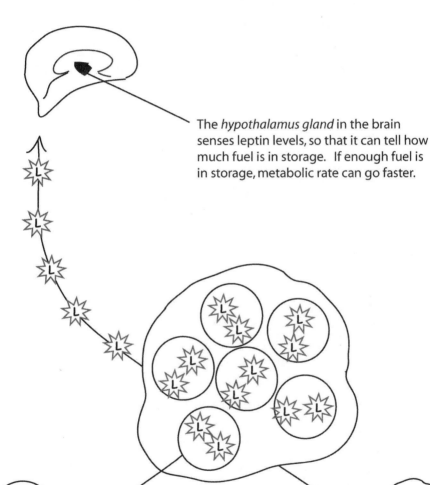

The *hypothalamus gland* in the brain senses leptin levels, so that it can tell how much fuel is in storage. If enough fuel is in storage, metabolic rate can go faster.

Fat cells produce the hormone leptin, which is sensed by the brain.

W*hite adipose tissue* contains fat cells that store fat and release fat when energy is needed.

mouse. It also becomes type II diabetic and has great difficulty reproducing. Scientists figured out that this mouse was missing a signal to stop eating, and leptin turned out to be the missing hormonal signal.

Since the discovery of leptin in 1994, intense scientific research has been carried out around the world in order to figure out exactly how leptin works. As it turns out, the issue is incredibly intricate. With each passing month, the jigsaw puzzle takes on new complexity. Enough is known to force a revolution in the entire scientific basis of medicine.

To understand why this is the case, let us back up and go through the story a bit slower, placing it in the context of natural balance and proper body weight.

ENERGY BALANCE

The energy needs of the human body are critical to the function of every cell, to every body part, and to humans as a whole. Thus, establishing adequate energy and maintaining energy balance are fundamental to survival.

Generally speaking, a person is going to be in one of three situations regarding energy balance and food intake:

1) **Energy Deficit** – Not enough intake of energy in the form of food relative to the need for energy. Examples include malnutrition, starvation, anorexia, bulimia, and low-calorie diets employed in an effort to lose weight *(figure 2)*.

2) **Energy Excess** – The consumption of too much food. This frequently promotes the storage of calories as fat.

3) **Energy Balance** – Body weight stays the same because the amount of calories consumed is about the same as the amount metabolized into energy. The person may be overweight or normal weight.

A primary purpose of the hormone leptin is to coordinate the metabolic, endocrine, and behavioral responses to starvation.[20] This hormone has a powerful influence on your subconscious mind which

Leptin Function when Dieting

Figure 2

 When on a low calorie diet, the body goes into a survival mode and slows the rate at which stored fat is used for energy.

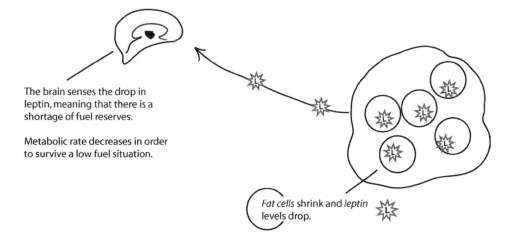

The brain senses the drop in leptin, meaning that there is a shortage of fuel reserves.

Metabolic rate decreases in order to survive a low fuel situation.

Fat cells shrink and *leptin* levels drop.

is programmed at a genetic survival level. Your subconscious mind will completely take over eating patterns if, from its point of view, the circumstances dictate that it should.

In our genetic evolution, there were many times when there was not enough food. This induced an energy-deficit state. In order for us to survive, calories stored in fat are broken down and used as fuel. When this happens, leptin levels drop and metabolism slows down to conserve stored energy. This slower metabolic rate is implemented to match the limited supply of food.

In our evolution, when food was found we would resume eating a higher amount of food. The amount of food a person eats in one meal cannot restore depleted fat reserves from a prolonged period of reduced calorie intake. However, after we eat a number of meals, the fat cells begin to replenish their reserves and the hormone leptin begins to increase. Once the leptin levels rise to a certain point, the fat cells are replenished. The message goes out to stop eating so much. The hormone leptin is key to the survival of our species. It is very powerful (figure 3).

So far, this seems like a relatively straightforward proposition. When leptin is low, we will be hungry and want to eat. When enough food is eaten over a period of days or weeks, then leptin will be higher, signaling the brain to reduce appetite.

The ob/ob mouse does not make any leptin due to a mutation of the gene that synthesizes leptin; thus the mouse is always hungry and eats endlessly. When the ob/ob mouse is given leptin, it quits overeating and loses weight. Indeed, this is how leptin works in our bodies when we are in a good and healthy state of natural balance.

This sounds like the weight-loss miracle everybody is awaiting. Why have the drug companies not made a leptin pill and given it to every overweight person? It seems like an ideal drug. It would certainly appeal to the quick-fix mentality of the American public. It would appeal to the cause-and-effect thinking of Western medicine. A blood test could check for leptin; it could be given as a prescription until the blood level is normal and the person no longer wants to overeat. Everyone's

Leptin Function when Food is Available

Figure 3

 When food is available, it heads to fat cells to replenish depleted reserves.

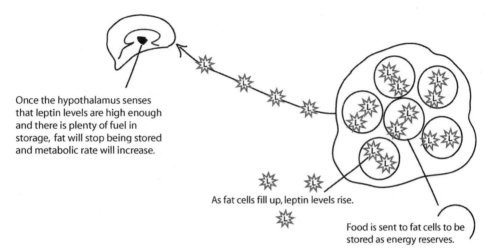

Once the hypothalamus senses that leptin levels are high enough and there is plenty of fuel in storage, fat will stop being stored and metabolic rate will increase.

As fat cells fill up, leptin levels rise.

Food is sent to fat cells to be stored as energy reserves.

weight-loss problem would be solved. Rest assured, the drug companies wish it were that easy.

EFFICIENCY AND RESISTANCE – DOMINANT HEALTH PRINCIPLES

Almost all overweight individuals have high leptin levels. That is right – most overweight people have too much leptin!

When a person gets thrown out of natural balance, the brain does not sense leptin levels correctly, literally building up resistance to the hormone (figure 4). This problem steadily gets worse as you get older.[21]

The main target for the leptin message is the hypothalamus gland of the brain. In overweight people who have difficulty controlling the amount of food they eat, their body is insulin resistant and their brain is leptin resistant. There are too many of these hormones circulating, and they are not productive.

In a normal situation, the white adipose tissue is trying to make a phone call to the brain. The message traveling over the phone line is a hormone called leptin. The amount of leptin in the phone message tells the brain how much fat is in reserve, much like the fuel gauge of a car indicates how much gas is in the tank. This information allows the brain to regulate energy for the rest of the body.

Virtually all overweight people do not make this phone call properly. There is plenty of leptin; it just does not get through to the brain. The fat cells make repetitive phone calls, and the brain does not answer. The net result is that the brain thinks the body is still starving and continues to order fat storage, even though there may be plenty of fat already in storage. This is like having a tankful of gas with the fuel gauge stuck on empty.

The problem is not having too much or too little of the hormone leptin; the problem is that leptin is not working efficiently. So how is the problem of leptin resistance corrected?

A drug company tries to follow the cause-and-effect sequence of leptin activity in the brain in order to locate a receptor or some other change in signal that leptin induces. A drug may be formulated to target

Leptin in Overweight People

Figure 4

 Leptin resistance occurs in overweight people. The brain thinks there is not enough fat in storage and continues to fill fat cells with fuel.

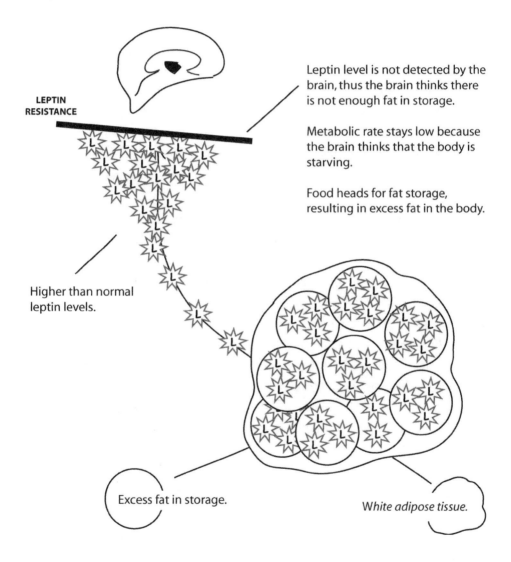

LEPTIN RESISTANCE

Leptin level is not detected by the brain, thus the brain thinks there is not enough fat in storage.

Metabolic rate stays low because the brain thinks that the body is starving.

Food heads for fat storage, resulting in excess fat in the body.

Higher than normal leptin levels.

Excess fat in storage.

White adipose tissue.

something closer to the "cause" of the problem. Drug companies are currently in a mad race to the market with drugs that affect neuropeptide Y, melanocortin receptors, and leptin receptors.[22]

These drugs will seek to reduce the desire to eat. There is no doubt this will be the next class of "hot" weight-loss drugs appealing to our quick-fix mentality.

There is also no doubt that such drugs will have many side effects that disrupt natural balance and will cause numerous health problems in individuals who use them.

If individuals are truly interested in managing their own health, they will ask a few basic questions: Why do I have leptin resistance? How did the problem get started in the first place? Can I eat in such a way that will improve the condition? What options do I have that will fix the source of the problem and thus forever change my weight issues and health risks.

These types of questions go against the grain of traditional Western medical thinking. For example, obesity is considered a disease. A primary cause of obesity is leptin resistance. However, leptin resistance cannot be surgically removed. It cannot be medicated out of existence. It is a functional problem of homeostasis; a problem of the natural balance system in the body gone awry.

Furthermore, obesity causes other diseases such as heart disease. Thus, a primary cause of the number-one killer in America is a problem in energy homeostasis. It is also clear that leptin resistance is a direct contributor to cancer, the second-largest killer in America. The leading causes of death in America are primarily the result of disruption of natural balance in the human body.

The answers to these questions about leptin resistance are not simple. However, with the current science that is available, it is possible to have a major impact on these issues. There is no quick fix; leptin is not a quick-fix hormone in the first place. But time invested in learning about its function may be a life saver.

BASIC WEIGHT LOSS

Let us take individuals who have eaten too much and have gained a few extra pounds. These people may be able to cut back on eating, increase exercise, and take off the extra weight. It really was not that difficult. As long as they keep up a reasonable amount of activity and do not go overboard with eating, they maintain their weight and do not have to think too much about it. Their energy level is good, and they feel healthy.

Such people do not have a significant problem with leptin resistance. When they gained their extra weight, they were pushing the leptin system into a condition of imbalance, but their health was good enough that they got things under control by watching food intake and increasing exercise.

As we get older, leptin resistance becomes much more of an issue. It provokes insulin resistance, in a somewhat chicken-and-egg manner, and the two lock each other into place. A third problem develops – resistance of fat cells to the stimulation of the sympathetic nervous system, a problem called adrenaline resistance. The metabolism of the fat cells becomes sluggish, making it easier for them to accumulate fat and more difficult to eliminate stored fat.

Fat cells have a tendency to become larger in size and to readily multiply as we age, and leptin resistance fuels this undesirable state of affairs. In this situation, we keep gaining weight. We can follow a diet for a while, but we find that it is all too easy to eat and gain the weight back, sooner or later. When this happens, there is a major problem with leptin resistance. This is typically reflected as being fifteen or more pounds above an ideal weight. While this happens more easily as we age, aging is no excuse.

THE PERSON WHO EATS LITTLE AND STRUGGLES WITH WEIGHT

Another example of leptin resistance can be seen in people who have a history of struggling with leptin-resistant weight issues and now eat very little in an effort to maintain a more optimum body weight. Such people may be at a reasonable weight, from their point of view, but they have low energy and poor immune response. They live in a state of energy deficiency. They frequently sleep all day. Their entire metabolism is in slow motion. They are prone to fatigue and have abnormally low energy.

They maintain their body weight by hibernating. They may force themselves to exercise, but it does not feel refreshing. They are afraid to eat because they know they will get fat. This forces leptin levels to be lower, for the time being. In some cases, this can develop into full-scale anorexia. However, when they do eat, the tendency is to gain back excessive weight. Unless they learn the secrets of leptin management, this pattern continues.

On the other hand, there are people who eat very little and cannot lose weight. Such individuals may go into rapid weight gain when they eat moderately. They can be significantly overweight and unable to lose weight even on a relatively low-calorie diet. Their body thinks it is starving even though it is not; therefore, their metabolism slows down.

In essence, they are also hibernating. If they try to reduce their calorie intake to a very low level in order to lose weight, they run out of energy, just like the person described in the previous paragraphs. When they start eating again, they gain even more weight.

These types of individuals often think they have thyroid problems. In some cases they do. However, in the majority of cases, the thyroid problems, or low-thyroid symptoms, are caused by leptin resistance and improperly functioning leptin signals. The thyroid gland is simply experiencing the brunt of the problem with poor leptin function.

SUMMARY

It is a survival instinct to replenish the supply of fat. This will never change. The primary problem that people get into and cannot get out of is a major breakdown in communication between the white fat cells and the brain. This problem is called leptin resistance.

The subconscious brain does not know what a person looks like in the mirror. It sets body fat levels by its perception of leptin, just like the fuel gauge in a car communicates the amount of gas in the tank.

Leptin resistance means that the brain cannot correctly judge when stored fats are at a proper level. It can keep a person significantly overweight because the subconscious brain is not sure there is enough fat on hand. Worse yet, the brain may be enforcing orders on a subconscious basis to replenish the fat, even though the stores of fat are overflowing.

Under the influence of leptin, a primary role of white adipose tissue is to act as a fuel reserve. Leptin controls how the body restores fuel after a period of food deprivation or illness. The fact that fat is much more than a storage bin is quite fascinating. Fat cells talk directly to the brain, and, in response, the subconscious brain commands eating behavior. In some cases, this may completely override willpower.

Fat cells carry out many types of communication. This makes understanding them a more complex issue. In addition to leptin, scientists have identified at least fifteen other major communication signals coming out of fat cells.[23] We will discuss this later. At this point, we know that fat is involved with immune function, cardiovascular function, kidney function, liver function, reproductive function, thyroid function, adrenal function, and toxins. Its involvement in these issues is not a passive one.

Due to this new understanding, the status of white adipose tissue has gone from being merely a storage bin to being a primary player in eating behavior, metabolism, cardiovascular disease, and cancer. White adipose tissue is a major endocrine organ in human metabolism. Leptin is the most important hormone discovered to date.

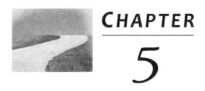

CHAPTER
5

How Fat Communicates

THE BRAIN remains commander and chief of the human body and the prime regulator of communication going on in the body. The brain relies on accurate perception of leptin to set the appropriate metabolic rate.

It has been known for many years that the sympathetic nervous system is the primary stimulant to the metabolic activity of white adipose tissue.

The sympathetic nervous system is the aggressive side of the nervous system. In a positive sense, the sympathetic nervous system enables an individual to be focused, communicative, and motivated toward a goal.

Sympathetic nervous system activity correlates to the "left brain" view of the world: more orderly, organized, and assertive. The left brain handles five to nine pieces of data at a time; it is time and sequence oriented. The classic Type-A personality is driven by sympathetic nervous system activity.

However, many individuals who have a dominant left-brain orientation to the world are not classic Type-A personalities. Such individuals are usually direct and straightforward with communication so as to organize and implement plans. Typical left-brain stress responses are anger, frustration, agitation, and irritation. Generally, these feelings are expressed.

By comparison, the more relaxed side of the nervous system is called the parasympathetic nervous system. It correlates to the "right brain" view of the world, more spatial and adaptive in nature.

The right brain handles millions of pieces of data at once and sees relationships among data. This side of the brain likes pleasure and sensory stimulation and tries to avoid or deny pain. The classic Type-B personality is driven by parasympathetic nervous system function. Typical right-brain stress reactions include sadness, guilt, resentment, and denial. These feelings are frequently not expressed.

SUBCONSCIOUS ACTIVATION

Under stress, the sympathetic nervous system takes over, at least on a subconscious basis. This is called the fight-or-flight response. A classic Type-A personality is more likely to fight, whereas a classic Type-B personality is more likely to be afraid or flee. Regardless of personality type, the release of sympathetic nervous system adrenaline is a survival impulse.

For example, a person is driving down the street and someone pulls out, almost causing a collision; the reaction is to quickly avoid the accident. The heart races and the body is jittery. There is no time to stop and think about what to do. A perceived threat to survival enters the conscious awareness, which is monitored by the hypothalamus gland in the brain, the bridge between the conscious and the subconscious. In the presence of perceived danger, the hypothalamus gland takes control of the body. It causes nerves to release adrenaline, stimulating the metabolism and body into fast reaction for survival. This is an example of how the subconscious brain takes over control of conscious thought processes in order to facilitate survival.

LEPTIN IS A SUBCONSCIOUS PERCEPTION

The perception of leptin occurs on a subconscious basis. It is "hardwired" into survival calculations, especially stress-related issues. It controls metabolic rate, the use of energy, and eating behavior.

When the hypothalamus gland perceives leptin correctly, then metabolism can run at a proper pace and stress can be handled in an appropriate way. When leptin is not perceived correctly, major problems with energy and metabolism occur.

LEPTIN AND THE STRESS RESPONSE

While some emergencies only last a split second, others last for longer periods of time. A person needs to be able to maintain energy long enough to deal with the stress. This is one reason why white adipose tissue is metabolically stimulated by the sympathetic nervous system. Under such stimulation, white fat cells begin to release their stores of energy so that an emergency demand can be met over a prolonged period of time. This mechanism of white adipose tissue stimulation has been recognized since 1929.[24]

Since this early time, scientists have shown that there are different types of receptors in fat cells for adrenaline. For example, fat around the midsection has more of one type of receptor than fat in other areas. This is why some people gain weight around the midsection and others gain it on the hips and thighs. When a certain type of receptor has trouble getting the message, fat accumulates more readily in that area of the body as the metabolic rate of those specific fat cells slows down.

We have mentioned that leptin is a long-term regulator of body-fat reserves, acting to restore fat reserves in an effort to recover from starvation or calorie restriction. When leptin is low, a person wants to eat; when leptin is high, a person does not want to eat, assuming everything is working properly. This is a longer-term issue, gauging fuel supply over a period of weeks or months.

Leptin is also under short-term control of the sympathetic nervous system. This is because the 911 call that goes out for the emergency need of the body takes priority over long-term storage goals. Thus, a quick burst of sympathetic nervous system activity depresses leptin production.[25]

The main point to understand is that the sympathetic nervous system drives the metabolic rate of white adipose tissue. This is a direct line of communication from the nervous system to fat. This communication is directed by the hypothalamus gland in the brain, the subconscious control center and the overall 911 commander and chief of the human body.

FAT COMMUNICATES

The primary hormone made by white fat cells is leptin. Leptin talks directly to the hypothalamus gland of the brain. When leptin levels are high in the properly functioning person, this tells the brain to decrease food intake and increase sympathetic nerve activity, thus increasing metabolic rate and stimulating white adipose tissue to break down stored fat.[26]

As sympathetic nerve activity increases and metabolic rate increases, leptin is lowered, signaling the need to accumulate more stored energy. This completes a circle of communication between fat cells and the brain. This is how metabolism works when a person's body is in a state of natural balance. It is an example of a homeostatic system in the human body relating to the natural balance of energy. It has its own built-in checks and balances. The ebb and flow of these communication signals are fundamental to having an appropriate appetite.

A BREAKDOWN IN COMMUNICATION

When there are problems with leptin, there is a breakdown of proper communication. Low leptin levels cause a person to have no appetite, resulting in too much weight loss and the loss of bone density. High leptin levels cause a person to eat frequently or to rapidly gain weight from whatever is eaten.

This is the opposite of how the hormone behaves when it is working properly. There is a disruption of the normal communication between the brain and fat cells. Not only does this cause confusion about eating, but there are major consequences for the rest of the body as well. It is not a desirable state of affairs for white adipose tissue, a primary endocrine organ, to be in a state of poor communication.

In addition to the daily eating patterns, this circle of communication can be viewed in the context of how a person does on a month-to-month basis. If not enough food is consumed, then leptin tends to stay low, decreasing sympathetic nerve stimulation and metabolic rate and increasing appetite. This results in the hibernation effect that enables humans to survive prolonged periods of reduced food availability. Metabolism consequently slows down to conserve body fat for survival.

When enough food is consumed, the leptin level rises, telling the brain to quit eating and increase metabolic rate. This enables the body to have an energetic metabolic drive. There is a higher level of leptin, meaning there is adequate fuel on hand so that the body can work at an optimum rate and does not need to be in starvation mode. This is how the leptin hormone behaves when it works correctly, as opposed to how it functions during times of leptin resistance.

When there is leptin resistance, the brain does not hear the phone call from fat cells telling it there is enough fuel in storage. Consequently, the fat cells keep accumulating weight because neither the brain nor the fat-cell troops have a sense of what is actually happening *(figure 4)*.

In an effort to stimulate metabolism, the brain releases adrenaline. This is magnified by too much stress. Such adrenaline should stimulate fat cells to release energy which in turn should cause weight loss. However, when adrenaline is too high too often, fat cells develop adrenaline resistance. From a fat cell's point of view, it is like being yelled at too often. After a while, the fat cells go numb to the adrenaline, and adrenaline resistance develops. This causes metabolism of fat cells to stay locked in a "hibernation metabolic rate." It also causes weight gain around the middle, high blood pressure, and sleep problems *(figure 5)*.

TIMING AND LEPTIN

In addition to communication between the brain and fat cells, leptin levels follow a daily pattern. Leptin levels are highest during the first few hours of sleep and fall to their lowest level in the morning.[27] They peak before the adrenal steroid cortisol which is highest at 6 a.m., and they are not tied to cortisol production.[28] A person who is in a good rhythm and pattern will not be hungry before bed because the brain correctly senses the higher level of leptin; thus the appetite signal is turned off and food cravings are absent.

A person who craves food before bed has leptin resistance, meaning that the brain does not sense the leptin signal to not eat even though leptin is naturally highest at this time. A major clue that a person is

Adrenaline Resistance

Figure 5

1. Sympathetic nerves release adrenaline based on normal behavior, exercise, and stress.
2. Under excess stress or leptin resistance, there is excess adrenaline released by the sympathetic nerves.

Normal Adrenaline Release

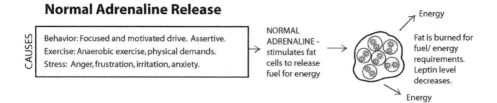

CAUSES

Behavior: Focused and motivated drive. Assertive.
Exercise: Anaerobic exercise, physical demands.
Stress: Anger, frustration, irritation, anxiety.

NORMAL ADRENALINE - stimulates fat cells to release fuel for energy

Energy

Fat is burned for fuel/ energy requirements. Leptin level decreases.

Energy

Excessive Adrenaline Release

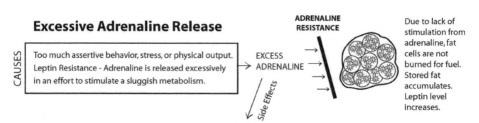

CAUSES

Too much assertive behavior, stress, or physical output.
Leptin Resistance - Adrenaline is released excessively in an effort to stimulate a sluggish metabolism.

EXCESS ADRENALINE

Side Effects

ADRENALINE RESISTANCE

Due to lack of stimulation from adrenaline, fat cells are not burned for fuel. Stored fat accumulates. Leptin level increases.

1. Weight gain around the middle.
2. Cardiovascular distress, including high blood pressure.
3. General inflammation, wear and tear.
4. Difficulty sleeping.

heading down a pattern of leptin resistance is out-of-control eating after dinner. Eating after dinner seriously disturbs healthy leptin function.

Furthermore, a meal that has too many carbohydrates or sweets can cause the normal night pattern of rising leptin to occur seven to nine hours earlier than it should, completely throwing the body out of proper rhythm.[29] In other words, eating too many sweets will cause leptin levels to rise at the wrong time. Once a person has leptin resistance, this leads to overeating, especially at night. For example, if a person has a sweet roll, muffin, or orange juice for breakfast or too many cookies at lunch, there will commonly be a leptin-resistant urge to eat after dinner that evening.

THE BRAIN SETS LEPTIN RHYTHM

It is interesting to note that the control of the daily pattern of leptin secretion comes from the biological clock in the brain.[30] Even though the hormone itself is produced in fat cells, it responds to a rhythmic signal coming from the brain. Previously, we have described how the sympathetic nerves are involved in communication to fat cells and how fat cells talk back to the brain. Now there is an additional feature of this communication system: there is a daily timing pattern essential for proper leptin function. This daily timing pattern is under control of the brain, which functions like the conductor of an orchestra.

Malfunctioning leptin patterns opens the door to understanding why leptin is the cause of so many health problems. Leptin levels are crucial to survival instinct, the fundamental core level of energy. Without fuel, nothing in the human body works. Leptin is the most important hormone signal gauging fuel supply. Just as we alter our driving patterns to go to a gas station when the car's fuel gauge says empty, so it is that leptin levels command powerful urges relating to food consumption.

When the rhythmic pattern of leptin secretion is disrupted, the brain has trouble with energy regulation in general, and other timing patterns in the body are thrown out of natural rhythm. There are numerous examples in this book that show that major health problems involve the loss of proper leptin timing, not necessarily related to the amount of leptin. Leptin levels in the blood could be at a "normal" amount; they are simply not doing what they are supposed to be doing at the right time. This is a very important point. A lab test for leptin in the blood does not reflect these problems.

LEPTIN TONE AND ACTIVE METABOLISM

In addition to the normal nighttime rise in leptin, there also occurs a pulsing regulation. In a twenty-four-hour period, there are as many as thirty-two pulses of leptin activity. These relate to circulating adrenaline levels.[31] This is believed to act as a sort of tension in the regulatory system, providing the ability of the hormone to fluctuate on a gradual basis, rather than in blatant on-and-off patterns. This leptin and adrenaline tension is essential for fast-action response to stress, as more fuel is needed to produce energy in the case of an emergency demand.

In essence, this leptin and adrenaline tension provides an "energy tone," much like the muscle tone we feel when we are in good physical shape. The opposite of this "energy tone" is a fatigued or washed-out feeling.

The dominant factor that influences leptin production is the sympathetic nervous system. There is a cycle of communication between fat cells and the brain. They talk to each other in an effort to figure out the fat storage needs on a long-term basis. This long-term plan can also be put on hold for short-term energy needs to deal with stress.

REVIEWING PRIMARY LEPTIN REGULATION

The brain determines other hormone activity in the body based on the perception of leptin. The brain controls the leptin rhythm. Leptin is the most important hormone in helping the brain determine energy use in the body.

Leptin is under short-term regulation, daily regulation, and long-term regulation. It is central to body rhythms, because timing is fundamental to your brain's calculation of how much energy it can spend for any particular situation. There is a tremendous amount of complexity in this system, which enables your body to elegantly distribute energy so that it can survive.

These points alone explain why drug therapy will not work to solve leptin resistance. Drugs will simply block transmission and cause a blatant off-or-on function. They will interfere with the natural trend of the twenty-four-hour pattern and will interfere with the proper leptin tone in circulation. Drugs will also handicap the stress response and depress immune function.

Only in the case of a true genetic inability to make leptin will leptin drugs have any value, which at this time affects only a handful of people in the world.[32] The great majority of overweight and fatigued Americans do not suffer from such a genetic problem; they suffer from serious leptin mismanagement.

LEPTIN AND INSULIN

Leptin from fat cells and insulin from the pancreas also communicate with each other. This is similar to two department heads in a company talking to each other. Insulin production stimulates leptin production.[33] Leptin receptors are present on the insulin-producing B-cells of the pancreas, demonstrating the ability to turn off insulin production.[34]

In normal physical function, leptin and insulin have a balancing effect on food intake, energy storage, and a stable energy level. Once leptin resistance sets in and leptin levels are high, then the pancreatic B-cells do not respond to the signal from leptin to stop making insulin.[35] However, insulin keeps stimulating leptin production at the same time that insulin promotes calories to store as fat. Furthermore, the high circulating insulin causes cells throughout the body to be resistant to insulin. Thus, we see that leptin resistance sets the stage for insulin resistance, and the two problems continue to play off each other and make each other worse *(figure 6)*.

THE KEY TRIAD OF PROBLEMS

Hence, we see the triad of leptin resistance, insulin resistance, and adrenaline resistance as the main cause of any problem of excess weight *(figure 7)*. For example, when the fat cells in the abdominal area become

Leptin Resistance Causes Insulin Resistance

Figure 6

Leptin resistance not only occurs in the brain, but occurs in the pancreas as well.

Normal Leptin Function in the Pancreas:
Self-regulatory loop between leptin and insulin.

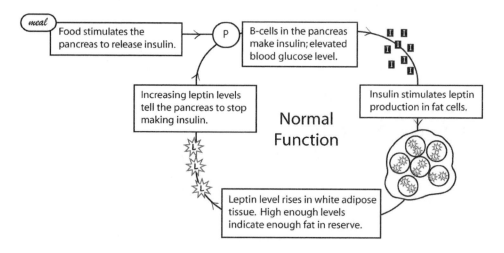

Leptin Resistance in the Pancreas, Causing Insulin Resistance
Impaired regulatory loop due to communication breakdown. Causes excess fat accumulation.

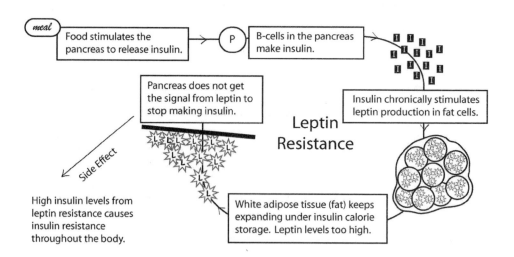

The Key Triad of Problems
at the Root of Weight Gain

Figure 7

There is always abnormal fatigue or lack of energy with this triad of problems.

Leptin Resistance:

The brain can not sense leptin, so it keeps metabolism slow and calories heading for storage. The pancreas can not sense leptin, so it keeps making excess insulin, setting the stage for insulin resistance.

Insulin Resistance:

Excess insulin production leads to insulin resistance throughout the body, as well as erratic or no energy from food.

Adrenaline Resistance:

The normal nervous system signal to stimulate fat cell metabolism is no longer received by fat cells. This causes weight gain especially in the abdominal area, the type of weight gain most associated with cardiovascular disease and reproductive organ cancer.

resistant to adrenaline, then the individual begins to gain weight around the middle. This is a common area for weight gain in men; it also happens to women who struggle with menstrual irregularities and women at menopause. This type of weight gain around the middle is the worst kind of weight gain, the type most associated with cardiovascular disease.

More is explained about insulin resistance in chapter 16. We mention it here to emphasize the issue of efficiency and metabolism. Individuals struggling with body weight have a key triad of efficiency problems. The common denominator is that the hormonal signals cannot get through to their targets; there is resistance. It is like trying to call someone on the phone and they do not answer. The messages in the phone calls contain adrenaline, leptin, and insulin. There are various reasons why the phone calls are not answered, all of which fall under the general category of the body being out of natural balance.

Expensive lab tests are not needed to prove there is a problem. A person just has to look in the mirror and then take note of his or her level of energy. The problem slowly and progressively gets worse as a person gets older.

THE ONSET OF DIABETES

If the problem is not solved, the body may just give up trying to solve the problem. Now a person has type II diabetes. Leptin levels may or may not be elevated in type II diabetes, because regulation is really messed up. Once diabetes sets in, the body is no longer able to bounce back in terms of regulating blood sugar; homeostatic energy balance is broken. The leptin levels are no longer able to correctly regulate the body. This is a poor state of affairs that is worse than leptin resistance.[36] Solving leptin issues and restoring natural balance is possible for many individuals with diabetes; however, it is a more difficult problem to fix. With diabetes many warning signs of poor metabolic function remain unresolved. It indicates a major problem with natural balance.

SUMMARY

Leptin is the main communication signal coming from white adipose tissue. One of its primary functions is to regulate the longer-term fuel supply of the body, ensuring that reserves are adequate for survival. Your brain does not "see" body weight in the way that you do when looking in the mirror; it knows by sensing the leptin levels. This system is fine until leptin resistance sets in and fat cells continue accumulating fat, and your subconscious brain does not know you're overweight or storing too much fat.

As health deteriorates, especially as one is prone to gain weight and unable to get back to an ideal weight, there arises a triad of problems. These involve leptin resistance, insulin resistance, and the resistance of fat cells to stimulation from the sympathetic nervous system – adrenaline resistance.

Unlocking this triad of problems, especially leptin resistance, will solve the actual cause of the problems and return the body to normal metabolic function. Taking effective action is essential before the problem spirals into more serious issues such as diabetes and increased risk for cancer and heart disease. The cause of the problem is in the homeostatic systems of the human body, the natural energy balance systems, not in disease or germs.

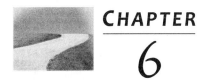

CHAPTER
6

Why Dieting Does Not Work

LET US ASSUME that some individuals are simply overweight, not gaining or losing any weight, just too heavy. Such people at their heavier weight will have a faster metabolism than they would at a lighter weight. They can eat two thousand to three thousand calories a day at their heavier weight. They are able to metabolize that amount of calories, possibly not gaining any more weight, but they also cannot lose any weight because they are eating too much. As they begin to cut back on calories, two things happen:

1) Initially they begin to burn stored fat for fuel because their metabolism is still set to burn the higher calorie amount.
2) As the diet continues, leptin levels begin to drop, initiating the genetic response to starvation. This in turn slows down the sympathetic nervous system stimulation of fat cells so that the body can conserve fuel. Metabolism slows down and weight loss stops.

As less food is eaten and weight is being lost, the tendency of metabolism is to slow down under the influence of less leptin and thus less sympathetic nervous system stimulation. There will be a point where no more weight loss is possible with the current diet plan because metabolism has slowed down to the new lower level of calories being consumed. Individuals may hit a plateau that is fifteen to twenty-five pounds from their goal, even though they are almost starving on a very low-calorie diet.

PREVIOUS DIETING EXPERIENCE

Such dieting problems become more severe the more often people have attempted calorie-restriction diets in the past. This is especially true for people who have gained and lost weight a number of times.

Their bodies can detect a diet a million miles away; even the thought of going on a diet may slow down their metabolism. Their bodies do not trust them anymore. The feast-and-famine principles of their genetics are in full force. As soon as there is a reduction in calories, the body slows down and starts to conserve.

People with more serious leptin resistance have an even more difficult time. They may be quite overweight, but they may already be eating a low-calorie diet, usually twelve hundred to fifteen hundred calories. Their weight will not budge. If they cut calories, they may lose a few pounds, but they run out of energy right away. If they increase their calories, they can start a weight gain process that they may not be able to stop. In this more serious case of leptin resistance, the body thinks it is starving, even though it may be significantly overweight.

There is only so much that can be done with diet and weight loss in the conventional sense. Once metabolism slows down to coincide with the reduced number of calories in the diet, weight loss stops. Some individuals do not lose any weight, others lose a few pounds, and others may lose quite a few pounds before this happens. However, it is quite common to encounter a weight-loss plateau before the goal weight has been achieved. Furthermore, as soon as a person starts to eat more food, leptin commands that calories go in the direction of fat storage.

It is a current fad in weight-loss clinics to increase drug stimulation when this plateau is hit. This is not only incredibly dangerous; it addicts the person to medication. As soon as the medication is stopped, leptin rises and weight comes back.

Keep in mind that leptin is in this for the long haul. It is the survival hormone that enabled our species to go for months at a time with very little food. Leptin will not be conquered by a diet plan that is designed to last for only a few months. Unless strategies are learned for mastering leptin and applied as a lifelong skill, failure to reach and/or maintain the goal weight is inevitable.

GAINING IT ALL BACK, AND THEN SOME

Eating little and not getting anywhere becomes frustrating. Now these individuals start to think they will just go back to eating as they did before. So, they eat more. This increase in food intake signals the end of the starvation mode, in turn causing the release of leptin. A primary survival goal of leptin is to replenish the fat stores.

The direct channel of food heading for fat storage is now opened nice and wide. The fat cells that had shrunk in size under the influence of starvation are more than willing to fill back up and even stretch to new levels of expansiveness. In fact, they readily multiply so that additional food can be stored as fat. The older a person is, the more difficult the issue becomes. Fat cells keep expanding and multiplying. If only our brain cells and muscles could perform this feat!

In a recent study with obese teenagers, those who had the lowest leptin at the end of the weight-loss period were the most likely to relapse and gain their weight back.[37] This is because the manner in which they dieted induced a starvation response, a clear sign that when even a moderate amount of extra food is eaten, it will head straight back to fat storage.

Leptin seems to possess some sort of "sixth sense" about the individual who diets. This is especially the case the more times the dieting approach is tried and the yo-yo factor has occurred. It is quite common for people to gain back more weight than their original diet starting point. This means that leptin is making sure that if another "diet" occurs there will be adequate stores of fat to deal with the apparent threat to survival.

Leptin has not had enough evolutionary time to figure out what to do with individuals who tend to overeat on a regular basis and then try to restrict themselves to a reduced-calorie diet. So far, its initial evolutionary response seems to be to store more fat.

Once the leptin management system of the individual has decided enough fat is in storage, the body starts to metabolize faster. However, for a period of time, the body is dead set on putting extra calories back into fat storage. All the weight that was lost is back, frequently along with another ten to twenty pounds. This is weight-loss misery, something very real to millions of people.

EMOTIONAL UPS AND DOWNS OF LEPTIN RESISTANCE

The previous section defines what happens to those people who are able to start a diet in the first place. People with a severe case of leptin resistance cannot stay on a diet at all. Frequently, they make it through part of the day eating fairly well, but nighttime is usually their downfall.

During leptin resistance, there are high levels of leptin but they do not communicate; thus, the brain does not receive the signal that there is plenty of stored fat, even though the fat cells are trying to tell the brain that they are all filled. The brain still thinks it is in some form of starvation mode; therefore, metabolism runs quite slowly.

At the same time, the brain commands the individual to eat in order to recover from the falsely perceived condition of "starvation." It is a vicious circle, and it leads to bizarre and erratic behavior around the subject of food.

One symptom of leptin resistance is that individuals may not have a real interest in starting a diet in the first place. They know from experience that they cannot beat the leptin problem. Frequently, they are just happy not to be gaining more weight. Then they get a poor medical report; blood pressure, cholesterol, or triglycerides are too high, or a knee replacement or back surgery that will be needed if some weight is not lost. This is a motivational jolt into reality that seems to be more painful than the idea of dieting. They are stuck between the anxiety of dieting and the painful consequence of what will happen if some weight is not lost.

THE LEPTIN-RESISTANT PERSONALITY TYPE

Leptin-resistant individuals who try to lose weight can become true diet schizophrenics. They have one personality that is associated with being on the diet and doing fine. This is usually apparent for at least several hours a day and quite commonly all day until about four to six in the evening. Then the other personality starts to come alive. The first signs of this are a grumpiness and irritability accompanied by a distinct lack of energy in the head.

This internal uncomfortable feeling then becomes the excuse for going off the diet and getting some kind of quick fix to make the head or energy level better. These issues have little to do with willpower; the urge to eat is driven by a misguided sense of survival. This confused survival instinct is under the influence of leptin.

This results in abnormal behavior and cravings for food. These individuals will sneak food. They attempt to hide what they are eating from anyone who tries to help them. They may concoct elaborate plans to get to the food they think they need. The need to get this food fix is as desperate as the craving for drugs.

There is no stopping the "bent out of shape" leptin impulse. It is a powerful survival urge, one that is extremely confused. There is no reasoning with people who experience this problem; all they want is food. Once they have eaten, they go back to their rational personality type. They even agree to try much harder on their diet starting tomorrow.

In this upside-down situation, leptin throws the entire body out of natural rhythm. Not only does this make weight loss difficult, it increases risk factors for numerous other health problems. Leptin that is not communicating properly is a prime cause of disruption of natural balance for the rest of the body.

THERE IS MORE TO FAT THAN MEETS THE EYE

White adipose tissue is composed of thirty percent immune cells. White adipose tissue is not just stored fat; that is, stored triglycerides. The more white adipose tissue there is, the greater the number of fat-related immune cells. Having extra immune cells sounds like a good idea, but given how uncomfortable too much leptin can make a person feel, it becomes plain that these extra immune cells may not be on the same page with the rest of the body.

In fact, these extra immune cells inside of white adipose tissue frequently secrete extra amounts of TNFa (tumor necrosis factor alpha). TNFa in the right amount at the right time is a powerful cancer-destroying compound. However, when the body is out of balance, TNFa is another example of homeostasis gone awry. Excess TNFa contributes to cancer, heart disease, arthritis, and numerous other problems by provoking a highly inflammatory state of affairs.

It is quite common for people to have ten to fifteen extra pounds of fat, and frequently much more. Thirty percent of the cells in this fat have the potential to send out highly inflammatory communication signals. These inflammatory signals set the stage for internal wear and tear and the onset of the diseases of aging. This is a serious issue.

Individuals with leptin resistance are in dire need of fixing themselves, not only to reach a healthier body weight but also to prevent these life-threatening conditions. Even individuals who have this problem to a lesser degree need to take steps to regain their body's natural balance.

SUMMARY

The ability to go on a diet and successfully achieve an optimum weight and maintain it implies that an individual has been able to overcome issues with leptin.

Most people under the age of thirty can just cut back on what they eat and exercise more and their body returns to natural balance. Leptin did not kick in as a major factor. After the age of thirty, leptin becomes a significant issue for anyone trying to lose weight. Minimally, leptin causes metabolism to slow down as one tries to lose weight, and it is the main factor that causes weight to be gained back once the diet is over. This is basic leptin survival genetics dealing with starvation issues.

More serious problems with leptin wreak havoc with weight and eating issues. On a subconscious basis, the body thinks it is starving, even though it may be quite overweight. When individuals with leptin problems attempt to diet their addictions and compulsions relating to food become obvious, as they are often unable to follow a diet for any length of time.

Progressively worsening problems with leptin cause a significant increase in other health problems, many of which are serious and life threatening.

Leptin problems are the cause of dieting failure. They are at the root of yo-yo dieting, of eating little and not losing weight, and of gaining weight back once a diet is over. The only solution is to learn to master leptin.

CHAPTER 7

Addiction, Alcohol and Candida

ADDICTIVE BEHAVIOR is another major problem in our society. The *Journal of the American Medical Association* had a New Year's message for the public. One study stated that alcohol consumption and binge drinking were going up at an alarming rate.[38] Another study announced that the obesity epidemic is continuing to worsen and is a major problem for our society.[39] Their message is clear: America is getting fatter and drinking more.

It has been our observation over the years that many individuals who struggle with significant leptin resistance have a history of excessive alcohol and/or drug use. Thus, it is not at all surprising that these two trends are occurring at the same time.

Individuals recovering from alcohol abuse do not like to be hungry because it triggers the cravings for alcohol. Certainly, a great deal of addictive behavior is shared by individuals who have significant food-related leptin resistance or some type of substance abuse. Since food is not illegal, we tend not to think of it in terms of addiction, but the similarities are obvious.

Our observations lead to these interesting questions:

- **Does leptin resistance put a person at higher risk for alcohol or drug use?**
- **Does alcohol or drug use put a person at higher risk for leptin**

resistance?

- **Exactly what is the relationship between food cravings and other drug/alcohol cravings?**

LEPTIN AND ALCOHOL CRAVINGS

Researchers are discovering that there are clear correlations between leptin levels and alcohol cravings. In experiments with mice, leptin administration enhanced the motivation to consume alcohol following a period of deprivation.[40] The same researchers found that in humans going through alcohol detoxification, those who craved alcohol the most had the highest levels of leptin.[41]

Other researchers demonstrated that leptin levels were higher in people with chronic alcoholism, independent of nutritional status, the amount of fat they had, or the state of liver disease. The data simply shows that the longer a person has consumed alcohol, the higher the circulating levels of leptin.[42] This indicates that leptin precedes other health issues caused by alcohol and may very well be the subconscious driving factor that reinforces alcohol cravings.

This also means that excess food consumption is fueled by alcohol consumption and vice-versa. The cravings for each share a common signal of excess leptin due to leptin resistance. This leads to misguided behavior wherein the brain thinks, on a subconscious basis, that alcohol is essential for survival. Literally, this means that the need for alcohol is being confused with the need for food.

In healthy people who do not have leptin resistance, alcohol consumption lowers leptin, thus stimulating appetite.[43] Therefore, alcohol consumption, especially at night, can fuel overeating even in healthy people, sending them into leptin resistance. This is a way to gain weight as well as gain an addiction to alcohol. Many young people heading off to college in good health find that too much alcohol quickly adds pounds they did not have before and gets them stuck in a rut of addictive patterns.

This also means that people with a history of leptin resistance may be prone to overeating at night even with mild alcohol consumption, such as having a glass of wine with dinner. Many times such individuals will have weak willpower about eating a proper-sized meal. Add a little alcohol and it is easy for them to overeat.

STRESS, LEPTIN, AND CRAVINGS

Remember, the hypothalamus gland of the brain is where this leptin signal is being processed. The hypothalamus gland is the "old brain." It seeks to regulate the chemical reactions in the human body from the neck down. In computer terms, its circuitry is more like hardware than software. Its computer program is based on survival.

Any perceived threat to survival causes a sense of instability and a stress-alarm reaction. During our genetic evolution, the scarcity of food was one of the most significant stressors on a day-in and day-out basis; thus, the body's genetics are hardwired to deal with these issues.

In a twisted, leptin-resistant way, the consumption of food and alcohol seem to have a direct effect on satisfying a subconscious threat to survival. Anytime a person starts feeling stressed or threatened in some way, there is a risk for excess food or alcohol consumption, resulting in "emotional" eating or drinking. Such cravings are directly wired into the subconscious hardware. Unfortunately they are incorrect and distorted perceptions due to pre-existing leptin resistance.

A person who has never had a problem with overeating or excess alcohol consumption is much less likely to experience these cravings. Conversely, any person who has struggled with food and alcohol cravings knows that these issues intensify dramatically under stress.

A true road to recovery from alcohol abuse would mean that a person solves leptin problems. That is to say, the individual will reach and maintain a healthy body weight, and leptin issues relating to food will be fully under control. This is an important key to permanent addiction recovery.

LIVER DAMAGE

Alcohol-related liver damage is a huge problem in our society. Excessive amounts of alcohol cause liver inflammation resulting in the "cooking of the liver structure." Eventually, the liver may look like a piece of fried bacon. By the time individuals suffer alcohol-induced cirrhosis of the liver, they have markedly elevated leptin as well as other inflammatory markers, such as C reactive protein, that induce the liver damage.[44]

Leptin is a major player in the causative mechanism that induces liver damage. This is why women, who naturally have higher amounts of leptin than men, are more sensitive to liver damage from alcohol. As we have pointed out, leptin is elevated in alcoholics regardless of the state of liver damage. It is not liver damage that causes elevated leptin; rather, excess leptin helps to cause liver damage.

In the previous chapter, we pointed out that elevated leptin causes an increase in immune-cell activity among immune cells that are part of white adipose tissue. One of these primary immune signals is called TNFa, a highly inflammatory signal. It has long been known that TNFa is elevated in liver disease and is a major part of the progression of the disease.

Researchers have proven in mice that regular alcohol consumption turns up the general production of TNFa and tilts the stress response to excessively make TNFa, not only in the liver but also in white adipose tissue.[45]

This data means that regular excess consumption of alcohol turns up extra production of TNFa. We already know that TNFa is generated by excess leptin. Therefore, the current data on excess leptin and TNFa indicate that they work together to generate inflammation that causes the liver damage. Conversely, this means that if leptin and TNFa can be lowered and brought into a state of natural balance, then liver damage can be prevented and possibly even reversed.

In addition to the issue of liver damage, the most recent study on this subject confirms the link between excess TNFa, leptin, and consequent ongoing cravings for alcohol, which results in continued consumption and further liver damage.[46]

INTRODUCING NF-KAPPAB

NF-kappaB is the 911 switchboard for each cell in the body. By comparison, the hypothalamus gland in the brain is the 911 switchboard for the body as a whole. NF-kappaB is typically dormant inside of cells, especially when everything goes along in a routine and generally nonstressed manner.

Under the influence of cellular stress, NF-kappaB is activated. It goes to the DNA of cells and tells the cell what proteins to make to meet the emergency needs of the stressful situation so that the cell can survive. Without NF-kappaB, cells would not be able to tolerate any type of stress, and we all would have perished long ago.

In some cases, this essential component of survival gets hijacked and starts working against the body. As we have explained, TNFa fortifies chronic inflammation that is a primary cause of cancer, heart disease, and many other diseases of aging.

Excess NF-kappaB and TNFa coexist in the majority of serious health problems. In cases of alcohol-liver inflammation, the problem is fueled by excess production of NF-kappaB and TNFa.[47] Further, in order to induce liver damage from alcohol, the NF-kappaB level must rise prior to the initiation of liver damage, meaning that it is a prime causative factor.[48] This damage to the liver occurs faster in women than in men, because women generally have a higher percent of body fat. This means they tend to have more leptin and can set off excess TNFa and NF-kappaB overproduction more easily than men can.[49]

There is clear-cut science showing why the herb silymarin is so good at protecting the liver. Silymarin directly lowers the production of NF-kappaB, specifically addressing the cause of the liver problem. Silymarin is gaining worldwide recognition as a powerful remedy for liver disease.[50]

CANDIDA ALBICANS

The issue of *Candida albicans* is as a great example of the function of natural balance involving the immune response. It is our opinion that an epidemic of *Candida albicans* infection, induced by the use of prescription antibiotics and the overconsumption of refined sugar, is a large factor in the obesity epidemic in America today.

Candida is yeast that is a normal part of the three to five pounds of foreign contents, including many strains of bacteria that comprise the natural fermenting environment of the gastrointestinal tract. In a state of natural balance, Candida appears to be involved with garbage recycling functions and the absorption of heavy metal poisons. Its population is kept in check by the other bacteria and your immune system; which, when in healthy balance, are aiding digestion and the production of needed nutrients.

An adverse side effect of taking antibiotics is the destruction of too many good bacteria in the GI tract. Antibiotics are poisons that are generally derived from yeast, thus they do not kill yeast. When antibiotics disrupt the natural balance of power in the GI tract, then yeast can "overgrow," reaching a population size in excess of normal.

It is now proven that a chronic Candida overgrowth drastically increases the production of TNFa,[51] and it induces general immune suppression for other infectious agents. This makes a person much less resistant to infection.[52] This problem is so serious that in immune-compromised individuals, for example, those with AIDS or in cancer treatment, the onset of Candida frequently pushes the situation into a life-threatening problem.[53]

As Candida spreads, it is an irritant to the surrounding tissue. The first response to the spreading Candida is for the endothelial cells of the mucosal lining of the GI tract to try to kill the Candida. They do this by shooting a blast of TNFa at the yeast, in an effort to kill the yeast.[54] This is a vital initial reaction that must take place in order to prevent the yeast from setting up shop and spreading as an infection.[55,56] This illustrates the efficient use of TNFa by the immune system to kill an infection, demonstrating proper natural balance.

If this initial TNFa response is inadequate, then Candida can take hold. One characteristic of an inefficient immune response occurs when the body is stressed. In this situation, the healthy TNFa release to kill a Candida infection does not occur.[57] Another example is inflammatory arthritis, where excess production of TNFa is already involved with the destruction of cartilage. This, in turn, stresses the immune system into inefficiency. In this stressed and inflamed state the immune system cannot fight Candida.[58] Another obvious source of excess TNFa is that coming from extra pounds of fat. Thus, a person who is overweight, especially one who has emotional stress, is much more susceptible to a yeast infection that will spread.

Interestingly, Candida itself produces TNFa[59] in an effort to destroy and weaken mucosal tissue so that it can spread and live in the weakened tissue. In fact, the primary damage done to the body by Candida has now been demonstrated to occur through the excess production of inflammation during battle.[60,61] It is like the shootout at the OK Corral. If the good guy fires first and wins, then Candida is stopped. If the good guy is stressed out and can not shoot first, then Candida loads its TNFa shotguns and fires away.

Medical researchers are now finding that turning off the excess production of TNFa is essential for getting rid of a yeast overgrowth.[62,63] How is a person going to do that who is overweight and chronically generating excess TNFa from fat cells?

An overgrowth of Candida directly relates to the tendency to become overweight. This is because Candida craves sugar in order to survive. When a person with an overgrowth of Candida eats sugar, especially between meals, Candida consumes the sugar and ferments it, producing an alcohol-based toxin called acetaldehyde. This is the same toxin that is produced as the liver metabolizes alcohol.[64,65,66] This toxin crosses the blood-brain barrier and damages brain cells, just like alcohol. It typically leaves a person feeling foggy, spacey, fatigued, prone to depression, and experiencing out-of-control cravings for sugar.

These symptoms tend to flare up whenever a person gets into an excess sugar-consumption pattern. Unfortunately, yeast infections can live in the GI tract or sinuses for decades, ebbing and flowing based on sugar and alcohol consumption patterns, constantly inducing wear and tear to metabolism. Candida induces sugar addiction.

The desire to eat sugar is also a hallmark of leptin imbalance. Excess sugar consumption fuels inappropriate leptin production and consequent leptin resistance.[67] This leads to a problem of excess weight accompanied by Candida overgrowth. Both problems generate excess inappropriate TNFa, leading to accelerated wear and tear and increased risk for disease.

SUMMARY

Addictive patterns, whether they involve excess alcohol, excess sugar, or over consumption of food in general, involve the excess leptin signal. This is as a driving subconscious force that makes these issues difficult to manage. It is quite likely that excess alcohol, toxins from Candida overgrowth, and food cravings share common pathways in the brain to the point that the "need" for alcohol or excess sugar is confused with the survival instinct of eating.

Alcohol consumption, excess sugar consumption, and extra pounds of fat work together to generate too much inflammatory activity, especially in the liver. This sets the stage for liver damage. The liver is the metabolic factory of the human body. Disrupting the function of the liver cripples healthy metabolism.

Too much inflammation leads to the "overheating" of cells, promoting the excess production of NF-kappaB. Chronic, inappropriate overproduction of NF-kappaB is a turning point in cellular health, tilting the tables in favor of disease.

The problems of extra pounds of fat, alcohol consumption, and/or excess sugar consumption magnify one another. They synergistically fuel one another in path toward rapidly declining health.

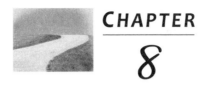

CHAPTER

8

Drugs and Leptin

ELEVATED NF-KAPPAB is a prime factor involved in the withdrawal from morphine addiction.[68] Inducing starvation as a form of stress causes animals to once again crave heroin after they have been through a prolonged drug-free period. The cravings are directly related to leptin fluctuation.[69] The mechanism of neurotoxicity from methamphetamine (METH) involves the excess production of NF-kappaB, which causes inflammatory nerve damage.[70]

This information sheds light on the true nature of drug addiction, as well as on how it accelerates the onset of, and increases the risk, for any disease of aging, especially brain damage resulting in cognitive decline.

Amphetamine-based diet pills, known to suppress appetite, have been around for a long time. The stimulative effects of cocaine are also well known. The brain actually makes small amounts of these substances, and they have a natural stimulant effect.

The cells in the brain responding to this stimulation are called CART (cocaine and amphetamine regulating transcript). Not surprisingly, CART is a favorite target of pharmaceutical company research. CART activation suppresses appetite by interacting with the hypothalamus gland.[71] In normal and healthy metabolism, as leptin goes down, so does CART. This is because lower leptin in the brain always slows down metabolism, including CART.[72]

Diet pills and cocaine work by stimulating metabolism and depressing leptin, interfering with the leptin signal to regulate the fuel needs of the body.[73] These drugs are a dangerous way of bypassing normal brain regulation of energy systems. They force stimulation on the core subconscious brain and bypass the natural breaks that prevent the brain from overheating from inflammation.

It has been found that leptin controls CART, and that problems with leptin resistance can lead to excess CART stimulation.[74]

Addictive craving patterns are likely to exist when there are leptin problems and cocaine/amphetamine addiction, because leptin and cocaine/amphetamine communicate with one another in the hypothalamus gland of the brain.

Excess CART activation causes too much stimulation, leading to anxiety (part of the paranoia of drug addiction).[75] If an addict has an appetite, eating food will turn off the anxiety by increasing leptin. This creates a reciprocal and cross-related addictive pattern among drug ingestion, anxiety, and food consumption – one massive confused state of addictive patterns in the subconscious mind.

This issue is further complicated by the fact that CART-related drugs, including stimulant diet pills, have no restraint to keep them out of the brain. In leptin resistance, leptin cannot enter the brain in proper amounts, even though the levels are high in the blood. Cocaine and amphetamine readily enter the brain, where they can directly wreak havoc with leptin.[76] No matter what quantity of the drug is consumed; it will always enter the brain.

CART is a normal neuropeptide. In normal circumstances in nondrugged individuals, it is under leptin control. When cocaine or amphetamines are consumed, they bypass genetic control and exert direct regulation on core issues of survival. While this may induce a temporary high, the consequence for the nervous system and overall body-fuel regulation, as well as for numerous other health issues, is profound. This is due in part to the neurotoxicity of the drugs and their stimulation of NF-kappaB, and in part to the drugs causing leptin problems.

The data on methamphetamine toxicity is quite alarming. The addictive nature of cocaine and amphetamine is becoming clear. Damage caused to regulatory centers in the brain and nerves in general sets the stage for lifelong problems with mood, memory, and metabolism.

CONCERNS ABOUT RITALIN

Ritalin is in widespread use in our schools as a psychotropic drug that stimulates brain function in an amphetamine-like manner. It is known to have direct effects in the same brain pathways as drugs of addiction. Thus, it is not surprising to find that it interacts with brain regions in ways similar to cocaine.

In fact, a recent animal study showed that rats fed Ritalin early in life were much more prone to self-administer and desire cocaine later in life. Researchers concluded that Ritalin changed brain neurons in a way consistent with increased addiction risk.[77] In another recent study, Ritalin was given to former cocaine abusers. Brain imaging reflected patterns of brain activity consistent with addiction stimulation, desires that were not linked to conscious control.[78]

This information shows that alcohol and drug-addiction tendencies could be fueled by early life use of Ritalin. Since food cravings are involved in the same brain pathways, it is quite likely that Ritalin could make a person more susceptible to overeating.

This is partly because the mechanism of amphetamines suppresses leptin in the hypothalamus gland of the brain – evoking the starvation response. This means there is a much higher risk for weight gain once Ritalin is stopped. And partly it is due to change in the structure of brain neurons so that the desire for pleasure is excessive, leading to excess food consumption. This is consistent with patterns of recovering alcoholics, who can not control the subconscious drive to overeat, simply shifting one addictive tendency to another.

Other studies in mice raise additional concerns about the long-term consequences of Ritalin and brain damage. One study showed that mice fed Ritalin in younger years had inappropriate depression in response to stress challenges in older years. This reflected some type of change in brain chemistry persisting into adulthood.[79]

Another study showed that Ritalin exposure in developing years resulted in significant behavioral changes as adults. These changes were reflected by a depression-like lack of interest in normal pleasure and an excessively sensitive response to stress, characterized by excess anxiety and an exaggerated secretion of corticosterone.[80] As we discuss in chapter 29, the rise in corticosterone, along with the existing leptin problem, fuels excess abdominal weight gain – the type of weight gain most associated with disease risk. Thus, animal studies with Ritalin show a change in stress response that fuels the mechanism by which adults gain disease-associated fat.

It would be relatively easy for parents and schools to help solve both the apparent need for Ritalin and the general obesity epidemic in our youth. Parents could ensure that their children eat a good breakfast, one with a good protein base and devoid of sugar-sweetened cereals. Schools could replace morning snacks with morning exercise and forbid snacking before lunch (except with instructions from a medical doctor). These simple changes would drastically change the prevalence of what is now being called ADD/ADHD and the rampant increase in obesity in our youth.

Considering the number of children taking Ritalin, it is a shame that there are not more studies to elucidate the precise reason for brain damage, which is noted in animal studies. However, it is easy to predict from existing scientific literature the likely mechanism, as we explain in the next section.

A BREAKTHROUGH FOR PARKINSON'S

The correct amount of leptin entering the brain turns out to be incredibly important in protecting the brain. One of the many roles of leptin is that it seems to help body tissue grow. This applies to bones,[81] cartilage,[82] the GI tract,[83] skin,[84] and the fetus during pregnancy,[85] to name a few.

It was recently discovered that adequate leptin protects the dopamine system in the brain and is an essential component responsible for brain plasticity.[86] In fact, leptin appears to be essential for protecting the brain from excess excitation that induces toxicity, especially protecting against damage to the NMDA receptor, the receptor that is damaged in Parkinson's.[87]

An experiment in which the neurotoxin methamphetamine was given to *ob/ob* mice and to normal lean mice showed that the methamphetamine killed the *ob/ob* mice but not the lean mice.[88] Remember, the *ob/ob* mouse has no leptin in the brain, thus no dopamine brain protection from chemical toxins.

This information shows that strategies to normalize leptin levels in the brain could become a primary treatment for Parkinson's patients. Throughout this book we discuss numerous ways to normalize leptin. One key factor we will explain is calcium. High-quality calcium, in the dose of 2,000 to 3,000 milligrams per day, is likely to become an integral part of the nutritional program for helping individuals with Parkinson's.

This information raises another question about the safety of Ritalin, especially when given to an overweight child. Since overweight children have leptin resistance, and thus less leptin in the brain, their brains are more susceptible to damage, not only from environmental toxins but also from any ingested amphetamine.

We see that leptin is involved not only in regulation of food intake and craving issues; a proper amount of it is essential for the protection of the brain against damage.

SUMMARY

Food addiction, alcohol abuse, and drug addiction share a common communication signal gone awry – leptin resistance or leptin signals that have been destroyed. These leptin problems fuel addictive behavior by confusing the subconscious brain into believing that these substances are essential for survival.

Stress that makes a person feel unstable in some way is likely to trigger addictive behavior patterns. In part, this is because normal CART function is related to the anxiety stress response. Anxiety problems can easily be manifested in food, alcohol, or drug abuse. They can either lead to addictive patterns or occur as a result of substance abuse.

In order to return health to a state of natural balance, it is essential to have leptin levels under control and in working order. Having the right amount of leptin working properly is the key to a healthy metabolism.

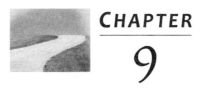

Are You Destined to Be Fat?

LEPTIN SCIENCE has yielded groundbreaking information regarding leptin, pregnancy, and the risk for obesity being programmed into a child shortly after birth. This means that good parenting takes on a whole new meaning: ensuring that one's children have a better chance of not becoming overweight as they grow older, as well as reducing health risks for the mother.

We have known for a while that environmental programming influences how leptin is set up in an individual's metabolism. These factors come courtesy of one's parents. If parents are overweight, their children are at a higher risk for developing leptin resistance. This is due to programming that took place while the children were still in the womb.[89,90]

Children born to such parents may develop problems early, or they may not manifest until middle age. This means that parents who get in better shape before conception – meaning that neither one is suffering from leptin resistance at the time of conception – are helping increase the chances for a better quality of health in their child.

Additionally, it has been reported that overeating in infants sets the stage for later-life obesity, high blood pressure, and heart disease.[91] This is especially true of bottle-fed infants, who are prone to getting too many calories.

This factor is alarming, because pediatric advice for many years has been to fatten up an underweight baby. In the past, as standard medical advice, low-birth-weight babies have been forced to eat more than normal. This advice turns out to be wrong because it programs leptin resistance into the developing brain at a very young age, setting the stage for later-life problems.

The explosion of new information about leptin, healthy pregnancy, and obesity can help many individuals avoid needless and serious health problems.

HEALTHY PREGNANCY

Mothers entering pregnancy with leptin resistance and borderline thyroid issues are at much higher risk for problematic pregnancies. This is because of the metabolic demand placed on the mother to grow another body inside hers; it is like working overtime in the construction business. If there are pre-existing problems with energy regulation before pregnancy, then it only stands to reason there will be a higher likelihood of problems when there is an increased and intense energetic demand such as pregnancy.

New studies show that leptin problems directly increase the risk for gestational diabetes,[92] preeclampsia (gestational high blood pressure and protein loss in the urine),[93] placental insufficiency and dysfunction,[94] increased inflammation (excess TNFa production),[95] increased risk for a low birth-weight baby,[96] and premature delivery.[97] Obese mothers are at high risk for all manner of serious pregnancy problems.[98]

Furthermore, women who experience leptin-resistant induced preeclampsia during pregnancy have a greater risk for heart disease later in life.[99,100]

Clearly, not having a leptin problem before pregnancy is a good idea. This means that a woman should get to a normal body weight and be healthy prior to conception. A woman who has never had a leptin problem and does not have a family history of leptin problems is much less likely to have complications during pregnancy. If a woman has struggled with leptin problems during her life (even if she is in good shape now) or if there is a family history of leptin problems (her mother or father), then the metabolic demands of pregnancy may push leptin issues into the problem category.

Preeclampsia is a common and serious complication of pregnancy, but there are workable solutions that can significantly improve the quality of health for the mother and newborn. If a woman is lacking in magnesium, she has twice the likelihood of developing preeclampsia. Magnesium is known to lower high blood pressure and is commonly used in Europe to help reduce the problem of preeclampsia.[101]

It has now been demonstrated that women with preeclampsia pregnancies also have insufficient antioxidants.[102] Even very conservative antioxidant support during pregnancy (1000 mg vitamin C and 400 IU vitamin E) has been shown to significantly improve this problem.[103] The most recent study on this topic showed that women with preeclampsia were lacking co-enzyme Q10 and vitamin E.[104]

These particular antioxidant deficiencies are highly relevant to any overweight person; it is simply that their lack during pregnancy creates major problems. We will explain in the next few chapters the newly discovered science that sheds light on why these antioxidants are not only vital for healthy pregnancy but also important in helping to correct leptin resistance.

At this point it is very safe to say that any pregnant woman who is overweight, struggles with low-thyroid symptoms, has a history of weight-loss issues, or has a family history of weight problems (mother or father), also has a vital need for antioxidant supplementation during pregnancy. This information is every bit as important taking folic acid during pregnancy to prevent neural tube defects.

LEPTIN'S CHANGING ROLE

New scientific breakthroughs center around the changing role of leptin shortly after a child is born. Leptin's role during pregnancy is different than its role after birth. During pregnancy, leptin promotes the growth of the fetus, is secreted by the placenta, and does not regulate body-fat deposition as it does following birth.[105] Leptin facilitates the uptake of nutrition into the fetus; it does not restrict uptake in any known way.

If the fetal environment is influenced by abnormal food cravings and binge tendencies of the mother, the developing fetus is at risk for imbalanced brain development while in the womb. This leads to a tendency toward excess food cravings and cardiovascular risk later in life for the unborn child.[106,107]

Following birth, leptin must switch gears. Instead of allowing the unrestricted food intake of pregnancy, it must now change into its role of appetite regulator. New studies show that a critical time for this programming is right after birth, especially within the first six hours. In essence, at birth the hypothalamus gland of the brain has a blank blackboard with regards to leptin's control of appetite.

The scientific breakthrough came when researchers were able to demonstrate that a surge of leptin following birth writes a message on the blackboard, saying, "You will have a proper appetite-regulation system and body-weight set point." The researchers showed that this message was embedded in newly formed brain circuitry stimulated by this leptin surge. If the message does not get written in the first few hours following birth, then appetite control is dysregulated and the person is destined to struggle with excess food cravings, hibernation metabolism, and high risk for obesity later in life.[108,109,110]

If you are wondering where a surge of leptin comes from in newborns, the answer is in the first milk colostrum of the mother.[111,112,113] Ensuring that an infant receives this first milk colostrum within the first six hours of life is an extremely important event. If for some reason a mother is medically unable to give her child this feeding, first milk colostrum from cows is an alternative. An appropriate leptin-hormone replacement drug would be another option, if one becomes available.

This initial leptin surge is vital for properly wiring the subconscious brain's relationship to food for an entire lifetime. If the proper wiring does not occur in the developing brain in its "programmable state," then this opportunity is forever lost. Furthermore, a baby left in a low-leptin state or born prematurely with low leptin, is at high risk for complications over the first fourteen days. This is because adequate leptin is also vital for the high energy cellular demand of rapid growth and adjustment to an environment that is twenty-five to thirty degrees colder than the womb.[114]

Now that we know this is a major health issue as well as a primary factor that will contribute to the obesity epidemic and heart disease in our society, every effort should be made by health officials to inform women of the importance of healthy pregnancy and this initial feeding of colostrum following birth.

MSG POISONING

Health officials should do the general public a service and ban MSG from the food supply, especially in light of this new information regarding the evolving appetite-control system in the subconscious brain of the newborn.

Scientists have known about the MSG problem for quite a while. They frequently study obesity by poisoning rats with MSG until they become obese. Naturally, this animal is called the MSG obese rat. There are over one hundred studies on this rat in scientific literature.

MSG causes glutamate neurotoxicity. It produces an obese rat because the glutamate toxicity destroys the leptin message written on the blackboard in the subconscious brain that directly controls appetite. In some cases it destroys the blackboard so no message can be written.[115] Thus, the MSG obese rat is very similar to a human who never got a proper leptin message following birth.

Ingestion of MSG by a pregnant[116] or nursing mother[117] can seriously compromise the infant's appetite-control center. Scientists have been sounding the alarm on this for a while; nobody is listening.[118] With the new discoveries regarding the programming of the brain directly after birth, this MSG data is of utmost importance.

These MSG damaged rats serve as a great lab test to observe what will likely happen to humans who have similar problems. A clear issue is that the MSG obese rats cannot properly adapt to stress, because they have elevated cortisol that is not in harmony with a normal stress response.[119] This is exactly the same effect as damaging the brain from cocaine, methamphetamine, and Ritalin. It results in hypersensitive stress responses and an eventual fat stomach with high risk for disease. Female MSG damaged rats have great difficulty reproducing later in life, in addition to becoming obese.[120]

Children and adults consuming MSG, especially in large amounts, can create a neurotoxic brain response in the appetite control center which could easily tilt them toward obesity. MSG should be completely avoided by everyone.

IS ASPARTAME SAFE?

The NutraSweet Company would like you to believe that aspartame poses no health risk, even with ongoing daily consumption for a lifetime.[121] The American Dietetic Association has recently published a position paper supporting the use of aspartame every day for the rest of a person's life.[122] They believe that it is not possible to consume enough aspartame for it to pose a toxic health risk, even at "abuse" levels. Their science is mainly based on studying the potential toxic effects of aspartame in isolated systems (not the real world) and by failing to find health problems in large groups of users (which statistically hides many subgroups who are most at risk).

Our response: What is the health risk to specific individuals? What happens when aspartame is consumed by an individual whose detoxification systems may already be overburdened from common pollution? How do people know if they are having a problem?

For example, there are case reports in the scientific literature of fibromyalgia patients who failed to make any recovery until they eliminated MSG or aspartame from their diets.[123] Aspartame is both a nerve stimulant and a producer of methanol (commonly referred to as wood alcohol) as it is metabolized. Methanol, when consumed like alcohol, is extremely toxic, causing blindness and brain-stem damage. Nobody ever gets this much methanol consuming aspartame: but how do people tell when the amount they are ingesting is contributing to a health problem?

Methanol produces formaldehyde in metabolism. This aldehyde-based poison shares common detoxification pathways with alcohol,

Candida albicans toxins, common pollution (all major metropolitan cities have higher-than-safe levels of formaldehyde in the air), cigarette smoke, nail polish, and some perfumes. Individuals who notice sensitivity to any of these chemicals already have pushed their detoxification capacity to the limit. In such individuals, aspartame simply adds to an already overburdened system.

In a less obvious way, aspartame can induce irritating symptoms even in the absence of toxic-overload issues. It is a known trigger for migraine headaches for many people, especially children.[124] The toxins produced by aspartame are known to have specific immune-depressing effects.[125,126] This means that if individuals who consume aspartame are getting sick too easily, they should avoid aspartame to see if it makes a difference to their immune response. In almost twenty years of clinical experience, we see that discontinuing aspartame frequently improves all manner of digestive-related complaints. It is our conclusion, based on science and experience, that aspartame may be a health problem for any individual with immune depression, headaches, GI tract problems, or chemical sensitivity. In order to establish what one's personal problems with aspartame might be, a reasonable strategy is avoidance, and then noting changes to one or more of these key areas.

The American Dietetic Association would like all pregnant women to think aspartame intake is perfectly fine. Do you trust their advice? The Surgeon General has warned against drinking any alcohol during pregnancy. Alcohol detoxification and methanol detoxification from aspartame share the same common aldehyde-based detoxification pathways in human metabolism. The placenta has no defense against fat-soluble, aldehyde-based toxins. This means that these toxins cross into the placenta and affect the fetus just as easily as alcohol crosses into a person's brain. How dangerous it is depends on a mother's specific detoxification capacity and health status. While healthy pregnant women may have no trouble at all in detoxifying a certain amount of aspartame, why push one's luck?

SUMMARY

The health of the subconscious brain is vital in determining a correct appetite and body set point for proper weight. Pregnancy and early life are crucial periods. How they are managed can have long-lasting effects. If these periods are managed correctly, a person is much more likely to have a healthy life. If not, a person is much more likely to struggle with body weight and heart disease.

Since unborn children have very little to say about these issues, and the decisions of others will affect them for the rest of their lives, it is the responsibility of parents and health officials to do as good a job as is possible to help our future generations get started on the right foot.

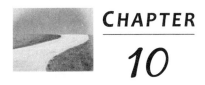

CHAPTER

10

New Fat-Burning Discoveries

A COMPLETELY NEW MECHANISM of leptin control has now been discovered involving leptin regulation of muscle energy production.[127] This is different than the primary control of leptin by the subconscious brain.[128]

Primary leptin control determines overall energetic metabolism for your body as a whole. The hypothalamus gland in your brain is in charge of overall leptin control, just as it is in control of the overall 911 stress response you use to meet an emergency demand.

We have already mentioned that each cell in the body has its own 911 stress-response capability, controlled by NF-kappaB. There is no way that your brain can directly determine the exact needs are for any specific cell; thus, local control for stress demands is delegated to NF-kappaB.

In a similar fashion, there is no way that leptin acting in the subconscious brain can determine the precise energy-production status of a specific cell. The new scientific discoveries have uncovered a new method of leptin operation, wherein leptin acts locally inside of cells to regulate energy production and consequently the antioxidant defense system of the cell.

UNCOUPLING PROTEINS

Mapping of the human genome has identified five primary metabolic uncoupling proteins (UCP). A UCP disconnects normal cell-energy production and turns calories into one hundred percent heat. In essence, this is a method of completely disposing of calories.

A well-known example of this is the metabolism of brown adipose tissue, or BAT. This type of fat tissue is totally different from the white adipose tissue that stores extra fat. It has many nerves flowing into it, as well as a blood supply, thus giving it a brownish color and its name. It is the only tissue in the body that contains UCP1.

UCP1 allows this tissue to turn a calorie into one hundred percent heat. Normal cell energy production makes thirty-five percent heat and sixty-five percent energy in the form of ATP. ATP is like cellular money: as it is made, it sits in the purse or wallet until it is needed. Upon activity, ATP is called into action so that a person has energy to do something, whether mental, physical, or emotional. By comparison, a UCP produces no energy at all, literally wasting potential energy by making heat.

Activation of BAT is naturally stimulated by an individual's need to adapt to a colder temperature, and the hallmark of its activation is the shiver response. This BAT response is essential for a newborn child in adapting to an environment that is colder than the womb. BAT is also stimulated by nerves, especially adrenaline. Since the 1980s, nerve stimulation of BAT has been a favorite target of many weight-loss strategies that employ ephedra, caffeine, stimulant drugs, or some other type of nerve stimulant. The idea is that by stimulating BAT, extra fat calories will be melted away in the form of heat production.

We now know that this type of weight-loss strategy is risky and prone to relapse. First of all, there are serious cardiovascular and kidney side effects from this type of excess and ongoing nerve stimulation. It is also likely to induce the problem of adrenaline resistance that we discussed earlier. Second, this type of nerve stimulation depresses leptin in the brain and induces the genetic response to starvation. This means it is highly likely that any weight lost from this strategy will be regained as soon as the excess nerve stimulation is stopped.

The new discoveries center on the operation of UCP3, which is under the influence of leptin and thyroid control. UCP3 is dominant in muscle cells.[129] Like the UCP1 in BAT, UCP3 has the ability to shift a cell out of regular aerobic energy production of ATP and into heat production. Interestingly, UCP3 is also found in BAT, and leptin can stimulate BAT without any nervous-system input. Accessing this pathway would be a very safe way to lose weight, although it is not practical.

For example, a low-protein diet will stimulate BAT because leptin is trying to figure out a way to dispose of extra fat and glucose that it can not burn normally, due to the lack of protein (protein drives normal liver metabolism).[130] Another problem with BAT and weight loss is that it shrinks in size as a person gets older because it is infiltrated by deposits of white fat that clog its function.[131] A much better way to lose weight is to master the healthy activation of UCP3, which significantly increases the ability of your body to burn off excess fat.

FROM A MUSCLE CELL'S POINT OF VIEW

Pretend for a moment you are a muscle cell. You need to make energy in order to perform. The greater the activity, the more energy you need. You plan on producing energy from calories. You prefer to use carbohydrates or fat for energy production; however, you are at the mercy of whatever your master has been eating. When the food calories enter your cell, you give instructions on what to do with them so that they can be burned for fuel. Carbohydrates go directly into your muscle cell's Krebs-cycle engines and crank out ATP; fats go through beta oxidation on their way to ATP production. In other words, you have strategies for converting any type of calorie sent to you into energy.

Let us assume for a moment that you are a well-conditioned muscle cell, like that of an elite athlete. Basically, you are as good as it gets. Fuel comes in, and you efficiently make energy out of whatever type of calorie it is; your cell energy production systems are top notch. Tests on elite athletes show this to be the case; there is no significant activation of UCP3, even during intense muscle activity. This is because a well-conditioned muscle is very effective at using any type of calorie to make energy. Even high fat intake does not cause UCP3 activation.[132]

Needless to say, this elite athlete is not overweight.

Let us say you are a muscle cell from an average fit person who is generally healthy. You get involved in some aerobic exercise requiring ongoing production of energy. At first, energy output is adequate; there was no trouble making energy from the sugar that was already stored in the muscle and from the extra sugar "care packages" sent by the liver as exercise continued. After a half hour or so, all the available sugar is gone and now you have to burn fat for fuel. However, efficiency is not anywhere near as good as in the elite athlete muscle. In fact, more fat is coming into your cell than you know what to do with. No wonder the muscles are getting tired. Now UCP3 activates in order to dispose of fat.[133] Why?

The new discovery is that the cell's decision to turn on UCP3 and dispose of fat calories as heat is mostly controlled by leptin, especially by a lack of leptin resistance occurring throughout the body. When leptin is working efficiently it is really smart. It reasons, "There is more fat coming into this cell than it can use. If it is not going to get used, it will pile up in the cell, clogging the cell with excess fat, literally poisoning the cell with fat. To compensate for this problem, I will turn on a backup system that will dispose of this extra fat." Thus, leptin activates UCP3 to defend the cell against fat poisoning. In so doing the cell now burns off the fat, making one hundred percent heat (and no energy).

In athletes, the point at which muscle cells start activating UCP3 is the point where they start losing muscle energy performance and increasing heat production. If it is also hot outside, the combination can push a person into heatstroke. For the first time, we can now understand the precise mechanism by which this happens. This is why so many professional sports teams struggle with health issues at the beginning of training camp. Professional athletes come in with out-of-shape muscles and then try to push performance, resulting in excess UCP3-driven heat production.

Let us assume for a moment that one has sluggish and tired muscle cells, part of an unfit person who is most likely overweight. These cells struggle to make muscle energy (ATP), which is reflected in weak and unfit-feeling muscles. Fatigue, a tired or irritable head, and a lack of sustainable energy through the day are commonly experienced symptoms. Due to low energy, the individual craves food and eats plenty. As the calories come in, insulin rises and brings them to the cell's doorstep. Insulin rings the doorbell and asks if the cell would like some calories. The cell politely says no thanks. However, insulin is under delivery directions to drop off forty percent of the calories in muscle cells. Insulin is very persistent and forces some of the calories into muscle cells. If insulin cannot get calories into the muscles or the liver, they are heading for fat storage.

For a muscle cell, this is a stressful situation. Here are these calories that need to be used. If a person is too inactive there is no need for them. If the extra calories are sugar, it is like spilling honey on the counter and letting it sit there for three days. This is a problem called caramelization, wherein sugar cements the cell and eventually kills it. If the calories are fat, they simply pile up inside the cell and clog its function.[134] It is a no-win situation.

Out of necessity cells try to burn some sugar in their Krebs-cycle car engines in an attempt to produce energy. This works to some degree, but the efficiency of the car engines is lacking. The engines actually start clanking, and there is black smoke coming out of the exhaust in the form of lactic acid and free radicals. Since trying to make energy is now poisoning the cell with exhaust fumes, it decides to switch to fat burning – after all, the fat is beginning to pile up. In order to do this at all, there must be a leptin control message to activate UCP3. Unfortunately, just as leptin resistance affects the brain, so it affects muscle cells. The leptin message is not getting into the cell at a rate it should, and thyroid activation is lacking too. Thus, UCP3 only partly works, meaning there is no way to dispose of the extra fat – it piles up.

We now have a muscle cell that is being poisoned by sugar, fat, and its own exhaust fumes. This is what fibromyalgia feels like. It is also how an elite athlete feels the day after intense exercise. The elite athletes will most likely recover from the strain of the excess exercise.

The individuals with fibromyalgia never did any exercise; they are more concerned about how they are going to have any energy to get through the day without their muscles aching everywhere. Even if they overdo it just slightly, their muscles will feel ten times worse the next day – as their ability to recover is severely compromised.

In the process of sliding down into this abyss of poor health and dysregulated muscle function, muscle cells earnestly begin to reject insulin's attempt to deliver calories. When insulin rings the doorbell to drop off calories, the muscle cell locks the door and throws away the key as a self-defense mechanism. This problem is called insulin resistance. At the same time, leptin resistance develops in relation to the muscle cell. Now the muscle cell cannot activate UCP3 and fat cannot be disposed of as heat.

THE LEPTIN KEY

A primary function of efficient leptin operation is to prevent fat from being deposited in cells that are not designed to store fat.[135] It does this by activating UCP3, which in turn burns off the excess fat by converting it to heat. It works in harmony with thyroid hormone. Low thyroid also reduces UCP3 activity.[136] This is a survival defense system. Once leptin resistance develops, then leptin does not activate UCP3 at an optimal rate, and fat accumulates.

The mechanism relates to muscles, heart, arteries, liver, brown adipose tissue, and other body tissues. As fat accumulates in the wrong places, it seriously alters the healthy function of that specific tissue. Developing fat in all the wrong places is a clear path to disease. The actual cause of this problem has now been identified as leptin resistance resulting in deactivation of UCP3.

A key sign that a person is headed down this path directly relates to muscle performance. A person either has a fit and vibrant feeling in the muscles or is headed into some state of fatigue or lessened function. As weight is gained in combination with a poor energetic feeling in the muscles, it can be accurately predicted that fat is being deposited in places that cause health risk – in addition to the extra pounds that are in white adipose tissue.

Another telling symptom of this problem is a person's heat response to increased physical activity. Many overweight people notice that they sweat easily upon exertion, yet this is not associated with any pleasant energy production, such as normal sweating during refreshing exercise. This occurs because the body has become very ineffective at burning sugar and has shunted the calories into heat production via UCP3, as a defense mechanism.[137] This causes an abnormal overexpression of UCP3 and UCP2, which in turn directly damages the pancreatic beta cells, eventually causing diabetes.[138]

Some overweight individuals never sweat. Some elite athletes do not sweat that much during exercise because they are so efficient at making ATP (sixty-five percent energy, thirty-five percent heat) that they never get into the one hundred percent heat production of UCP3. They usually sweat after they are finished, as they are cooling down and dissipating heat. Compare this to the overweight nonsweater who struggles to make ATP and thus does not even get thirty-five percent heat and cannot do normal sweating from increased ATP synthesis during exercise. This reflects an inability to burn sugar and fat – classic insulin and leptin resistance. Calories just pile up in the blood (sugar, triglycerides, and cholesterol) as this person heads toward type II diabetes.

In both situations the adrenaline resistance sets in, causing blood pressure to rise. This explains the path to metabolic syndrome X from a muscle's point of view, with an individual's increased risk for becoming one of the 400,000 people a year who are dying from obesity-induced disease.

THE EXERCISE SOLUTION

In part two, *The Leptin Diet*, we explain how to eat in order to unravel this problem. At this time it is worth pointing out a few tips regarding exercise and fat burning.

Based on the newly discovered function of leptin in muscle, the necessity of consistent exercise to maintain health has never been more important.[139] People who have been in a consistent exercise program and have slipped out of the pattern will notice that this was an adverse turning point in their health. Conversely, people who get into a good exercise pattern notice an improvement in health.

Individuals with more serious muscle problems like fibromyalgia have trouble exercising, even if they want to. Their path to recovery is slower but can be accomplished. Gradual improvement in exercise progressively disposes of junk fat that is clogging body function.[140] Consistency is always more important than intensity, in terms of how to exercise in order to solve a more serious metabolic problem.

The following information applies to a person who is fit enough to do some exercise and wants to maximize the burning of fat for weight loss. We are in favor of a wide variety of exercise types involving strength, flexibility, and aerobics. This tip is specifically about aerobics.

Ideal aerobics for weight loss needs to be done at least three times a week, for one to two hours in duration. How fast a person goes or what a person does is based on current level of fitness and preferred form of exercise. For most people, even people who have a degree of fitness, long walks are best for the purpose of weight loss, primarily because most people are not fit enough to jog for an extended period of time and get a good response (jogging is better if you can do it).

When exercise is too intense, it produces tiredness during, following, or the next day. This typically involves water-weight retention to cool off the tissues that were overheated by the exercise. When this happens, no weight loss will occur. A person may dump two pounds of fluid with the exercise, but with the next meal all the weight will be back because the body insists on holding onto water to cool off the wear and tear.

This problem is typically experienced by individuals in their thirties and forties who used to be in better shape. They think that by going faster they will burn more calories and lose weight. Obviously this is not working, because the scale is not moving down – in fact it may even move up! Going faster is fine for those who know what they are doing and are getting a good response.

To maximize fat burning during exercise, new science supports the following:

1) Do aerobics between meals or first thing in the morning before eating. When you have not eaten for a few hours, exercise will begin to liberate fatty acids and turn on UCP3 within a half hour.[141] If a person has eaten high carbohydrates prior to the exercise, UCP3 activity will not activate or will activate only slightly, thus drastically-reducing the fat burning potential of exercise.[142]

2) It is more important to go longer than faster. The goal is to find an accelerated muscle pace that can be sustained. After about fifteen to twenty minutes muscles will feel like they have "clicked into a gliding pace." This is reflective of entering a fat-burning mode. If you are going too fast, meaning your legs are getting heavy and tiredness is setting in, fat-burning mode has stopped. Slow down; within a few minutes you should feel better and fat burning will resume. The goal is to maintain this gliding-along feeling for one-two hours. The fat-burning UCP3 can be increased up to seven times its resting value by prolonged aerobic exercise.[143]

3) After exercising, do not eat until there is a hunger signal. Conversely, be sure to eat when there is a hunger signal; otherwise, your body will go into a stressed state. The hunger signal may happen five minutes after you are done or it may not happen for several hours. Once you have clicked on this UCP3-driven fat-burning mode, this is prime weight-loss time. It may last for several hours at an accelerated pace as your body continues to burn fat even though the exercise is over. This mode is reflected by a clear head and good energy feeling. When in this mode, do not eat anything. Water is okay. Eating will raise insulin and send all the fatty acids that could have been burned off by UCP3 back to storage. However, if you are hungry you should eat; otherwise your body will shut down and there will be an inflammatory response from the exercise which may cause weight gain.

A good response to such an exercise time will typically result in a half pound of actual fat loss, not just a drop in water weight. Amazingly, a healthy response to increased UCP3 activity actually improves the antioxidant status of cells.[144,145,146] If a person does this three times a week this can equate to one to two pounds a week of healthy fat loss from this fat-burning time. There are other fat-burning times related to how a person eats, which we will discuss in our next section. The good news is that when all of the healthy fat-burning techniques are put into place, it is technically possible to lose three to four pounds a week of actual fat in a healthy way.

NUTRITIONAL SUPPLEMENTS AS TOOLS FOR HEALTH

Nutritional supplementation can significantly enhance the production of ATP and the function of UCP3, enabling more efficient weight loss. Activating UCP3 is a safe and effective way to lose weight and reduce obesity.[147] How do people know what they need?

Our government lags ten years behind the clear-cut science about using vitamins to fortify a given health need, and often actively tries to suppress you from knowing what your options are. If individuals were told how to activate UCP3 with nutrition, it would help many to lose weight and reduce their risk for diabetes and heart disease.

Politically, drug companies are terrified of natural solutions for health. Many people use vitamins instead of drugs to naturally improve their health – thus vitamins are a direct competitor to drug sales. Additionally, people who feel better or get better do not then need drugs. The pharmaceutical companies are constantly trying to regulate supplements to control this competition and suppress health options other than their own; and they trash individual freedom of choice in the process.

Medical doctors are generally a useless source of help when it comes to employing nutrition. People with doctors who understand nutrition, or who are at least open minded about nutrition, should count their blessings. But they still should not expect much actual help other than some encouragement.

Government recommendations for nutrient intake do not offer any assistance. These guidelines are for preventing nutrient deficiency disease. They have nothing to do with helping to improve metabolism in an overweight person.

One commonsense way to establish a personal nutritional support program is to base it on a definable response to some type of need. In the case of muscles, UCP3, and weight loss, this would mean using nutrition to help produce or fortify the desired response of actually burning fat from exercise.

People who follow our guidelines for eating and the exercise tips for fat burning just given above, who feel great and are consistently losing weight, do not need extra nutritional support for the specific purpose of weight loss. Extra support may make weight loss go faster or make it easier, but that is different than a true need.

By comparison, take overweight individuals with fibromyalgia. Their doctor tells them to go out and exercise to lose weight. They think to themselves, "Easy for you to say, hard for me to do." As they try to exercise they hurt more and are actually increasing the damage in muscles while trying to fulfill the doctor's request. The doctor gives them pain pills, antidepressants, and sleeping pills. They still cannot exercise. The source of their problem has nothing to do with pain pills, sleeping pills, or antidepressants. From the muscle cell's point of view, this is a problem of being poisoned by sugar, fat, and its own exhaust fumes while trying to make energy. Here is a real need for extra nutritional support. As such people gradually improve, they will eventually be able to do the long walks. Enough nutritional support for them is whatever it takes to start heading in the right direction. If they can get three to six months of consistent progress under their belts, then they can get back to a level of health that most people simply take for granted. We know – we've helped thousands of people with fibromyalgia.

It has recently been discovered that coenzyme Q10 is required for the function of UCP3.[148] It has also been discovered that a lack of antioxidants, in general, stresses out UCP3 and causes it not to work well, since UCP3 actually helps coordinate a cell's antioxidant defense system in harmony with antioxidant nutrients.[149] Virtually all overweight people are low in antioxidants.[150]

It has long been known that B vitamins, Krebs-cycle intermediates

- especially malic acid, magnesium, and coenzyme Q10 – are needed for cellular energy production (ATP synthesis).

Thus, one strategy for weight loss is to ensure that there are enough B vitamins and magnesium for energy production. These could be taken at meals or before exercise. Specifically to enhance the fat burning during exercise, an individual could take 100 to 300 milligrams of coenzyme Q10 and a multiple antioxidant just before exercise. This increases the likelihood that the UCP3 system will work better to burn off fat more efficiently.

An athlete could use these strategies to enhance performance. An average fit person could use these strategies to enhance weight loss. A person who is stuck at a particular weight could use these strategies to start the scale moving in the right direction. A person with fibromyalgia could use these strategies to be able to take a ten minute walk and get started back on a path of health.

Any person getting older has a higher need for nutrient support because the entire UCP system works less efficiently with aging.[151] The purpose for using nutrition is based on the ability to get a desired result. The "desired result" varies from person to person, based on their existing health and what they are trying to accomplish. Sometimes extra nutrient support makes things easier; sometimes it is the only way a person can get moving in the right direction.

A NOTE ON PREGNANCY

Preeclampsia is a common and serious complication of pregnancy. It can be life threatening to the mother and can cause a variety of health issues for the unborn baby. This problem is diagnosed by a medical doctor when blood pressure rises during pregnancy and protein spills out into the urine.

A mother who enters pregnancy free of leptin resistance and in good health is much less likely to have this problem. Becoming pregnant is a huge metabolic demand for the mother. In many ways, it is the same as a five-mile run or eight hours of construction work a day, on top of whatever the mother is already doing.

When individuals exercise too much, they have the option of recovering or doing less the next time. When a woman becomes pregnant, there is no such option. If she enters pregnancy with inefficiently functioning leptin and borderline muscle fitness, the daily high-energy demands of pregnancy can push her body into a state of leptin resistance. In the leptin-resistant condition, excessive amounts of TNFa are generated, a highly inflammatory signal. This is what drives up blood pressure, damages the kidneys so protein leaks out into the urine, and induces drastic wear and tear throughout her body.

Now it makes sense why women with preeclampsia have low levels of coenzyme Q10, vitamin E, and vitamin C. By using nutrition to enhance cell energy production and the function of UCP3, the problems of preeclampsia can be reduced or prevented. Thus, the mother can more efficiently keep up with the constant metabolic demand of building another body.

Common sense tells us that any woman wanting to become pregnant should do everything she can to gain good muscle fitness and proper body weight. Keep in mind that preeclampsia is a problem defined by a progression of leptin issues that have reached a serious level of risky blood pressure and severe kidney stress.

Many women will experience lesser degrees of this problem during pregnancy. It may not manifest as a serious health problem during pregnancy, but it takes a significant toll on the mother. This is why many women never physically feel the same after having kids; pregnancies are an adverse turning point in their health.

Key symptoms of such wear and tear of pregnancy are the inability to lose weight following pregnancy, excessive weight gain during pregnancy, and the internal feeling of wear and tear that has not been repaired. If a woman gets pregnant again without fully recovering from the previous pregnancy, then these effects become more pronounced. Getting weight off after pregnancy and fully recovering from the pregnancy are vital for any mother wishing to maintain her quality of health, especially if she wants to have more children.

SUMMARY

Science has made incredible progress uncovering the exact nature of health problems faced by many individuals. This opens the door to solutions that can enhance fitness and lower body weight for many people who are either stuck or have given up. This information can also help generally fit people avoid the weight gain that is common in the third and fourth decades of life. That way, when the high-risk-for-disease decades are reached, individuals will not find themselves in the high-risk category.

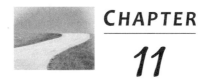

CHAPTER

11

The Cause of Heart Disease

SCIENCE NOW DEMONSTRATES that leptin problems are an independent and significant risk factor for cardiovascular disease and metabolic syndrome X. On the other hand, the healthy function of leptin directly prevents cardiovascular disease. There is no such thing as "good leptin" and "bad leptin." It is entirely a matter of leptin efficiency and the restoration of natural balance of leptin function. Indeed, leptin is the king hormone of natural balance.

It is well known that leptin problems are a major cause of obesity and obesity is a major factor causing heart disease. In order to prove that leptin problems are a cause of heart disease, it is necessary to prove that they cause heart disease independent of extra pounds of body fat.

Scientists have now shown that leptin causes heart disease, demonstrating that leptin problems directly induce insulin resistance, high cholesterol, and high blood pressure, and not as a result of the amount of extra fat.[152] This has now been proven to be the case for healthy older women, regardless of their weight. Leptin problems stand out as the top heart-related risk factor issue when compared to all the other traditional markers of heart disease.[153]

On the encouraging side, just getting weight loss moving in the right direction reduces the stressful and problematic side of leptin that causes heart disease.[154] Simply getting into a better diet pattern reduces TNFa up to fifty percent.[155] Statistically, a five percent initial weight loss places a person in the category of lower risk for heart disease.

When a trend of weight loss is maintained then the same risk reduction is associated with a ten percent initial loss of body weight.[156] These findings are very encouraging because they mean that just getting started on the right path and making some progress automatically puts a person in a lower risk category. Continuing on that path consistently over time will further reduce risk and actually eliminate the extra pounds of fat that reflect a potential problem.

INERTIA IN THE MEDICAL COMMUNITY

The studies referred to above, published in April of 2004, actually point out the main cause of cardiovascular disease. How long will it take the practicing medical community to grasp their meaning and implement something useful in day-to-day medical practice?

Most doctors have established a comfort zone around cardiovascular care and are under high pressure to prescribe various drugs in the name of prevention. High blood pressure gets this drug, high cholesterol gets that drug, sticky blood gets a different drug, to name a few. Along with this goes some generic advice about eating a low-fat diet and exercising more. What doctors are allowed to do and how much time they can spend with any one person is heavily influenced for them by administrative systems that control cost.

Almost no attention is given to the meaning of adverse side effects of these medications in the short term, and even less attention is paid to changes in natural balance that invariably occur as a result of using the drugs in the long term. Numbers on paper from lab tests result in the dispensing of a drug, with a reduced priority on truly understanding the person who is taking the medication. And in the world of controlled-cost medical "care," there is never any time to work with individuals to actually return their body to a state of natural balance.

Even when a new risk factor such as CRP (C-reactive protein) is clearly identified patients have to argue with their doctors to order the test. Why? Because there is no convenient drug to administer for poor scores on such a test, and until there is such a drug doctors won't give the test. The CRP reflects the inflammatory problems induced by leptin, because elevated TNFa drives up CRP. The CRP test is backed by overwhelming scientific agreement to support it as a useful marker for heart-disease risk. However, Western medical strategy will be to find a drug to knock down CRP without addressing the actual cause of the problem. The *Health Asset Manager* will be smarter than this; working to change health issues at the root of inflammation and thereby solve the source of the problem. To the *Health Asset Manager* lab tests are sign posts to help mark progress and implement solutions.

For most people leptin blood tests are not important in order to understand whether they have a problem with leptin. All they have to do is look in the mirror, a rather inexpensive test. Blood levels of leptin are typically high when a person is really struggling with food cravings and eating too much. After several weeks on a good diet, as the cravings go away the blood tests will show normal, which only means that surplus leptin has been cleared out of the blood. You have problems with leptin until you are energized and normal body weight and can maintain that weight for a number of months. This is a real-world test – and for most it is all that matters.

Blood tests are not necessarily going to reflect leptin resistance in the brain, liver, pancreas, or muscles. Thus, a normal blood score does not rule out a problem and is not as accurate as the mirror test. However, elevated leptin levels in the blood may relate to heart-disease risk in individuals who are not overweight. A leptin blood test is most relevant for those who are normal weight yet concerned about their cardiovascular health. Any overweight person doesn't really need a test as they obviously have a problem.

HIGH BLOOD PRESSURE

Elevations in blood pressure are directly correlated to increased leptin and body weight.[157] Healthy leptin function enhances the membrane fluidity of cells in the circulatory system through the proper function of nitric oxide (NO). Properly functioning NO throughout the circulatory system is vital for correct vascular tone and relaxation, and consequently for normal blood pressure.

In leptin resistance, a feature of the accompanying high blood pressure is that platelets change and become less fluid and more prone to stick together adversely.[158] When leptin resistance is induced in mice, the systolic blood pressure rises thirty percent, free radical production is drastically elevated, and NO levels are decreased by fifty percent (seemingly due to depletion counteracting the excess production of free radicals). At the same time, sodium is retained in the kidneys.[159]

This study demonstrates that leptin resistance induces high blood pressure by several mechanisms, one throughout the entire circulatory system as a form of stress to arteries and blood vessels, and another by inducing kidney dysregulation. This is consistent with the information we have provided about adrenaline resistance, wherein sympathetic nerves try to stimulate fat cells that have gone numb to stimulation. Even though the fat cells have gone numb to stimulation, the kidneys have not. This leads to direct stimulation of high blood pressure from kidney distress.[160]

This information documents that excess leptin generates high blood pressure by two distinct methods. A vicious side effect of this problem, which locks it into place, has now been identified. Obese women with high blood pressure have significantly elevated levels of NPY (neuropeptide Y) compared to normal-weight individuals with normal blood pressure. Oral glucose challenge in these individuals provokes an exaggerated insulin response.[161]

NPY is an appetite signal involved in the desire for carbohydrates. Improper elevations cause excess carbohydrate cravings. Normally, excess NPY is controlled by leptin entering the subconscious brain. In overweight individuals leptin is not getting into the subconscious brain and NPY stays excessively elevated. Improper carbohydrate cravings result in further overeating that works against healthy blood pressure.

Every time the carbohydrates are eaten the person feels better for a brief period of time, but the exaggerated response to insulin makes insulin resistance, leptin resistance, and adrenaline resistance worse. This in turn acts to lock in the metabolic syndrome X and high risk for heart disease.

Blood pressure medications act in one way or another to de-energize your circulatory system. This may make the number look better but it does not fix the reason blood pressure is elevated and may make problems worse as time goes along as the flow of nutrition anywhere in one's body is adversely affected by any long term use of blood pressure medication. Unfortunately, when doctors treat numbers instead of the person, they think everything is now fixed and the drug should be taken indefinitely. Granted, the more fragile the health of the individual, the greater the need for medical attention and medication management. However, a great majority of people taking blood pressure medication are not in this true drug-need category.

If the actual cause of the high blood pressure is repaired, then there is no need for medication. Leptin resistance has now been identified as a primary cause of high blood pressure. From a health professional's point of view, solving this problem is labor intensive, with no shortcuts. Individuals who wish to solve it will need to take a lot of initiative on their own.

HIGH CHOLESTEROL, LOW THYROID, AND LEPTIN

The liver is recognized as the primary metabolic factory of cholesterol production in the human body. The liver will make cholesterol even if little is consumed in the diet. As it turns out, snacking between meals is like punching the liver in the nose: the liver responds by making extra cholesterol.

This is a primary dietary mistake leading to improper cholesterol elevation, which we fully explain in part two, *The Leptin Diet*. The statin drugs, now being widely promoted for lowering cholesterol, work by interrupting the liver's effort to make cholesterol. There are pros and cons to this class of drug, but the main point is that it is an effort to get the liver not to make so much cholesterol.

Reasonable questions to ask in order to really understand this problem are: Why is the liver making extra cholesterol? Is it part of a defense system, or is it part of an imbalance? For that matter, how does the liver know to make cholesterol in the first place? What is LDL cholesterol actually doing in the human body, especially in a specific person with high cholesterol? These simple questions have many answers, far beyond the scope of this book. We will simply point out that doctors seldom think about the unique needs of any individual before giving out statin drugs for high cholesterol.

We have already cited a number of studies indicating that high cholesterol is associated with leptin problems. Now a new study confirms that leptin problems cause high cholesterol. Researchers were able to lower cholesterol by injecting leptin into the brain of rats, and they documented the direct down regulation of liver enzymes that make cholesterol as a result of the brain injection.[162]

This is a major finding, because humans with leptin resistance do not have a proper amount of leptin getting into the brain. Leptin resistance creates an improper signal to the liver, telling the liver to make extra cholesterol. When a person overcomes leptin resistance, then a normal leptin message can go into the brain, which in turn promotes a more normal synthesis of cholesterol.

A concurrent factor is the presence of poor thyroid function induced by leptin problems. Low thyroid slows down the rate that cholesterol can be cleared in normal metabolic processes. Blatant hypothyroid problems as well as subclinical thyroid problems are associated with elevated cholesterol.[163] The *Journal of the American Medical Association* recently published a study of issues relating to individuals with subclinical thyroid problems. Their research confirmed such individuals are likely to have high cholesterol, but any benefit from treatment with thyroid hormone was inconclusive.[164] That is because the low thyroid tendencies are caused by leptin problems.

The precise mechanism of thyroid hormone control by the subconscious brain has now been discovered.[165,166] Yes, the problem is caused by low leptin in the brain, part of the genetic response to starvation. Low leptin in the brain produces a signal to slow down metabolism so that we do not perish from a lack of food. Higher leptin in the brain says metabolism can go faster plenty of food is being consumed. Leptin resistance means there is too much food being ingested, but the brain is not getting the message.

There is now proof that leptin signals the specific production of thyroid hormone; consequently, when there is leptin resistance thyroid hormone will be less active everywhere in your body. A low thyroid condition produces a three-fold lowering of UCP3 in muscle.[167] As we have discussed, this directly turns down healthy fat burning by muscle, which in turn contributes to obesity.

Taken together, the new science shows that leptin-induced elevated cholesterol occurs by two mechanisms working synergistically together in the wrong direction:

1) Low leptin in the brain signals the liver to make extra cholesterol.
2) Low leptin in the brain slows down thyroid hormone, in turn reducing normal cholesterol clearance from the body.

Fixing leptin resistance fixes the source of both problems and returns the body to a state of natural balance.

ARE STATIN DRUGS SAFE?

Heart disease is the number-one killer in the world, a serious health problem. Statins are a widely used drug for lowering cholesterol and attempting to reduce the risk for heart disease. They are obviously a large profit center for drug companies, with billions of dollars at stake.

Let us focus on the key side effect that is a potential problem – that of muscle damage. The public is being told by major medical journals that the benefits of statins far outweigh the risks, and that the incidence of side effects is low, ranging from one to five percent, depending on the health of the individual taking them, the amount taken, and their combination with other drugs.[168,169] Patients are told to report to their doctors any muscle pain, muscle fatigue, or other muscle problem that may be experienced while taking them.

Do you believe the safety proclamation? After all, women were told for years that the benefits of estrogen far outweighed the risks, only to find out the opposite was true. And now there are serious side effects of antidepressants, so that suicide warnings are now placed on their labels – how safe are they?

This safety proclamation about statins comes even though nobody has been able to figure out how they cause muscle problems or who is really at risk. It is hard to believe in the risk/benefit safety assurance when the cause of the problem is unknown. Keep in mind, we are talking about muscle problems. We just spent the previous chapter explaining that healthy function of muscle is essential to proper weight loss and health.

Also, keep in mind that the one to five percent risk is based on serious muscle damage, not on reports of feeling crummy while on the medication. The number of individuals experiencing adverse muscle changes from statins is over thirty-five percent. There are no studies on statins and UCP3 function. We have known since 1996 that statins change healthy muscle function adversely in almost every individual, as reflected by a clear increase in lactic acid and pyruvate measured in the blood of those who take these drugs.[170] This means that normal energy production in muscles is shifted into a condition where excess exhaust fumes are produced, rather than healthy muscle-cell energy.

We also know that coenzyme Q10 is depleted by statin administration, as Q10 synthesis is based on cholesterol metabolism pathways.[171,172] Not only is Q10 vital for muscle function, it is vital for energy production in the heart.[173] It has also been discovered that statins are toxic to human immune cells, even in small amounts. This toxicity is based on the depletion of Q10 from the immune cells and can be prevented by Q10 supplementation.[174] Depleting Q10 is not a good idea, period.

Science supports the co-administration of Q10 with statins in all cases. Statins provide their benefit by lowering cholesterol. In many cases, the same could be accomplished by improving leptin and thyroid function and losing weight. Statin side effects work against the healthy response to exercise and may damage muscle function. Fixing leptin problems enhances muscle function and the health of muscle. Leptin management is clearly the first choice for prevention and long-term resolution. Statins, like all medications, will have an appropriate role in managing serious cardiovascular disease. The choice of preventive strategy is in the hands of the individual; it does take more work to be truly healthy.

SUMMARY

Groundbreaking discoveries have proven that leptin problems are the major cause of cardiovascular disease, from the point of view of internal body function that produces the disease. This is no longer an open question; it is proven. Improving the healthy function of leptin is the key to resolving cardiovascular risk factors. It is also the key to not developing them in the first place.

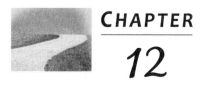

The Importance of *Mastering* Leptin

MANY RESEARCHERS, SCIENTISTS, HEALTH PROFESSIONALS, AND INDIVIDUALS have sought to uncover the keys to a healthy life. A great deal has been written about the lifestyles of healthy people. Despite all the research and personal explorations, no clear defining principle has emerged that explains the fundamental science behind optimum health.

Our new understanding of leptin marks the defining principle of optimum health. This is because leptin controls energy regulation in the human body. Without a proper energy supply, nothing can work correctly.

Understanding leptin and learning how to manage it will make a healthy life possible for many individuals who would otherwise suffer from poor energy and poor physical health. A failure to master leptin is a fast track to increased disease risk and accelerated aging.

Mastering leptin is the best chance our society has, on an individual basis, of solving the obesity epidemic, along with reducing the associated and overwhelming health costs. It is a shortsighted individual who believes that others harm only themselves when they eat poorly. The eventual costs, in terms of health care, lost productivity, and quality of life are a staggering burden.

We live in a world of temptation on every corner. Learning to master leptin is a true life skill. It is not easy. The reward is quality of health. It is a personal choice. It is the most important life skill of a

Health Asset Manager.

In the first part of this book, we introduced the scope of leptin. Leptin is the hormone secreted by fat cells in white adipose tissue. It communicates to the brain to let the brain know how much fuel is "in the gas tank." If there is adequate fuel, then metabolism runs along at a nice pace and everything works normally. If fuel is running low, then metabolism slows down in order to not run out of fuel and thus die of starvation. Leptin is truly the survival principle of the subconscious mind.

Overeating leads to excess leptin production and the eventual development of leptin resistance. Once this happens, the brain no longer perceives the true amount of leptin. The brain cannot judge how much fat is in storage. Typically, this causes a person to carry an extra five to twenty pounds that will not go away.

In more serious situations, the brain thinks the body is starving, even though there is plenty of leptin and lots of extra pounds of fat in storage. The individual is stuck in a pattern of leptin resistance, insulin resistance, and adrenaline resistance.

Many individuals experience problems with leptin at very young ages. Type II diabetes, formerly called adult-onset diabetes, is now common in adolescents. This is an alarming trend of society-wide leptin mismanagement.

It would be bad enough if the problems with leptin simply caused individuals to be overweight. That is only the tip of the iceberg. White adipose tissue also contains immune cells that, under the influence of leptin problems, generate massive amounts of inflammation. This sets the stage for all types of ill health, including the early onset of virtually all diseases of aging.

The fact that these risk factors and trends can be completely stopped, simply by learning to master leptin, is a major breakthrough in our understanding of optimum health.

In part two, we explain lifestyle essentials that form the foundation of leptin management. These are the important basics of how to eat so as not to upset the leptin apple cart. It is essential that individuals learn enough diet skills and lifestyle skills to maintain an excellent state of natural balance.

In part three, we explore numerous leptin issues in more depth. We explain how thyroid problems are almost always leptin problems; by solving the leptin problem, the thyroid problems tend to go away. We explain why leptin is essential for a variety of factors in healthy function, including healing, immunity, and strong bones.

We explain how nutritional supplementation can help individuals overcome issues with leptin resistance, insulin resistance, and adrenaline resistance. These are true solutions that open the door to good health for many individuals who would otherwise struggle needlessly.

We discuss how leptin relates to cardiovascular function and how leptin problems are a prime cause of cardiovascular disease. This opens the door to a new understanding of heart health, and it explains practical steps to change the actual source of the problem that makes cardiovascular disease the number-one killer in America.

We explain how the new understanding of genetic science demonstrates that disease is caused when the body's own natural defense systems are hijacked and turned against itself.

Not surprisingly, leptin mismanagement is key to fanning the flames of these gene-related problems. A lifetime of leptin mismanagement significantly increases cancer risk.

The factors behind how leptin relates to male and female hormonal function, growth hormone, stress hormones, and fibromyalgia are explained. This leads to an understanding of how leptin problems set the stage for male and female cancers.

The human body is complex. It takes some time to learn principles of leptin management and successfully apply them. The time spent is worthwhile; it more than pays for itself in extended lifespan and higher quality of health.

PART TWO

The Leptin Diet®

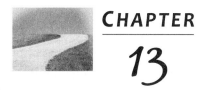

CHAPTER

13

A Lifelong Strategy

The Leptin Diet places a whole new emphasis on how to eat. The entire purpose of the diet is to eat in harmony with leptin. Doing so reduces the serious health risks associated with obesity, and it significantly improves energy utilization from food, even for normal-weight individuals. While a great many of our tips are directed toward overweight individuals trying to get back on track, the underlying principles of *The Leptin Diet* relate to everyone.

Leptin is a hormone governing energy expenditure. When it is working properly, energy is freely liberated. When people click into fat-burning mode on *The Leptin Diet* their energy will be much better. In general, this signifies extracting more energy from less food. People should never feel de-energized and struggling with hunger cravings for an extended period of time while eating less food. This signifies that the body has entered into starvation mode and leptin levels are being excessively depressed. Any weight that is lost in starvation mode is most likely to be regained later.[175]

Leptin balance is reflected in a natural desire for nonsweet food and a very slight, controlled desire for sweet foods. This is because leptin is in control of NPY in the subconscious brain; elevated NPY enforces cravings for sweet foods on a subconscious basis, like an addictive drug. Furthermore, sweet ingestion alters the perception of taste, causing leptin resistance on the tongue. This blunted taste response to the normal sweetness of food induces excess cravings for sugar and sweets and keeps the brain wanting more sweets. At the same time, it provokes brain levels of leptin to stay too low and out of balance, resulting in fatigue and clogged thinking.

This excess desire for sweets is further complicated by a digestive or sinus Candida overgrowth. This overgrowth is reflected by digestive gas and bloating following sugar consumption. It is also reflected in ongoing sinus problems. *Candida albicans* contributes to the excess sugar cravings. The toxins they produce from sugar ingestion make a person feel foggy and spacey, contributing to the overall fatigue present in any person with out-of- balance sugar cravings.

It is best to avoid all artificial sweeteners on *The Leptin Diet* because they flood the brain with sweet sensation in the absence of calories. This type of "sweet ingestion abuse" occurs nowhere in our genetic evolution.

Antiquated dietary guidelines recommend that individuals use these to lower calorie intake, in essence replacing sugar. However, both sugar and artificial sweeteners skew the taste and appetite systems in a way that tends to compromise leptin balance. Proper leptin balance is vital for energetic metabolism; it is a more important principle than whether or not a sweetener has any calories. Compulsive sweet cravings are invariably reflective of leptin imbalance. They go away when leptin goes into balance, a key sign of improvement. It is impossible to make a proper judgment on this improvement if a person is consuming artificial sweeteners.

All soda pop, regardless of the sweetener, should be avoided on *The Leptin Diet*. All high-fructose sweetened beverages should also be avoided. MSG is avoided on *The Leptin Diet* as it is a potent neurotoxin that damages the leptin message in the brain.

The Leptin Diet is designed to maximize fat-burning times. Understanding leptin metabolism enables an individual to increase the times during the day when fat burning is most likely to occur. The more of these times a person takes advantage of, the faster he or she is likely to lose weight in a healthy manner.

The Leptin Diet is a lifestyle of eating that produces significantly improved energy and clarity of thinking. When the diet is working right, an individual wakes up feeling good in the morning. When individuals diverge from the diet, they notice how much less energy they have the next day when they wake up. *The Leptin Diet* is a strategy for eating that can easily be followed for a lifetime.

The diet produces obvious results. It is capable of clearing up depression and a wide variety of body aches, allergies, and other problems, without doing anything specific to address such issues. A common side benefit of the diet is overall improved health and energy, even improvement in difficult or chronic health conditions.

The Leptin Diet is not a manipulation diet based on some weakness a person seems to be experiencing. If a person knows that a certain type of food is bothersome to them, that food can be avoided. However, the diet is not based on food combining, food rotation, or avoidance of food based on blood types.

The Leptin Diet is not based on calorie manipulation; it is based on more efficient calorie utilization. If we "manipulate calories" it is only to improve utilization. We do not want anyone to end up a carbohydrate cripple or head back into weight gain because that person finds it impossible to avoid something. The best way to maintain healthy weight over the long run is to efficiently burn calories and have a proper set point for body weight. *The Leptin Diet* is the key to attaining these goals.

The Leptin Diet is composed of five key principles of eating, called the *Five Rules*. These form a simple theoretical framework for leptin improvement. Each of the rules can be modified if a person understands what he or she is doing in relationship to leptin. For the majority, simply following the *Five Rules* is an easy way to go.

In a sense, implementing the *Five Rules* is like building up physical fitness in relation to eating. Although the rules apply to anyone, some people may not be quite fit enough to immediately employ them. Nevertheless, to move in the direction of the *Five Rules* is to move in a better direction. Modifications can be made to help individuals get started, with the eventual goal of implementing all the rules.

The specific effects of fats, proteins, and carbohydrates will be discussed in detail in the various sections relating to each of the *Five Rules*. This helps an individual gain a better understanding of what to eat and, just as important – when to eat.

SUMMARY

The Leptin Diet is based on current science relating to the hormone leptin. Eating and living in harmony with this hormone is the key to energetic vitality, youthful hormonal balance, optimum body weight, and disease prevention.

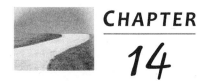

The *Five Rules*

The Leptin Diet consists of five key dietary rules. These rules apply to almost everyone. They are essential to mastering leptin. Individuals need to learn to implement the *Five Rules* on a consistent basis in their life. Doing so establishes a solid foundation for mastering leptin.

Rule 1: Never eat after dinner. Allow eleven to twelve hours between dinner and breakfast. Never go to bed on a full stomach. Finish eating dinner at least three hours before bed. This rule is explained in chapter 15.

Rule 2: Eat three meals a day. Allow five to six hours between meals. Do not snack. This rule is explained in chapter 17.

Rule 3: Do not eat large meals. If you are overweight, always try to finish a meal when you are slightly less than full; the full signal will usually catch up in ten to twenty minutes. Eating slowly is important. This rule is explained in chapter 18.

Rule 4: Eat a breakfast containing protein. This rule is explained in chapter 19.

Rule 5: Reduce the amount of carbohydrates you eat. This rule is explained in chapter 20.

WHY THESE RULES?

Traditional dietary advice focuses on the number of calories in food. Calories come in the form of fats, carbohydrates, and proteins. These substances can potentially become energy; however, if your body cannot metabolize them for one reason or another, they may become stored fat.

No progress will be made on weight loss or maintaining a high quality of health if your body is abused with too many calories or if consumption of calories is improperly timed. Any type of calorie can become toxic to your body if it is consumed inappropriately.

Defining inappropriate is no small task. One glance through the diet-book section of any bookstore quickly reveals that there are as many diets as there are possible food combinations. However, understanding leptin places a whole new perspective on appropriate eating. The *Five Rules* are fundamental to eating so as not to upset leptin balance.

It is certainly wise to eat fresh, organically produced, high-quality foods whenever possible. This includes foods free of chemicals, preservatives, food coloring, partially hydrogenated oils, hormones, antibiotics, and mold toxins that arise when food is stored too long.

THE IMPORTANCE OF THE *Five Rules*

The *Five Rules* are not a special diet in the conventional sense. Conventional diets rely on inducing starvation metabolism in order to lose weight. Their underlying principle is to eat less food and exercise more. Individuals with out-of-balance leptin seldom get to their goal weights in a healthy manner and stay there by following such diet guidelines. Yo-yo dieting is the common response to any weight lost using such an approach. *The Leptin Diet* is a lifestyle that promotes health. It is designed as an effortless dietary lifestyle to be used throughout life.

Some individuals can violate the *Five Rules* and seem to get away with it. This will catch up with them sooner or later. Minimally, this is like rowing a boat against the current. It is a harder way to go. The *Five Rules* are a safe and effective way to maintain a healthy eating pattern over the course of a lifetime.

Some individuals do not have the physical ability to follow the *Five*

Rules. This does not mean the rules are wrong; it simply means these individuals need to get in better shape. People know they should exercise. Some are physically not able to go; others do not find the time. Both leading to poor fitness. It is the same with the *Five Rules*. Working toward better "eating fitness" is essential for any person, so that they can eventually implement the *Five Rules* into their life.

There are ways to vary the *Five Rules* and still maintain healthy metabolism. Elite athletes may need to eat more often, simply to get the number of calories they need. Diabetics have nonfunctioning hormone switches and end up using food to compensate for a broken metabolism. There are a variety of special circumstances that require tailoring the *Five Rules*. However, the principles underlying the *Five Rules* are workable concepts to help keep one's body in natural balance and enhance the proper communication of leptin.

This is why an individual needs to learn to be a competent *Health Asset Manager*. People need to understand why a rule is a rule, so that they can think intelligently with the information and apply it to their life.

Oddly enough, the *Five Rules* are so helpful that eighty percent of the population could simply follow them without knowing why they work, and they would be healthier. This includes resolving long-standing issues with body weight.

Because our goal is to teach individuals to become a *Health Asset Manager*, this part of the book explains the *Five Rules* in great detail, including the science behind them.

WHAT DO CRAVINGS MEAN?

Once you are on the path to implementing the *Five Rules*, the next important issue is to stay on that path regardless of what happens in your life. A variety of factors induce food cravings, and these need to be managed effectively in order to stay on track.

There is tremendous knowledge and scientific research about food cravings, addictive eating patterns, and compulsions. Understanding how these factors relate to each individual and how to manage them effectively is a key skill of the *Health Asset Manager*.

In part two, we explain the fundamentals involved and solution strategies for stress eating and other craving issues. Part three offers additional information about disease, as well as more advanced strategies for stubborn patterns. These issues can and must be solved.

SUMMARY

Understanding and implementing the five key dietary rules for mastering leptin is the foundation of health and getting one's body into natural rhythm. It forms a stable frame of reference for other hormonal and energy patterns in the human body. The *Five Rules* are fundamental for efficiently extracting energy from food – being able to transform the calorie potential in food to real energy – energy that can be felt!

Master these rules and build the foundation of optimum health through dietary stability. This is not simplistic dietary information. These dietary principles are essential for healthy, disease-free living.

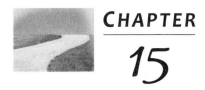

Maximize Primary Fat-Burning Time

WHEN LEPTIN is out of balance, it interferes with the ability of your body to burn fat for fuel. The number-one sign that there is a problem with leptin resistance is overeating at night. This is the single most important symptom indicating that leptin is really out of control.

It is common for people to do a fairly good job of eating correctly until about six in the evening. After that, the "other eating personality" takes over, the one driven by leptin resistance. This other personality is reinforced by alcohol consumption and/or stress – it craves either sweets or fats. The failure to obey the erratic impulses of this personality makes individuals feel tired, grumpy, and irritable. Only when they eat will they feel better – or so they think.

THE 24-HOUR LEPTIN PATTERN

In order to unravel this issue, it is important to understand what is taking place. Leptin levels rise at night. They follow a twenty-four-hour pattern of natural rhythm or natural balance. They peak in the evening hours and are the highest during the first two hours of sleep. They gradually fall during the night and reach their lowest level around noon; then they begin to rise again. Obese individuals have lost their leptin rhythm[176], which is the same as saying they have lost the ability to burn calories properly – that is how they became obese.

When leptin works properly, a high leptin level tells you that you are full; there is no desire to eat. Therefore, it is completely natural not to be hungry after dinner or before bed. There are a variety of reasons for this, one of which is that your body has functions other than digestion to carry out during sleep.

The person with leptin resistance, too, has higher levels of leptin at night, but the brain is not able to perceive the message. The result is that the brain thinks the body needs to store more fat in order to survive, a conclusion that is terribly incorrect. This aberrant conclusion is reinforced by core survival instincts stronger than conscious thought.

This is why people with leptin resistance have trouble looking in the refrigerator after dinner and not eating. It is why their conscious self may try to ensure that there is no food around the house. There is no way a person can win a direct confrontation with leptin-resistance urges. The only way to win this battle is to prevent leptin resistance from happening in the first place *(figure 8)*.

The first step is to understand what is supposed to be done and why. The next step is to implement various strategies to keep leptin under control and working correctly for optimum balance and health.

THE *Five Rules* – Rule 1

Never eat after dinner. Allow eleven to twelve hours between dinner and breakfast. Never go to bed on a full stomach. Finish eating dinner at least three hours before bed.

Any person with active leptin resistance finds this rule somewhat inconceivable to follow. Even people who do not have active leptin resistance may have a variety of reasons why they cannot follow this rule. Some examples include:

1) If I do not eat before bed, I cannot get to sleep.
2) If I do not have a nighttime snack, I wake up hungry in the middle of the night.
3) If I do not eat before bed, I wake up with a headache or feel queasy.

Just because someone cannot follow this rule does not mean the rule is wrong. Anyone who cannot follow this rule has a significant

Normal Leptin Function after Dinner

Figure 8A

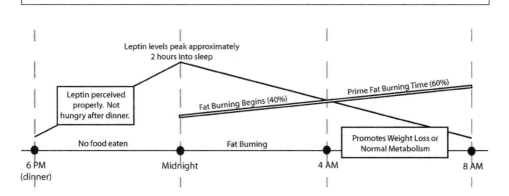

Leptin Resistance

Figure 8B

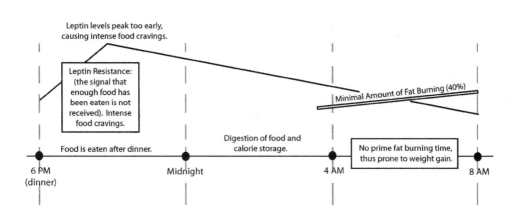

problem with blood glucose metabolism, liver function, and/or leptin resistance.

Most people agree that it is good to go for a long walk or a three to five mile jog. Many people do not have the ability to do this. Reasons vary and may include lack of energy, lack of desire or drive, or physical problems such as a knee problem, just to name a few. Regardless, if people are fit enough to do the exercise and get a good response, they will be healthier. The same principle applies to not eating after dinner and allowing eleven to twelve hours between dinner and breakfast.

There are many reasons why this is a key rule for weight loss and overcoming leptin resistance. It is fundamental for establishing healthy patterns of hormones in the human body. Improperly timed eating can disrupt thyroid hormone, growth hormone, adrenal hormones, sex hormones, and melatonin, and it throws the body out of rhythm, setting the stage for serious diseases.

If physicians or public-health officials informed people of the extreme importance of not eating after dinner, the health-care costs of our country would decline. It may be the most important and under-appreciated principle relating to any type of health problem.

PRIME FAT-BURNING TIME

Sleep is a prime metabolic time. It is when individuals can access the stores of fat that they wish to lose. This works well only when no food has been consumed for eleven to twelve hours and the quality of sleep is good.

In general, the body burns a certain amount of sugar and fat at the same time. When a meal is eaten, the sugar and fat are readily available from the ingested food. After three or so hours, the sugar entering the blood is produced by the liver. A certain amount of sugar is released into the blood, otherwise the brain will not function well and blood sugars will be low. This principle applies whether someone is awake or asleep.

Most of the fat burned during the day either comes directly from food that is consumed or is already in the blood. The majority of calorie metabolism during the day is mostly from readily available energy supplies.

During the night, your body gradually begins to burn a higher portion of fat for fuel. Nine hours after dinner it is quite likely that the readily available fats have been used, and your body will dip into the fat savings account. Therefore, nine to twelve hours after dinner are prime fat-burning hours, in terms of accessing the fat stores in the buttocks, thighs, and stomach.

If anything is eaten before bed, this prime fat-burning time is shut off! This principle is not going to change; it is a fact of biochemistry.

SUMMARY

In order to lose weight properly and healthfully, natural balance must be restored to the leptin communication system. Since leptin is highest at night, this points to nighttime eating patterns as a key indicator of health.

Individuals with significant leptin resistance are not able to control their eating at night. Their eating behavior deviates in the evening hours. The first step is to simply recognize that this is an important part of the problem.

Ideally, a person should not eat after dinner and should go eleven to twelve hours before eating breakfast. A person in good health feels satisfied eating this way and is in an improved state of natural balance.

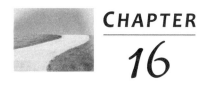

CHAPTER
16

Leptin and Insulin –
Birds of a Feather

INDIVIDUALS with leptin resistance also have problems with insulin resistance. This fact has been well established in scientific literature. It has been proposed that excess amounts of insulin are a prime contributing factor of leptin resistance that leads to obesity.[177] It is also clear that the triad of insulin resistance, leptin resistance, and adrenaline resistance lead to high blood pressure.[178]

Adrenaline resistance fueled by leptin resistance and insulin resistance must exist before a person has a breakdown of their blood glucose regulation ability and becomes type II diabetic – what is known as adult-onset diabetes.[179]

In order to reduce adrenaline resistance and leptin resistance, one approach is to reduce insulin resistance. Whatever a person does to improve any one of these three problems has a synergistic, positive impact on the other two.

There is so much confusion on the subject of insulin and eating that it is truly mind-boggling. The fact that so many health professionals and "dieting experts" recommend snacking and eating frequent small meals is a real disservice. Along with overeating at night, snacking is the primary reason why so many Americans are overweight. Even if the snack is low in calories or is a "healthy snack," such as an apple, it becomes a problem.

When you eat between meals it changes powerful hormonal signals which prevent the breakdown of fat, confuse your liver, and induce calories to head for fat storage. This is a primary feature governing how food can induce stressful problems with hormone balance. Taking the time to understand why this is the case is important for learning how to master leptin and become an effective *Health Asset Manager*.

HOW INSULIN WORKS

The pancreas secretes two hormones that regulate blood sugar: insulin and glucagon. These two hormones play crucial roles in how the body regulates fuel utilization. Imbalances in these two hormones cause vicious circles of hyperglycemia followed by hypoglycemia, resulting in the inability to lose weight.

Insulin is released in response to a rise in blood glucose from food that has been consumed. Insulin signals the body to refuel and possibly to store extra fuel in the form of fat. The primary function of insulin is to promote the storage of calories. The big question is – where will the insulin store the calories?

Normally, insulin is secreted in two phases. The first phase occurs when food is eaten; it is an initial burst of insulin for the first ten minutes from readily available insulin in the pancreas. This is followed by the second phase, where the pancreas synthesizes more insulin.[180] Insulin normally peaks about thirty minutes after a meal and then gradually returns to baseline over the next three hours. This is an important rhythm – it has a normal pattern, and this pattern is very important.

Beyond immediate energy needs, ideally the liver takes about sixty percent of the blood glucose from a meal and stores it in the liver as glycogen – fuel to be used later.[181] Insulin also promotes the storage of amino acids in the liver that are used to help sustain energy five to six hours after the meal.[182]

Muscles throughout the body, depending on how much they have been used, are also stimulated to take up blood sugar and store it as glycogen for future use. If muscle tissue breakdown has occurred, as from exercise, then insulin is also a key signal that enables muscles to take up protein to rebuild themselves. The use of muscle is essential for conditioning the body to use insulin and glucose correctly.[183] Thus, in an ideal situation, the other forty percent of calories are taken up directly by muscles and other body tissue.

In the ideal situation, insulin is promoting storage of calories into the liver and body tissues, especially muscle. It is not promoting excess calorie storage into fat cells.

When muscles are not used enough – a person is too sedentary or a meal is too large – then insulin facilitates the storage of extra calories as fat. Insulin helps carry glucose into fat cells, where it is converted into glycerol to help form triglycerides, the type of fat in storage. [184]

Insulin turns on the enzyme lipoprotein lipase, which tells fat cells to grab circulating triglycerides in the blood and store them in fat cells.[185] Insulin also inhibits enzymes that cause fat to break down.[186] Thus, overly high insulin levels are a primary reason why calories are stored as fat, and why fat is not broken down to be used as fuel.

If there is excess fuel from an oversized meal or from a lack of physical activity, that extra fuel is likely to be stored as fat.

HOW GLUCAGON WORKS

The counterbalance to insulin is another pancreatic hormone called glucagon. It is stimulated by the fall in blood glucose and is a natural defense against blood sugar dropping too much. It is the main fuel regulator that helps a person to go five or six hours or longer without needing to eat.

Glucagon orders the liver to quit storing fuel and to begin making fuel. The liver does this in two ways:

1) It converts the stored fuel called glycogen back to glucose, a process called glycogenolysis.
2) It makes sugar from other compounds, including protein; and it makes glycerol from stored fat and lactic acid, a process called gluconeogenisis. Glycerol may then be converted to glucose.

In the process of breaking down stored fat, fatty acids are liberated.

The liver does not generally take these up; primarily the muscles take them up directly to be burned as fuel.[187] It should be rather obvious that if muscles are not used, then there is no demand for these fatty acids. The next time the person eats, insulin rises and the fatty acids now circulating in the blood are turned back into triglycerides and put back in storage. To lose weight, one needs to exercise.

In a healthy person, insulin and glucagon take turns. It is all about timing. Insulin is used to refuel the body; glucagon helps sustain energy between meals. It is a survival system that ensures a steady supply of glucose to the brain and nervous system, essential to maintain energy and health *(figure 9)*.

Our survival genetics enable us to go for long periods of time with little food. There are enough carbohydrates stored in the liver and muscles to last only twenty-four hours. After that, the body breaks down muscle protein as the primary fuel, for up to a week.[188] Once skeletal muscle is significantly lost, then fatty acids become the primary fuel. This is why fasting for weight loss is not advised; too much protein is lost from the physical structure before the body ever gets to the stores of fat, a dangerous and unhealthy thing to do.

Factors that disrupt the balance of insulin and glucagon create major havoc in the body, setting the stage for weight gain. An obvious example is that of insulin-dependent diabetes mellitus (IDDM), or type I diabetes. In this case, the pancreatic B-cells that make insulin are destroyed for one reason or another. Since the rising level of insulin is the key signal that turns off glucagon, the liver is under constant orders to synthesize more sugar in the absence of insulin. This causes blood sugar levels to raise dangerously high, the condition known as diabetes.

A problem called type II, or non-insulin dependent diabetes mellitus (NIDDM), is much more common. This is often referred to as adult-onset diabetes. This is a situation of excessive insulin production due to insulin resistance. This type of diabetes now extends to teenagers because of their excessive dietary abuses and inactivity.

Any person who progressively gains weight and has trouble losing weight is at serious risk for developing type II diabetes. Before the

Insulin Pattern After Meals   Figure 9

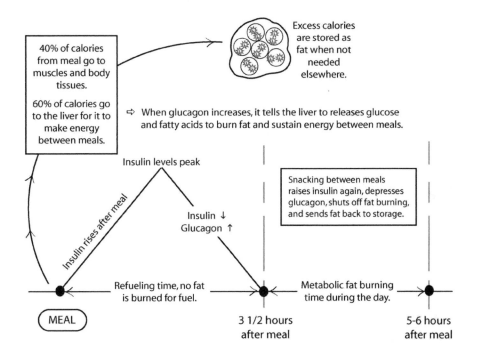

actual diabetes occurs, it is preceded by a condition known as insulin resistance.

INSULIN RESISTANCE

Insulin acts like a taxicab carrying passengers (glucose) to various destinations. Generally, the body synthesizes insulin whenever food is eaten and for as long as food is eaten.

Let us say that we overeat or eat between meals. Insulin, acting in its taxicab role, takes its passengers to the liver, muscles, and other places to be dropped off. However, the cells have no need for the fuel.

At first, they politely tell the taxicab to go someplace else. As time goes by, they see the taxicab coming and they lock the doors, literally turning off and, in some cases, eliminating the receptors for insulin on the membranes of cells. This is called insulin resistance.

Insulin resistance is a means of self-preservation for cells. If the cells did not reject the calories, they would enter the cell and cause the cell to become cemented. If sugar cannot be used, it caramelizes or hardens structures, similar to leaving spilled honey on the counter for a few days.

Over the years, insulin resistance causes major problems in the balance among insulin, glucagon, and fuel utilization.

LIVER INSULIN RESISTANCE

Like every cell of the body, the liver also develops insulin resistance. When this happens, the liver fails to store the sixty percent of fuel it typically stores from a meal. This means that the calories consumed head in the direction of fat storage.

This problem is magnified when a person eats too often. Not only does the liver fail to store calories properly, eating too often causes the liver to retain the calories it already has in storage. The bottom line is that frequent eating clogs the liver's fuel system. Fatigue is a common symptom for a person with a clogged liver.

When a person eats too often, especially meals high in sugar, the liver goes into a chronic stimulation of VLDL synthesis (very low density lipoproteins), the form of cholesterol most associated with cardiovascular disease. This delivers an excess of fatty substances to muscle, which clog muscle tissue and make it resistant to glucose. This is a typical way that many individuals start on the path to insulin resistance and elevated cholesterol,[189] and consequently leptin resistance. Thus, from a dietary point of view, the foremost reason for elevated cholesterol is snacking between meals, not the cholesterol content of food.

Liver fuel is the first fuel released under stress; it is essential to meet a current energy demand. If there is reduced storage of fuel in the liver, an individual is easily tired by stress and susceptible to irritability and moodiness. Individuals with insulin resistance typically have some level of fatigue and irritability.

Liver insulin resistance also makes it difficult for the person to go five to six hours without eating or to sleep properly through the night, as it is the liver's consistent release of stored sugar, under the direction of glucagon, that stabilizes blood sugar between meals and prevents hypoglycemia.

When there is insulin resistance in the liver, the liver decides to turn calories into fat at an increased rate, thus causing the person to become overweight.[190]

During leptin resistance and insulin resistance, the liver gets confused and misunderstands the messages. Excess leptin becomes involved with the normal pathway of insulin in the liver, confuses the liver about the state of fuel on hand, and has the net effect of turning down glucagon, the hormone needed to activate the liver's metabolic drive.[191] The result is that a person continues to gain weight, even with plenty of fat already in storage.

When a person has insulin resistance, the calories from a meal have a difficult time getting into muscles.[192] Such muscles are weaker, contributing to fatigue. Therefore, insulin resistance is a combination of a lack of physical fitness and a lack of liver fitness. Just as we know how it feels when our muscles get out of shape, fatigue and getting hungry too often are key signs of an out-of-shape liver.

HIGH BLOOD SUGAR

The extra calories which are not used need to go somewhere. In part, they are stored as fat, leading to progressive weight gain. Since blood sugar levels tend to stay higher than normal during insulin resistance (hyperglycemia), the flexible structures of the body are exposed to the caramelizing effects of sugar. This makes the body age faster. It causes the circulatory system to stiffen, leading to conditions such as high blood pressure. It causes capillaries in the eye to stiffen, leading to circulation problems of the eye, resulting in all manners of eye problems. It causes nerves to harden, leading to a variety of neurological issues, including mental decline and memory loss.

Properly functioning leptin is essential for normal glucose uptake and utilization in the liver, both in the fed and fasted state.[193,194] Leptin resistance causes high blood sugar following a meal, leading to hypoglycemia three to five hours after the meal.

SYNDROME X

It is quite common that insulin resistance results in the combination of weight gain, high cholesterol with low HDL, high triglycerides, and high blood pressure – a combination called Syndrome X. Syndrome X, also called metabolic syndrome, is recognized as a precursor to serious disease.[195] Leptin resistance is a prime cause of Syndrome X, a major factor in the onset of cardiovascular disease.[196]

Syndrome X is a serious problem because fat infiltrates structures that should not have excess fat; this includes the liver and heart. This sets the stage for lipotropic disease, meaning diseases of excess fat accumulation in all the wrong places.[197] Properly functioning leptin acts to burn off excess fat in body tissues such as the liver and heart, thus guarding against this serious health problem. Once leptin resistance sets in, then leptin no longer performs this function well, and concurrent insulin resistance speeds up the rate at which the liver accumulates excess fat. The first sign of this problem is weight gain around the midsection.

IS INSULIN BAD?

On the surface, it may appear that insulin is a bad guy. After all, it is the main hormone that helps the body store fat. When levels are elevated, a person is prone to increased risk of heart disease, hypoglycemia, hyperglycemia, and developing non-insulin-dependent diabetes. On the other hand, when there is no insulin, a person becomes diabetic in a hurry.

This apparent conflict emphasizes an important way in which the body works. Timing is everything. When insulin is secreted at the right time and in the right amount, the body runs like a fine-tuned engine.

As mentioned earlier, insulin is secreted in two phases. The initial phase comes from stored granules in the pancreas, followed by a second phase of insulin production by pancreatic B-cells. When a person does not eat between meals, the pancreas has time to prepare for a meal by getting some insulin ready. When the meal is eaten, this already prepared insulin is released and, in turn, tells the pancreas that more insulin is needed. This causes the B-cells to go into a high level of insulin production, which peaks about one-half-hour after the meal is complete.

As a person develops insulin resistance, the first phase of insulin secretion does not occur. Part of the reason for this is eating too often; therefore, the pancreas does not have enough time to prepare insulin for the next meal.

This sluggish initial insulin response to a meal is followed by a prolonged release of insulin in the second phase, leaving higher insulin in the blood for longer periods of time. This increases the storage of fat and prevents the breakdown of stored fat.[198] This inability to release insulin in the first phase response is considered to be the first sign that a person is on the path to becoming type II diabetic.[199]

The prolonged and inefficient insulin release suppresses glucagon from being released three to four hours after the meal, thereby blunting the healthy function of the liver and setting the stage for hypoglycemia. As blood sugar drops, the ability of the body to sustain blood sugar is suppressed, because the liver cannot synthesize blood sugar well enough to maintain normal energetic function. The individual then becomes hypoglycemic, or has low blood sugar symptoms, three to four hours after the meal. This sets up the vicious circle of hyperglycemia followed by hypoglycemia, leading to excess eating in an attempt to prop up the blood sugar.

In this common situation, a person uses food to maintain energy. This is not a normal reason to eat. Eating becomes a quick fix to solve the symptoms of out-of-balance insulin and glucagon. Even if a person feels better for a while, the body does not use the calories efficiently, and weight gain and a poor energy level are common results.

It is not that insulin is bad; it is an issue of the right amount of insulin at the right time. The problem of insulin resistance is an example of how poor timing throws one's energy level out of sync.

To make matters worse, it is not just insulin and glucagon that are in a state of imbalance. This out-of-sync fuel utilization has a negative domino effect on hormones throughout the body. There are problems dealing with stress; thyroid hormone is dysregulated; growth hormone is depressed; and estrogen imbalance locks in the problem. All these problems occur in a generally simultaneous way: in a more or less chicken-and-egg proposition, each problem makes another problem worse, and vice versa.

There may be no disease present, such as thyroid disease, that can be defined in traditional medical terms. Yet, a person may have the symptoms of hypothyroid function. The entire functional system of the human body becomes less responsive and less functional.

SUMMARY

Insulin and glucagon must function in natural rhythm in order to have an efficient metabolism. Developing and maintaining muscle and liver fitness is essential for preventing problems with leptin.

Individuals with insulin resistance are generally tired and hungry, often shortly after eating. Such individuals do not extract proper energy from the food they eat; instead, food acts as a block on metabolism because it forces hormonal signals into a state of imbalance. Even worse, more food is eaten at the wrong times in an effort to solve the unpleasant hypoglycemic symptoms that result from the out-of-balance situation.

These issues pose a huge metabolic Catch-22. No drug can fix the problem. Only a return of true health can set the body's systems back on track. It can be done. The *Five Rules* are essential ways to eat in order to avoid stressing the balance between insulin and glucagon. Rule 2, explained in the next chapter, is the functional test of insulin and glucagon efficiency.

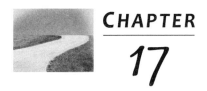

Space Meals for Maximum Benefit

EVEN THOUGH LEPTIN is primarily involved with long-term fuel issues, it still has a secondary communication system which supports short-term energy needs. We know that leptin and insulin are in a process of communication, similar to cross communication between two department heads, as opposed to a direct order from the boss/brain. Insulin production stimulates leptin production.[200] It has also been proven that leptin receptors are present on the insulin-producing B-cells of the pancreas, demonstrating the ability to turn off insulin production.[201,202]

This forms a circle of self-regulatory checks and balances that is another example of natural energy balance in the human body. In normal physical function, leptin and insulin have a balancing effect on food intake, food storage, and a stable energy level.

Once leptin resistance sets in and leptin levels are high, the pancreatic B-cells do not respond to the signal from leptin to stop making insulin.[203] Not only is the brain developing leptin resistance, so is the pancreas. However, insulin keeps stimulating leptin production while at the same time insulin is encouraging calories to be stored as fat. Developing leptin resistance in the pancreas has now been proven to be a fast track to type II diabetes.[204]

This is why leptin and insulin are frequently at high levels at the same time, with neither hormone working efficiently. A key step in avoiding this difficult problem is to follow Rule 2 of the *Five Rules*.

Unfortunately, many who provide weight-loss advice do not advocate adherence to this rule, a factor that contributes to the societal obesity problem.

The *Five Rules* - Rule 2

Eat three meals a day. Allow five to six hours between meals. Do not snack.

The first three hours after eating, your body refuels under the influence of insulin, like filling up at a gas station. Insulin is the carrier of calories to other locations throughout your body. During this storage time, weight loss is not possible.

Three hours after eating, insulin levels should be lower. As insulin falls, glucagon rises. This is a true fat-burning time. It is when your liver, which is the metabolic factory of your body, kicks into high gear. During this time, your liver maintains blood sugar through a combination of using its own stored sugar, called glycogen, and converting protein and fat to fuel as needed. Fats in the blood begin to burn, thereby clearing out stagnant calories.

Not eating between meals is a form of exercise for your liver; it is just as essential as exercising your muscles. Everyone knows how it feels to be physically out of shape. The same thing happens to the liver when there is snacking between meals. The liver needs to have time to generate energy. It needs to deplete its stores of glycogen. If a person eats sporadically throughout the day or has a series of consistent small meals, that process is blocked. This is a fast track to insulin resistance. It synthesizes excess amounts of cholesterol, even if the food eaten contains no cholesterol.

The majority of fat that is broken down between meals is taken up directly by the muscles; thus the importance of exercise. If a person does not exercise, the demand for fatty acid use in the muscles is negligible. Even if fatty acids are freed from triglycerides to be potentially burned for fuel, they are not used anywhere near the rate they could be if muscles were more active. The next time a person eats and insulin goes up, these free fatty acids turn back into triglycerides and head back to fat storage.

The "need" to snack, reflected by dropping energy levels between meals, is a sign of how out of shape the pancreas/liver/muscle system is. When a snack is eaten, insulin levels rise, fat burning is shut off, and calories go back to storage. True enough, some of that fuel will prop up the dropping blood sugar levels; but if the system were in proper condition, blood sugar levels would not have dropped in the first place.

Snacking causes the pancreas to become fatigued. Remember that insulin is released in two phases: the first phase is from stored granules of insulin in the pancreas. Snacking between meals is like a repetitive strain injury to the pancreas. The pancreas does not have time to get itself ready for the next meal; that is, time to prepare stored insulin granules for the first part of the insulin response to a meal. This causes an exaggerated second response. This means that insulin stays elevated past the three-hour point, in turn depressing glucagon and causing hypoglycemia. These two issues, no first-phase insulin response and a prolonged second-phase insulin response, are the hallmarks of insulin resistance. Eating too often causes them. Another cause is eating too much.

The prolonged insulin response shuts off fat burning so no weight loss is possible. Because the prolonged insulin response is inappropriate, it also interferes with the release of glucagon that is essential to get the liver into motion. As blood sugar drops, glucagon is not released because insulin is still too high. This causes the low blood sugar situation that makes a person want to snack. This is the vicious Catch-22. There will be no weight loss if energy crashes between meals or the person eats between meals.

Some individuals may need to gradually work their eating in the right direction. They may need to have four meals a day, four hours apart. As they increase their exercise and improve the condition of the pancreas, adrenals, muscles, and liver, they will gradually be able to move to the three-meal-a-day plan without their energy dropping between meals.

If five to six small meals a day are needed to maintain energy, the metabolic situation is not in good shape. Eating very small meals may cause some weight loss, but metabolism will likely slow down before the weight goal is achieved. Even a low-calorie snack increases insulin release; thus fat-burning mode ceases or never begins. Only by increasing the amount of time between meals will proper weight loss take place.

Many children, teenagers, young adults, intense bodybuilders, and athletes can seemingly violate this rule without any apparent consequence. This is because their demand for calories to aid body growth and repair is quite high. This genetic gift tends to disappear after age thirty. However, it is alarming the number of children who are overweight and too inactive, and who thus have hormonal balance problems that used to be present only in the over-thirty age group.

After age thirty, if this rule is violated there will be a tendency to slowly and progressively gain weight. If it is truly impossible for an individual to make it five hours without eating, the following may apply:

1) There was not enough eaten at the previous meal.
2) There were too many carbohydrates eaten at the previous meal.
3) There needs to be a gradual improvement in physical fitness.
4) There was poor digestion of the food eaten, so little or no energy was derived from it.
5) There are sluggish and congested liver problems, with weak adrenals. The gall bladder has commonly been removed by this time as well.
6) Metabolism is exhausted; the individual has fibromyalgia.
7) There are too many toxins clogging metabolism.
8) Normal blood sugar regulation is broken, meaning the individual is likely to be diabetic.

SUMMARY

The fundamental problems of day-to-day fuel regulation lead to a combination of insulin resistance, leptin resistance, and adrenaline resistance. This combination precedes the onset of high blood pressure and type II diabetes. There is a high risk for serious heart disease, cancer, and other disease as well.

The timing of the release of insulin determines if insulin is "good" or "bad." When meals are properly spaced, the pancreas has time to recharge and get prepared for an efficient insulin release following a meal. This initial insulin surge, followed by pancreatic synthesis of more insulin, enables a proper peak of insulin about half an hour after a meal is complete. It then gradually declines over the next few hours.

Insulin acts as a taxicab for calories taking them to places that need refueling, in the case of glucose; or that need repair, in the case of protein.

Once insulin returns to its baseline level, three to three-and-a-half hours after the meal, then your liver takes over to maintain your blood glucose levels in a healthy range. Your liver secretes glucose from sugars it stored from the previous meal or it synthesizes sugar from protein, fat, and/or lactic acid. This provides the base of blood glucose needed to fuel your brain, as well as providing the essential base of sugar-based calories needed for burning fatty acids. Proper function enables a person to avoid being hypoglycemic between meals.

When the next meal is eaten, rising insulin tells your liver to quit making sugar and start storing sugar. This is a natural rhythm of your body. Major body organs work in a particular way for a period of time and then get a break. The entire system has natural checks and balances, some that enable a person to get extra bursts of energy as needed to meet the demands of any type of situation.

This system slides out of balance when an individual eats between meals; even a "healthy" snack is a problem. It does not matter how many calories are consumed; the snack causes insulin to rise. This interrupts the liver's synthesis of sugar, causes the liver to become clogged with fat and develop insulin resistance, and causes fats that were breaking down to go back into storage.

Eating between meals also causes the liver to excessively secrete cholesterol and initiates insulin resistance for the whole body. Almost anyone who keeps stressing their metabolism by snacking will have this problem, usually by their mid-thirties. When this takes place problems with leptin resistance take hold. If nothing is changed after that, health rapidly declines.

Individuals who think they must eat between meals for their head to be able to function have significant liver, adrenal, and blood-glucose metabolism problems. The underlying problems need to be fixed so that eating patterns become healthy ones.

An apple a day may keep the doctor away, but not if it is eaten between meals. Snacking between meals or eating small, frequent meals is a counterproductive way to eat. Those who master leptin will learn to space meals five to six hours apart and eat nothing between meals.

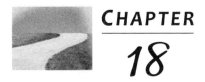

CHAPTER
18

Preventing the
Super-Sized Waistline

THE FASTEST WAY KNOWN to cause leptin resistance is to overeat.[205] Once there is a pattern of excess food consumption, leptin resistance and insulin resistance will be in hot pursuit. When they get locked into metabolism, it is difficult simply to use one's willpower to get on top of them. This is because their signals are core subconscious signals, programmed into the instincts for survival.

It is common scientific practice to feed high-fat and high-fructose diets to animals to make them diabetic so that they can be used in experiments. Apparently, we have many humans willing to conduct the experiment on themselves. High-fat junk food sources are obvious; high fructose corn syrup is found in soda and other sweet products, especially beverages.

Recently, scientists tried to figure out if it was the high fat or the high fructose that was most to blame. Their new research shows both diets caused major imbalances to sugar metabolism and leptin. The high-fat diet caused higher blood sugars because fatty deposits from high fat intake clogged the function of the pancreas and liver.

The high-fructose diet directly created leptin resistance and insulin resistance, leading to excessive formation of triglycerides.[206] Furthermore, animals fed high-fructose diets not only have increased insulin in their blood; they have increased amounts of free radical damage compared to the same caloric intake of complex carbohydrates.[207]

Recently, researchers analyzed ingestion patterns of high fructose corn syrup in America, noting that it is forty percent of the caloric sweetener used in our food supply. The use of this sweetener has increased by a factor of one thousand percent since 1970, far more than any other food source in the American diet. This increase parallels the increase in obesity in our country. The researchers hypothesized that because fructose dose not simulate insulin or leptin in response to a meal, as would regular white sugar, a person does not get a proper full signal and thus eats too much.[208]

These researchers did not know about the findings in the previous study. The previous study shows that a regular pattern of consumption drastically raises insulin and leptin. Thus, while one high-fructose meal may not raise insulin and leptin, a regular pattern of consumption induces both leptin resistance and insulin resistance, which directly causes obesity and overeating. With many Americans consuming 300 calories of high fructose corn syrup a day, that is an alarming piece of information.

A high-sucrose meal (white sugar) increases leptin secretion fivefold over normal.[209] Such meals directly induce leptin resistance. Unfortunately, any large dessert at the end of a meal creates "leptin stress." If a person is already overweight, even small desserts perpetuate and stimulate leptin resistance, thus shutting off fat-burning mode. This becomes especially frustrating for individuals trying to lose weight and having an occasional treat; the treat flares up leptin resistance which may knock out fat-burning mode for two to three days.

One of the natural rhythms of leptin is in response to the elevation of insulin in response to any meal. As insulin rises, leptin levels rise. Healthy leptin function does two things: it tells the subconscious brain a person is full, and it tells the pancreas to stop making insulin. This is a normal leptin fluctuation in response to a meal.

If the meal induces insulin resistance or leptin resistance, then these signals will not work correctly. The more a person starts to overeat, the more he or she continues to overeat, because the correct full signal does not get into the brain. This was recently proven in a restaurant setting;

researchers thought individuals would not continue to eat more food if given the opportunity. Using a variety of scientific monitoring options, much to their surprise, they found that individuals, regardless of body weight, constantly ate larger portions when given the opportunity, with almost no regard for the concept of an appropriate meal size.[210]

This confirms what many people already know when they find themselves in a leptin-resistant craving. Their meal or snack portion is not dictated by hunger but by packaging: a whole pizza, an entire bag of potato chips, or a super-sized meal.

Since two-thirds of Americans are overweight, it is safe to conclude that we are a nation of leptin-resistant food addicts. This is demonstrated by the clear tendency to eat whatever portion of food is served or ordered, easily ignoring an internal "full signal" if food is there to eat. Even worse, once the full signal is ignored, appetite regulation no longer applies to the meal; thus, dessert is frequently consumed long after a full signal was reached and ignored. This pattern is very conducive to weight gain.

Besides the obvious health costs related to this problem, the productivity loss – represented by the corresponding lack of mental clarity and physical energy – is staggering. Is it any wonder why de-energized and addictive personalities fritter away countless hours, mesmerized by their computer games and Internet compulsions?

There will come a time when employers realize that a job application should include an evaluation of BMI (body mass index). This relates not only to potential health-care costs, it also reflects the ability of many individuals to sustain productive and energetic output with clear-headed thinking.

The first two of the *Five Rules* place emphasis on the timing of eating and how improper timing fuels an out-of-balance situation that leads to overeating. That is why the first two rules are of extreme importance.

For most people the key time for leptin-resistance overeating is at night. However, because leptin-resistant people arrange their eating to fit their life, they may become excessive during the day if their schedule allows it or if they are under some type of stress. This brings us to the third of the *Five Rules*; another one to learn on the path to becoming an effective *Health Asset Manager*.

THE *Five Rules* - Rule 3

Do not eat large meals. If you are overweight, always try to finish a meal when you are slightly less than full. The full signal will usually catch up in ten to twenty minutes. Eating slowly is important.

The amount of food that should be eaten at any one meal depends on how active a person is that day. More food may be eaten by the physically active person and by the person who strenuously exercises. Most overweight people, however, eat meals that are much too large. Healthy meal sizes for the average active person fall into the 400 to 600 calorie range for women and 500 to 700 calorie range for men.

It is always best to predefine a meal amount before sitting down to eat, while the conscious brain still has some control. Commonly, leptin resistant individuals will not feel satisfied on a normal amount of food. These people will feel quite irritable and will think they won't have any energy until they eat more. This is because the message that leptin is elevating from the meal has not yet entered their brain.

Eating slower is very important. Take smaller bites, chew slower, and engage in some conversation. Shoveling down food does not allow time for the body to raise the leptin signal properly. A tremendous amount of excess food is easy to eat when a person eats too fast. Not only does this tend to upset digestion, it also tends to upset the digestion of any normal eater who happens to be watching. It is also an issue of manners.

The ability to get a proper full signal always improves as a person becomes less leptin resistant. People who start to improve will notice that they finally get the full signal, even though it may come ten to twenty minutes after they stop eating. When leptin resistance improves further, they will get a normal full signal as the normal-sized meal is finished.

It is incredibly important to get the subconscious brain to think that enough food has been eaten. Individuals who struggle with this may benefit from extra nutritional support that enhances the full feeling, without more food being eaten. This enables leptin to work more normally.

SHRINK AND TONE YOUR STOMACH

One reason that individuals eat too much is because the size of their stomach becomes stretched from large meals. Thereafter, they have to keep eating large meals to feel full.

In order to get on a healthy eating track, the stomach needs to become smaller. This cannot be accomplished if one eats a bag of popcorn as a snack, or a lot of bread with meals. These foods simply enlarge the size of the stomach. Even if it seems that popcorn is not such a bad "little meal" at night to satisfy food cravings, it makes one want to eat more at following meals because it stretches the stomach.

Start cutting down on portion sizes, especially carbohydrates. Skip extra bread with meals. Begin to train your stomach to shrink in size, it is a noticeable sensation and you can actually feel your stomach as smaller in size. Do some stomach crunches to obtain better abdominal tone.

When you are overweight stop eating before you feel full. If you are having a larger meal, have it at lunch when there is more time to metabolize it during the day. Also, try to restrict eating time to thirty or forty-five minutes whenever possible. This causes insulin to rise for a definable amount of time. Individuals who eat a meal and then eat dessert an hour later are more likely to get an excess insulin surge, which results in calories heading in the direction of fat cells for storage.

BIG MEALS CAUSE HYPERGLYCEMIA

If the meal is too large it does not matter what the ratio of fats, carbohydrates, and protein may be. A big meal causes excess secretion of insulin in order to deal with the excess calories. This results in hyperglycemia – high blood sugar.

Hyperglycemia from a meal that contains too many calories causes a person to feel fatigued within forty-five minutes of eating. Sometimes it even causes cravings for more food. If the meal was really overdone, this fatigue may be extreme and a nap is required or the head feels heavy. This is a common feeling after the classic Thanksgiving dinner. This issue is prevalent with many individuals all year long.

Hyperglycemia from a large meal is a major stress to the body. It usually results in a rebound hypoglycemia three to four hours after eating. The potential energy from food is derailed because the hormones regulating the ability to use that fuel are thrown into disarray by the large meal. The calories are headed for fat storage.

Individuals are frequently surprised to find that they notice increased energy from eating less food. This is because smaller meals help insulin and glucagon act on calories in the proper way, leading to energy production. This is a clear example of smaller being better.

American restaurants typically serve excessive portions, even offering super-sized options. These large portions are unnecessary and are detrimental to health.

SLOW DOWN

When you are out to dinner with a group of friends, look around the table and see who finishes their meal first; then look at their waistline. Nothing more needs to be said.

It takes ten minutes for your brain to receive the signal of being full. A lot of unneeded food can be eaten in those ten minutes.

Take the time to chew food well. This not only helps your digestive system immensely, it enables your brain to turn off hunger signals with less food.

Engage in conversation, relax, slow down, and enjoy the meal. If food is chewed for a longer time, there will be the same amount of pleasure in terms of taste, and much less food will be consumed.

If you are prone to being a fast eater, learn to take a five-minute break in the middle of the meal. The satisfaction of feeling full will be felt sooner. There is no need to eat as much.

Many leptin-resistant individuals cannot seem to inhale food fast enough. While some younger people can eat fast and get away with it, this will not last long. Leptin resistance is knocking at the door. After age thirty, eating too fast invariably involves eating too much, and metabolism cannot keep up.

SUMMARY

This point is simple but important in the road to mastering leptin: eat too much as a lifestyle pattern and be on the fast road to leptin resistance and increased risk for any disease. Meal size, including portion control, is essential for a balanced body free of leptin and insulin problems.

Eating slowly, relaxing during the meal, and having enjoyable conversation are all great ways to learn to eat less food.

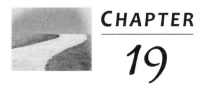

CHAPTER
19

Getting Off to a Good Start –
The Importance of Protein

EACH CALORIE is potential energy that can be extracted from food. Theoretically, protein and carbohydrates contain the same number of calories. They contain four calories per gram, whereas fat contains nine calories per gram.

If fuel regulation is inefficient, then the potential energy of a calorie does not become actual energy that is used; instead, it gets stored as fat. It is fine for people to be aware of the number of calories they eat; but it is equally important to eat in such a way that improves energy and enhances any type of food so that is can be used more efficiently.

Each type of food has a different effect on the liver, regardless of the amount of calories in that food. The liver is the metabolic factory of the body, the most important organ in regulating the use of calories. When the "liver factory" sees fats or carbohydrates coming, it does not need to change these substances much before they are useful to the body. Fats and carbohydrates increase the liver's metabolic rate by only four percent.

Protein, on the other hand, is a very complex food. Proteins form the backbone of the genetic signaling system. Everything in your body is made of protein. The liver must take proteins from the food and as-semble them for the various needs. Sometimes the liver will attach fats or carbohydrates to proteins, but it is the complexity of protein that drives the liver factory into action.

Dietary protein is the raw material that tells your liver to get in gear. Without adequate protein, the work cannot get started and metabolism will sit still. It is like a carpenter waiting for the nails and plywood to be delivered to the job site.

THE *Five Rules* - Rule 4

Eat a breakfast containing protein.

Metabolism can increase by thirty percent for as long as twelve hours from a high-protein meal, the calorie-burning equivalent of a three or four mile jog.[211]

A high-carbohydrate breakfast such as juice, cereal, waffles, pancakes, or bagels does not enhance metabolic rate. It may trigger a problem with insulin resistance because a lot of insulin is released in response to the carbohydrates, causing energy fluctuations and sugar cravings during the day. High glycemic carbohydrates can shift normal leptin release to earlier in the day. If there is leptin resistance, this fuels overeating throughout the day and especially at night. The two signs of a poor breakfast are:

1) Being unable to make it five hours to lunch without food cravings or crashing energy.

2) Being much more prone to leptin resistance later that afternoon or evening. This sets in motion strong food cravings, resulting in poor eating habits.

A high-protein breakfast helps metabolism turn on, and it stabilizes hypoglycemia or low blood sugar reactions later in the day. A high-protein meal helps prevent leptin fluctuations later in the day.[212] Protein enhances the release of glucagon, helping to blunt the excess insulin response that causes insulin resistance. Eggs are a good breakfast, just not smothered in butter and cheese. Cottage cheese is another high-protein breakfast food, and along with a serving of complex carbohydrate or fruit makes a great breakfast. Even a few tablespoons of peanut butter or almond butter (not half the jar) on a piece of toast could work well, especially for the person in a hurry.

We use high-efficiency whey protein for quick and easy breakfasts. Any lean protein can be eaten at breakfast along with a moderate amount of carbohydrates. Avoid fruit juice at breakfast; this is too much sugar for anyone who has a problem with insulin or leptin resistance.

Soy protein is potentially problematic, especially for people consuming soy protein drinks. It may lower thyroid function in many individuals. Pay attention: if you like soy protein but are getting tired and not losing weight, it may be problematic. If, on the other hand, soy protein is not getting in the way of progress then it may not be a problem.

Rule 4 becomes even more important as people age. This is because there is less ability to tolerate stress. A poor breakfast adds to the wear and tear of the body and induces an unstable energy level before the day is over. If people begin to pay attention to how they feel based on what they ate for breakfast, fatigue later in the day from a poor breakfast may be noticeable.

With children, there is some variance in this rule. Some children can do just fine on a high-carbohydrate breakfast. However, those with learning difficulties, ADD, ADHD, depression, mood fluctuations, and/or those who are overweight, do best eating a high-protein breakfast. This is especially true for children whose parents struggle with leptin resistance.

Eating no breakfast is an extreme version of a poor breakfast. This forces the body to run on energy reserves and tends to leave the liver struggling with a shortage of proper raw materials. Even for people who get through some of the day after skipping breakfast, it will not be long before this pattern catches up with them in terms of energy issues, mood swings, poor eating patterns, and overall increased wear and tear on the body.

Some individuals simply do not feel like eating breakfast. Their digestive system is too full of toxic waste from the inadequate job of house cleaning that was done the night before. It may be two or three hours before they can even think about eating a normal-sized breakfast. A bowl of oatmeal may work well for them, as it is a higher-protein grain. They may just have to have a little something in order not to feel queasy, and then eventually have the high-protein meal. This problem improves as their overall level of toxicity decreases.

PROTEIN AND FLUID RETENTION

Protein has a significant effect on fluid-retention issues. Adequate protein helps make a primary blood-transport protein called albumin. Many nutrients are carried on albumin. Albumin circulates in the blood. Blood pressure pushes nutrients and water out of capillaries and into the tissue, delivering oxygen and nutrition.

However, water must be drawn back into circulation; otherwise the body becomes dehydrated. This is accomplished by the osmotic force of albumin, which attracts water from tissues back into capillaries. If there is not enough protein, albumin levels drop and the body loses its ability to maintain water in circulation. Instead, water accumulates in the tissues, causing edema. Adequate protein intake helps solve fluid-retention problems by ensuring that there is a proper amount of albumin.

GRADUALLY INCREASE PROTEIN INTAKE

For people who have not been eating enough protein, it is best to gradually increase the amount of protein, especially for those in poor health or who are significantly overweight. It is also important to improve physical fitness at the same time that protein in the diet is increased. This is because muscles use protein to repair themselves. Additionally, the increased exercise stimulates the use of many enzymes that are protein dependent.

People in poor fitness who eat too much protein too fast will feel irritable and fatigued, because the liver, in a poor state of fitness, cannot process the protein efficiently. There is an important relationship between liver function, physical activity that results in improved fitness, and protein intake. This is especially important for individuals recovering from a prolonged period of poor health.

When individuals gradually increase protein and exercise, the liver is able to channel the consumed protein into a health-promoting direction. Muscle strength, muscle fitness, and the ability to exercise longer will improve, and the liver will be in better working order. Protein is the calorie that can wake up a sleeping metabolism, as long as protein is increased in a way that benefits health.

SUMMARY

It is not just the amount of calories that are eaten that influences the ability to lose weight. The type of calorie and the timing of eating are just as important. One essential principle is to eat enough protein to help the liver stay metabolically active.

Eating a solid protein breakfast provides a stable base for energy, mood, and blood sugar throughout the day and evening. It helps keep the body in a calorie-burning mode, a mode that can burn fat for fuel. When energy crashes during the day, frequently due to poor breakfast, then metabolism and weight loss come to a grinding halt.

A great number of metabolic problems can be solved or avoided by eating a breakfast that consists of ample protein.

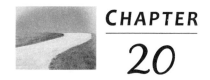

Eat Like a Pyramid, Look Like a Pyramid

THE FOOD PYRAMID places much too much emphasis on eating carbohydrates relative to protein. This leads to carbohydrate snacking between meals or eating meals that contain an overabundance of carbohydrates.

While the designers of this pyramid are certainly not in favor of overeating, the pyramid plan subconsciously causes individuals to overeat. This is because this style of eating causes imbalances in insulin and glucagon, in turn inducing leptin resistance and out-of-control overeating.

Thus, the pyramid designers can preach portion control all they want; they just cannot get individuals to follow their advice with this type of diet plan.

The *Five Rules* are far more important than what the food pyramid may have to offer. There is nothing very innovative about the food pyramid. There is agreement about eating a variety of food. Most would agree with not overindulging in fat, junk food, and sweets. These basics are already known.

The problem with the food pyramid is that the amount of carbohydrates in this diet plan causes individuals who are heading in the direction of insulin resistance and leptin resistance to worsen, especially when they get into excess refined-sugar consumption. This is because the extra sugar promotes excess insulin release, which in turn promotes fat storage and higher circulating insulin. This leads to insulin resistance and leptin resistance. Further, with the food pyramid there is no warning not to snack, an issue that really gets a person going in the wrong direction.

The food pyramid contributes to and, in some cases, directly causes problems with leptin resistance, especially for those age thirty and over. People are literally pulled down the dark alley of leptin resistance by inducing insulin resistance from consuming the amount of carbohydrates suggested in this plan. Even though the carbohydrates may have little fat, the liver becomes congested and synthesizes excess fat due to the pitfalls of the pyramid plan. Excess carbohydrates lead to elevated NPY in the brain, a condition inducing excessive cholesterol production – regardless of the cholesterol content of food.

Unfortunately, because this plan makes leptin resistance worse, it increases the onset of major diseases in our society, including obesity. This is not good public-health policy.

THE *Five Rules* - Rule 5
Reduce the amount of carbohydrates you eat.
Carbohydrates are easy-to-use fuels. Your body takes money from its purse or wallet – the food on a plate – before it dips into the savings account – the hips, thighs, buttocks, and midsection. Carbohydrates in the diet are the main signal for insulin secretion. If an individual has a problem with insulin resistance and leptin resistance, as is the case with most who are overweight, then cutting back on carbohydrates helps reduce the amount of insulin produced and tends to cool off the problem, as well as settle down the leptin resistance.

Some carbohydrates are needed in a healthy diet or the thyroid turns off, electrolytes become dysregulated, muscles weaken, growth hormone is not released correctly, fat is not burned efficiently, there is an unsatisfied feeling after a meal, the heart becomes stressed, and the digestive system goes on the blink. We certainly do not advocate a no-carbohydrate diet.

In general, many Americans eat twice the amount of carbohydrates they are able to metabolize, a main reason why more than fifty percent are overweight. Low-glycemic complex carbohydrates are the best type to consume in order not to aggravate a leptin problem.

When the amount of carbohydrates is reduced, the amount of fat or protein needs to increase in order for there to be enough calories to function. Finding the right balance for each individual takes time and paying attention to the body. Every meal of the day does not have to be the same. The goal is to be able to go five to six hours between meals with a good energy level and to be able to lose weight or maintain proper body weight.

EMPLOY THE 50/50 TECHNIQUE

In most cases, just getting the protein and carbohydrates into better balance goes a long way toward assisting weight loss. This is easily done with the visual 50/50 technique. Look at a meal and see a palm-size piece of protein (a four to six ounce portion for women; six to eight ounce portion for men). Try to keep the total physical size of the carbohydrate the same as the protein, a 50/50 visual. This way there is no calorie counting. Compare the protein (chicken, meat, turkey, eggs) to the carbohydrates (bread, rice, pasta, potatoes, fruit, etc). Eat any amount of vegetables; however, eat corn, carrots, and peas in moderation.

If dessert is on the menu, plan to skip most of the carbohydrates in the meal. Instead have a large salad or extra vegetables with the protein serving. If carbohydrates are eaten during the meal, then plan on only one bite of dessert. Those trying to lose weight should avoid all desserts; an occasional thumb-sized portion is acceptable as a person's metabolism begins to improve.

The consumption of too many carbohydrates causes leptin to rise too high at the wrong time of the day. For example, people with leptin resistance who eat a sweet roll, muffin, juice, or bagel for breakfast, with little or no protein, will have trouble with overeating later in the day. If such people eat too many carbohydrates at lunch, they will be ravishingly hungry by dinner.

Such individuals have a lack of energy later in the day and insist on eating a larger meal so that they feel good. In this situation, calories are not being used efficiently, and misguided leptin signals enforce eating behaviors. When these individuals quit eating the excess carbohydrates, they are amazed to find that they have a better energy level and mood.

SOME CARBOHYDRATES ARE IMPORTANT

Carbohydrates are a primary fuel source for your body. The other primary fuel source is saturated fat. A debate could easily be held over the preferred fuel source, but that issue is not critical to weight loss. The important point is that carbohydrates are easy to use for fuel.

Excess consumption of carbohydrates prevents the body from dipping into fat reserves for energy. Excess consumption also turns into fat quite easily, even though there are no fat grams in the carbohydrates. This is because under the influence of excess insulin, the body stores excess calories as fat. At the same time, excess insulin inhibits the breakdown of stored fat. When the liver also has insulin resistance, it is prone to directing calories to fat storage as well.

On the other hand, carbohydrates are especially important for muscle function. Without enough carbohydrates, muscles lose their water content and become dehydrated, weak, and/or develop cramps. As part of their role in maintaining proper hydration of the body, carbohydrates have a direct influence on electrolytes. Diets too low in carbohydrates can eventually lead to kidney and cardiovascular distress. A person with leptin resistance may already have strained kidney and cardiovascular function: thus, a diet too low in carbohydrates may aggravate these issues.

Physically active people who uses their muscles frequently have a higher need for carbohydrates and an increased ability to metabolize carbohydrates. If physically active people do not eat enough carbohydrates, they will have insufficient sustainable muscle energy. Performance suffers.

SUMMARY

The basic approach for weight loss is to visually balance the amount of protein (four to six ounces for women, six to eight ounces for men) with the amount of carbohydrates one eats. Generally, a certain amount of fats naturally occur in the protein.

Active individuals with no weight issues can certainly eat more carbohydrates than this amount, because they have an ability to metabolize them. As individuals lose weight and maintain a good weight for a period of time, along with a good level of physical activity and energy, the ability to metabolize carbohydrates improves.

In order to keep weight off after losing it, it is important to exercise and maintain the goal weight, while slowly increasing the carbohydrate amount. Too many carbohydrates too fast after losing weight causes rapid weight gain. Once there has been a problem with insulin resistance and leptin resistance, it is easy to get back in a poor pattern.

Being a *Health Asset Manager* means that one must pay attention to the trend one's body is in and learn to manage that trend effectively. A *Health Asset Manager* who has mastered leptin has the knowledge and life skills needed to keep weight off after losing it.

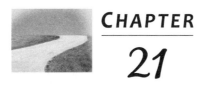

The Secrets to Accessing Fat-Burning Mode

THE ENTIRE PURPOSE of the *Five Rules* for mastering leptin is to create energy and metabolic efficiency in your body. You have the ability to correctly extract more energy from the food you eat. If you are overweight, employing the *Five Rules* helps normalize body weight. These rules also keep normal-weight people from gaining weight, especially as they grow older.

When the *Five Rules* are employed in an effort to lose weight, they help individuals enter fat-burning mode. This is a metabolic ability to dip into the stores of fat without the body slowing down into the hibernation mode because it thinks it is starving.

HOW TO ENTER FAT-BURNING MODE

Stored fat is called a triglyceride. It contains three fatty acids and one glycerol – a carbohydrate. In order to induce fat-burning mode, it is necessary for the body to break down stored fat, the savings account of stored energy. For this to occur, there must be a relative deficiency in the easiest-to-use fuels in the diet; these are carbohydrates and saturated fats.

If there is a deficiency in all fuels, metabolism slows down and stored fat is conserved. For most people, in order to lose weight, there should be slightly higher protein relative to fat and carbohydrate.

When you eat in accordance with the *Five Rules* and gradually reduce easy-to-use fuels, (that is, saturated fat and carbohydrates), you enter a fat-burning mode that can access fat from storage – not just burn off what is being eaten.

THE FLUID-RETENTION PROBLEM

If fluid retention is present, weight loss becomes difficult. When the body clicks into fat-burning mode, the first thing it does is dump three to six pounds of stagnant fluid, and only then does it get down to the business of burning fat.

When people lose weight or maintain their ideal weight, they do not have a fluid-retention problem. Individuals who struggle with weight loss may be two to four pounds lighter after a strenuous workout, but all they have done is dump the water that was embedded in their connective tissue. After their next meal or later that night, they are right back where they were prior to the exercise, as their body has regained the water it lost.

There is a simple test to help determine you have eaten too many carbohydrates. Stand on the scale first thing in the morning and then stand on the scale at night. If you weigh over two pounds more at night than in the morning, one of the *Five Rules* of eating has most likely been violated. If rules 1-4 were followed, then you may have eaten too many carbohydrates that day.

Gradually decrease carbohydrates in the diet until there is less fluid retention, and a fat-burning mode will begin.

ONCE YOU ACCESS FAT-BURNING MODE, STAY THERE!

Following the *Five Rules* and accessing fat-burning mode creates a wonderful feeling of energy and well-being. However, when individuals have been in fat-burning mode for a few days and feel great, it does not mean their underlying issues with leptin resistance are solved.

There may be numerous temptations that divert people from fat-burning mode. Such temptations cause them to violate one or more of the *Five Rules*. Beware: fat cells lurk in the wings, ready to refill themselves at a moment's notice.

While it may not seem like a big deal to occasionally go out of rhythm, unfortunately it is. If a person is in a good fat-burning mode and then violates one of the *Five Rules*, fat-burning mode will stop.

However, even if the individual goes back to the *Five Rules* the next day, it may take two to five days for fat-burning mode to resume. During that time, the individual will have to wrestle with the additional urges of leptin resistance and previous compulsive eating patterns that did not exist in fat-burning mode.

Unfortunately, when a person tries to lose weight and is in a good pattern, any violation of the *Five Rules* can slow progress for a few days. Sometimes extra exercise can get you back on track faster. Once in fat-burning mode, stay there!

SUMMARY

The purpose of healthy eating is not calorie restriction and deprivation. These approaches simply result in yo-yo dieting and endless problems with fluctuating leptin. The purpose is to improve the metabolic efficiency in response to food. Most Americans need to eat less; when they do it right, they will find they have more energy on less food.

The *Five Rules* prevent and correct insulin resistance, leptin resistance, adrenaline resistance, fatigue, and mood problems. They promote a metabolic balance that leads to relatively easy fat burning, even for those who have struggled with their weight.

People who can violate these rules and still maintain a healthy weight and good energy level are fortunate and blessed with good genetics. However, sooner or later they will not be able to eat in violation of the *Five Rules* and get away with it.

When individuals try to follow the *Five Rules* and are not able to, they need to work themselves into a better level of "eating fitness." A workable plan is to begin implementing some of the rules, and then as there is improvement, to work on all of them.

Even though there is tremendous individuality in terms of our biochemistry, the *Five Rules* are of fundamental importance to virtually everyone. This is because the rules are based on survival, and they facilitate correct signals in the body relating to survival. The *Five Rules* address the subconscious brain at a core level; this is a much more powerful principle than any diet based on metabolic type or blood type. The *Five Rules* are the essence of mastering leptin from a dietary point of view.

The single most important point about how to eat is eating in a way that does not confuse basic communication signals in your body relating to survival. If this principle is violated, minimally it will feel like rowing a boat upstream. More commonly, it feels like health is slipping away.

Following the *Five Rules* is the foundation of a healthy eating lifestyle – one that facilitates energy needs and helps keep the body efficiently metabolizing calories throughout life. This includes accessing fat-burning mode for the purpose of healthy weight loss. These simple eating rules are the keys to growing older healthfully. They form the foundation of being a competent *Health Asset Manager*.

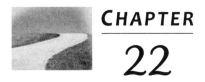

Conquering Stress Eating

LOOK AROUND. How many things do you have to get done? How many projects are on the backlogged "to do" list? How many demands are there today or this week? Many of these demands are responsibilities essential to living, such as working and raising children. There seems to be no end to how energy can be spent. Are the demands of life in any reasonable state of balance in terms of ability to recover? When can you make time for yourself?

Most individuals with leptin resistance have trouble balancing the demands of their life with their need to recover, relax, and have fun and enjoyment.

In terms of food, the fastest way to leptin resistance is to overeat. In terms of exercise, the fastest way to leptin resistance is to do none. In terms of lifestyle, the fastest way to leptin resistance is to stress out. When the "solution" to stress is eating, there is double trouble.

STRESS FUELS ADRENALINE EXCESS

Stress generates an adrenaline response to meet the demands of the stress. This is a survival trait to deal with increased demands or emergencies. In today's world, we have ongoing stress that is generally not life-threatening. These demands and pressures lead to excessive adrenaline production on a regular basis.

Excess adrenaline is behaviorally manifested in different ways. Some people feel anxiety or fear; others feel anger, irritation, and frustration. Some express these feelings; others internalize them. Regardless of how the excess adrenaline is manifested, the bottom line is that there is too much of it.

FALSE ALARM

Normally, the hypothalamus gland, the 911 control center in the brain, signals fat cells to release energy by sending an adrenaline message to them. This is a normal survival mechanism wherein adrenaline is associated with an increased energy need, and increased fuel is supplied to meet the emergency demand. This method of survival is certainly handy when one is confronted by saber-toothed tigers.

However, what happens when the body cries wolf? Maybe the stressors in life don't seem like crying wolf, but from a genetic survival point of view, the great majority of today's stressors are in the crying-wolf category. In essence, the survival instincts to deal with major stress are activated by relatively trivial issues. At first, your body behaves according to the genetic program. After a while, your body realizes that there is a false alarm.

The fat cells are no longer going to listen to the crying-wolf adrenaline release. The fat cells develop adrenaline resistance due to excess trivial stress; this, in turn, causes fat cells to become metabolically numb and slow down. Sluggish fat cells easily expand, causing weight gain.

Adrenaline resistance is one-third of the key triad of weight-gain issues, along with insulin resistance and leptin resistance. Once one of these three is in motion, the other two follow. True enough, people may overeat in response to stress. However, the main reason they gain weight from stress is because of adrenaline resistance.

STRESS CHANGES ENERGY NEEDS

Stress is the wild card that wreaks havoc with fuel regulation. Stress comes in many sizes and shapes. There can be major stressors such as accidents, surgery, chronic illness, or loss of a loved one. There can be emotional stressors such as conflict or other relationship issues that involve bad feelings.

There can be physical stressors such as living with pain, not getting enough sleep, physically demanding work, a flu bug, or intense exercise. There can be acute intense stressors such as a big argument or an unexpected change.

These various demands and challenges of life, regardless of their size and shape, are intimately connected with fuel-regulation systems in your body. The reason for this is easy to understand. When there is an increased demand, there is an increased need for fuel.

Too much stress not only upsets schedules and routines, it can upset the underlying fuel balance in the body. This causes food cravings, energy fluctuations, and fatigue. This is a fast track to weight gain, or it may cause disruption of a good weight-loss routine.

ONGOING STRESS

Managing acute or short-term stress is difficult enough, but what happens when stress is ongoing for a number of years?

The hormones released under stress are adrenaline and cortisol. Adrenaline is released by the nervous system; it is also secreted by the inside part of the adrenal glands, called the adrenal medulla. Cortisol is secreted by the outside part of the adrenal glands, called the adrenal cortex.

Adrenaline and cortisol are friendly with glucagon, but they are not as compatible with insulin. Since insulin works with food to help store it, it is not a good hormone to help make extra energy on demand. Conversely, glucagon is the hormone that synthesizes fuel from storage and helps protein and fatty acids to be burned for fuel. It makes sense that adrenaline, cortisol, and glucagon all work together to produce more energy in response to increasing demands, especially stress.

In the absence of stress, glucagon does its basic role of maintaining blood sugar between meals and setting the stage for consistent blood sugar support during sleep. It is much easier to maintain proper blood sugar during sleep if glucagon is not also having its volume turned up by adrenaline and cortisol.

In the presence of stress, the release of adrenaline and cortisol signal the liver to dramatically increase the supply of blood sugar. In essence, there is a synergistic effect among glucagon, adrenaline, and cortisol. The liver responds to this combined hormone stimulus by making fuel from stored glycogen and by synthesizing fuel from protein. Fatty acids may also be used, if the stress is prolonged.

On the one hand, this might sound like a great way to lose weight; unfortunately, stress hormones break down the protein of the body structure before they burn fatty acids for fuel. Stress-induced weight loss is debilitating to heath because there is a loss of physical fitness. The physical feeling of wear and tear is obvious.

STRESS EATING

Stress causes a rise in blood sugar; this is a hyperglycemic state. This means there is a higher than normal amount of blood sugar so that a person can either run away or go into battle. Genetically, this was for fight-or-flight purposes. This hyperglycemic response activates many subconscious behavior patterns associated with survival.

These patterns are not necessarily rational. Hyperglycemia drives violent and aggressive behavior. It also causes anxiety and fear, and, in the case of children, causes irrational and emotional outbursts and odd social behavior such as ADHD. If blood sugar rises before bed a person will have trouble getting to sleep without eating something, staying asleep, or sleeping restfully.

Hyperglycemia causes the body to run hot. The engines are hyper aroused, as if prepared for battle, whether real or imagined. One way to cool off a hot hyperglycemic reaction is to eat food. The higher the concentration of calories, the faster the stress reaction will cool off.

The reason this works is that eating food causes a rise in insulin. The fastest way to raise insulin is to eat fats and carbohydrates in combination. The rise in insulin causes a depression of glucagon, turning off the liver's ability to make excess sugar. This settles down the hyperglycemic reaction to stress, sometimes in a matter of minutes. When stress is more intense or has gone on for a long time and the hyperglycemia is more severe, then dense fatty/salty junk foods sound better than sweets.

This is why people stress eat; it is how excess food becomes an individual's best friend. It is a temporary solution for turning off unpleasant feelings. It has a short-term "workability," but with major adverse and long-term consequences. Regular stress eating is a fast track to leptin, insulin, and adrenaline resistance.

STRESS WHEN ALREADY FED

Let us say that something stressful happens after eating. In this case, insulin is already the dominant hormone in the system. The release of stress hormones upsets the digestive system, because they reduce peristaltic motion and take blood away from the digestive tract.

Additionally, insulin response is blunted by the stress hormones, which causes improper refueling. The liver does not want to store energy under stress; it wants to synthesize energy.

Therefore, stress in a fed state causes liver confusion and indigestion. This destabilizes energy and results in energy dropping either immediately, if stress tolerance is not good, or in several hours, causing food cravings between meals due to low blood sugar.

FIND ALTERNATIVES TO STRESS EATING

Instead of eating when there is a stress feeling in the body, do something physically active. Go for a walk, do some jumping jacks, briskly climb up and down the stairs ten times. This has the effect of putting the high blood sugar to use, at which point the craving for food will cease.

We frequently use extra nutritional support to boost energy in order to offset stress. This support is very helpful for people who feel worn down or eat in response to stress, especially when they notice that extra stress throws them into a poor eating pattern. Any type of nutrient support that helps a person to have a better mood and higher tolerance for stress is worthwhile. Use enough nutrient support, as needed, to not get derailed by stress.

The more stress a person is under the greater the importance of consistent relaxing exercise or activities. This helps build up the relaxed reserves of the nervous system, so that there is more tolerance for stress. Just getting in a good rhythm with the *Five Rules* can make a big difference. This will improve stress tolerance and create less likelihood for stress eating.

SUMMARY

Stress is one main factor that dysregulates the natural balance of insulin and glucagon, setting the stage for leptin resistance. If these hormones are already out of balance from food issues, then stress simply makes matters worse.

Eating and exercising in a good rhythm and pattern are the basic to handling and tolerating stress more effectively. Building a good "savings account" of relaxed reserves is essential for any person with a physically or emotionally demanding life.

In order for one to grow older with health intact, good eating patterns and stress management are essential components that exist alongside proper blood sugar control and healthy immunity.[213]

Finding comfort and pleasure in alternatives to stress eating, such as enjoyable walks, is an important solution for individuals prone to this behavior.

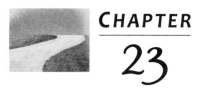

CHAPTER
23

Is Caffeine Good or Bad?

CAFFEINE is one of the most widely consumed and addictive substances in the world. It serves as an example of how a substance can be beneficial or harmful, depending on the person consuming it and that person's existing health situation.

The most basic view of caffeine is as a metabolic stimulant. It works by increasing sympathetic nervous system activity, which in turn increases metabolic rate.[214] The ability of caffeine to increase metabolic rate is the opposite of the slow and "perceived starvation" metabolism of the typical overweight person; thus, it has been incorporated into various weight-loss plans.[215,216]

In some circumstances caffeine can suppress the excess insulin production of leptin, which could be a handy weight loss tool since many people suffer from this exact problem.[217] A recent study shows that the weight-loss stimulating effect of caffeine is enhanced by antioxidants.[218] Antioxidants appear to protect cells from the friction generated by nerve-related caffeine intake, thus enabling caffeine to stimulate fat burning for a longer period of time without producing cellular distress.

Conversely, this means that individuals who are sensitive to caffeine (in terms of it producing anxiety or other uncomfortable symptoms) are most likely deficient in antioxidants. Since all overweight people, statistically speaking, are lacking antioxidants, it is a very good idea to supplement a basic array of antioxidants if you consume caffeine.

Caffeine has been found to increase the rate of fat burning in the liver, enhancing the burning of fat for fuel.[219,220] It has been hypothesized that caffeine, by means of its increase in sympathetic nerve activity, can help reduce abdominal weight gain – the type of fat most associated with cardiovascular disease.[221]

Caffeine may even help protect the liver from damage.[222] Caffeine consumption reduces the risk of gallstones by helping the gall bladder to contract and thus move along its contents more efficiently.[223] This is why coffee enemas have been in use for over a hundred years. Caffeine also helps the bowels move along, promoting a better elimination and rate of overall toxin clearance.[224] When caffeine works in a friendly manner in the body, it helps to depress leptin.[225,226]

It was recently reported in the Lancet that individuals drinking seven cups of coffee per day had half the chance of developing type II diabetes compared to individuals who had two or fewer cups of coffee per day.[227] This study of Dutch coffee drinkers did not compare coffee drinkers to healthy non-coffee drinkers; thus, while this study made national media headlines, it is misleading.

Navy Seals, intentionally sleep deprived and placed under intense physical stress, had significantly better cognitive function and performance with the assistance of 200 milligrams of caffeine.[228] It is safe to assume that because they must be very physically fit most Navy Seals do not suffer from leptin resistance. This study shows that individuals in good physical fitness may benefit from caffeine stimulation when under stress. This is a short-term response to caffeine stimulation.

The cognitive effects of caffeine seem most prominent in individuals who are deprived of caffeine and then consume some. These improvements tend to be lost with regular caffeine consumption.[229]

In a rather interesting experiment, researchers tested the accuracy of timing perception in individuals who consumed no caffeine, less than 135 milligrams a day, and more than 135 milligrams a day. The moderate-caffeine-consumption group had the best timing perception. Those with higher caffeine consumption or no caffeine consumption did not score as well.[230] Since body rhythms are a matter of proper timing and being in sync, this study provided evidence that a moderate amount of caffeine may be helpful for some individuals in achieving natural balance. Whether caffeine actually has this effect depends largely on the amount consumed and the existing health of the individual.

CAFFEINE PROBLEMS

Individuals with eating disorders are known for their overconsumption of caffeine and other metabolic stimulants such as nicotine.[231,232] Caffeine excess can lead to very serious health problems in these individuals, including psychosis[233] and heart attack.[234] Individuals with eating disorders attempt various strategies to suppress leptin out of existence so that no weight gain is possible, then they get stuck in the problem and cannot get out.

Caffeine can be used to facilitate this misguided behavior; it is an example of too much metabolic stimulation in an individual who is already malnourished. Such individuals frequently live on diet soda and cigarettes as their primary "nutrient" intake.

The other side of the coin is people who are over nourished, even though their body may think it is starving. While consuming caffeine can potentially benefit such people, this is frequently not the case. For example, instead of getting improved bowel function, such individuals simply get heartburn or a sore stomach from consuming caffeine, especially when they exceed a small amount.

Even in healthy individuals, caffeine can tilt metabolism in a manner that begins to induce insulin resistance.[235] As a healthy person begins to run on stimulants, the natural balance in the insulin system is disrupted. Every individual has a different tolerance level for this shift, meaning that some individuals are able to consume more caffeine than others.

At some point, however, overstimulation with caffeine begins to create insulin resistance. Once insulin resistance occurs, leptin resistance and adrenaline resistance are close behind. When a person who consumes caffeine is gaining extra weight, the fact of resistance is impossible to deny. At this point, caffeine has crossed the line.

In our experience in observing overweight individuals who consume caffeine, it is common that caffeine disrupts leptin timing. Instead of hitting its highest level during sleep, leptin's timing is moved forward. This results in excess cravings for carbohydrates between meals, overeating at night, and/or poor quality sleep. In essence, it causes an individual to violate the two most important rules of eating properly.

People who are overweight need to reduce caffeine intake to no more than two servings per day. People who notice that they crave carbohydrates with caffeine consumption, or shortly thereafter, are overstimulating the liver and nerves into a friction response. The craving for sugar serves to cool off or prevent the overheating effect of caffeine. Such an individual needs to cut back or completely eliminate caffeine.

Some individuals may need to eliminate caffeine in order to wake up their sluggish fat cells that are adrenaline resistant.

Caffeine has a natural tendency to slightly elevate blood pressure (about four points) as part of its nerve-induced metabolic push. In men, this is due to increased vascular resistance; in women, it is due to increased cardiac output.[236] Individuals with cardiovascular disease should avoid or minimize caffeine.

If caffeine raises blood pressure more than four points, contributes to weight gain around the middle, and/or there is great trouble following the *Five Rules*, then it can be assumed that caffeine intake is excessive. This is because excess sympathetic nerve stimulation causes a numbing effect on fat cells in the abdominal area. This leads to excess weight gain around the middle. In such situations, caffeine is making adrenaline resistance worse.

The excessive amount also has a stimulating effect on the kidneys, leading to high blood pressure and over-reactions to stress.[237] Therefore, the overcaffeinated individual is irritable, hyper, prone to high blood pressure, has trouble sleeping, has insulin resistance, and is gaining weight around the middle. Such individuals are also fatigued and think they must have caffeine for energy stimulation.

Caffeine issues are complicated with a coffee shop on every corner. Many drinks ordered in these shops contain excess sugar and fat calories along with the caffeine. Caffeine contains 10 to 20 calories per serving.

Adding one tablespoon of cream to coffee adds 50 calories. A latte is 200 calories and a mocha with whip cream is around 270 calories.

When such drinks are consumed between meals, they count as a snack, directly unbalancing the *Five Rules*.

SUMMARY

If a person has a moderate amount of caffeine, sleeps well at night, sticks with the eating pattern of the *Five Rules*, has normal blood pressure, maintains an optimistic mood, and is losing weight or maintaining optimum weight, then caffeine may actually work toward improved health and metabolic fitness. At least it is not noticeably detracting from health.

The problem for most individuals who are leptin resistant is that they are prone to compulsive or addictive consumption patterns. This easily leads to excess intake of caffeine, which wipes out any benefit it may have had.

Individuals with a history of weight issues, leptin resistance, and any type of drug/alcohol abuse need to be quite wary of falling into the trap of excess caffeine consumption. Any person consuming more than two servings of caffeine a day is on the edge of, if not already in, a significant problem with energy and metabolism.

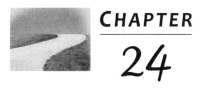

Brain Cravings

WHEN ALL IS SAID AND DONE, people will eat when they are hungry. Hunger sets in motion powerful subconscious survival instincts.

The key issue is whether the hunger signal the person is experiencing is a proper hunger signal or one that is misguided. The abnormal hunger signal leads to excess weight gain and serious health problems as the years go by.

The issue of leptin resistance is the key factor for a truly misguided hunger signal: the brain cannot properly sense the amount of fuel stored in fat; therefore, it enforces a hunger signal. The result is that the eaten food keeps being sent into fat storage.

Insulin resistance and adrenaline resistance work together with leptin resistance to lock in eating patterns that are erratic. Individuals with these issues are lacking in stress tolerance, and they try to use food to cool off or settle down emotional feelings. The result is an emotional eater who locks in the problems of leptin, insulin, and adrenaline resistance.

In virtually all situations of inappropriate eating that are due to a faulty hunger signal, the individuals feel better for a few minutes or a few hours after eating. However, there is no stability in their daily energy, mood, eating patterns, or sleep patterns. Any benefit from the improperly ingested food is easily offset by the consequences to energy level, weight gain, and overall natural balance.

We are learning more and more about the science behind food cravings. It may help people to combat food cravings if such science is more thoroughly understood. However, the bottom line is an issue of staying in natural balance. The better this is done, the fewer improper hunger signals they will experience.

NEUROPEPTIDE Y

The hypothalamus gland in the brain is the subconscious command and control center for the entire body. It is the part of the brain that senses the amount of leptin on hand. When it senses the correct amount of leptin, it means there is plenty of fuel in storage, so it turns off appetite and enables a faster metabolism.

If there is truly a lack of food or if there is leptin resistance, then the hypothalamus will keep hunger signals elevated in an effort to motivate the person to gather more food.

Neuropeptide Y (NPY) is the key hunger signal in the brain. This signal must be turned off for an individual to feel satisfied from food. If this signal stays elevated, then eating continues *(figure 10)*.

Leptin and NPY are opposites. As leptin levels rise inside the brain, NPY levels fall. Unfortunately, when there is leptin resistance, leptin does not enter the brain at the proper rate. NPY levels stay high, causing individuals to eat more than they need before the brain gets the message that they are full. Diabetics and obese individuals have the highest elevations of inappropriate NPY.[238]

DOPAMINE AND NEUROPEPTIDE Y

As we have pointed out, leptin is closely related to sympathetic nerve function. The primary neurotransmitter relating to leptin is dopamine. Dopamine is involved with reward behavior. The fastest way to increase dopamine is to eat fat; this in turn raises leptin and shuts off NPY.

This makes individuals feel rewarded on a subconscious basis; they feel satisfied. The primary protein needed to make dopamine is the amino acid tyrosine, found in animal proteins and cheese. Therefore, high-tyrosine and high-fat foods, such as a steak dinner, pizza with

Food Cravings

Figure 10

Stress places demands on the nervous system. When stress is not managed well or when stress is too great, then food cravings will intensify. When a person eats in response to stress, it sets the stage or locks in the problems of leptin resistance, insulin resistance, and adrenaline resistance.

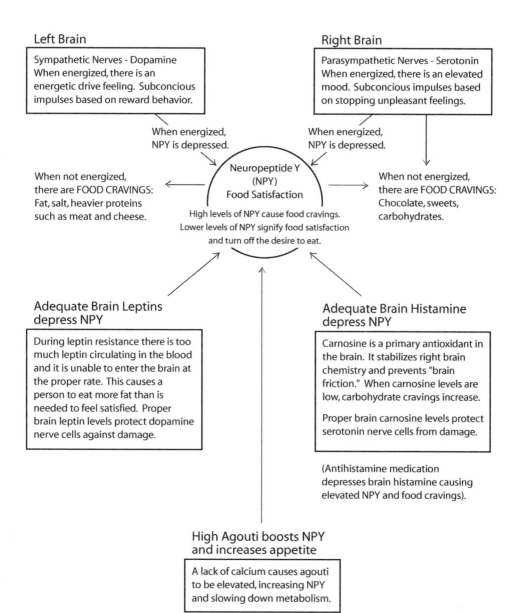

Left Brain

Sympathetic Nerves - Dopamine
When energized, there is an energetic drive feeling. Subconcious impulses based on reward behavior.

Right Brain

Parasympathetic Nerves - Serotonin
When energized, there is an elevated mood. Subconcious impulses based on stopping unpleasant feelings.

When energized, NPY is depressed.

When energized, NPY is depressed.

Neuropeptide Y
(NPY)
Food Satisfaction

When not energized, there are FOOD CRAVINGS: Fat, salt, heavier proteins such as meat and cheese.

When not energized, there are FOOD CRAVINGS: Chocolate, sweets, carbohydrates.

High levels of NPY cause food cravings. Lower levels of NPY signify food satisfaction and turn off the desire to eat.

Adequate Brain Leptins depress NPY

During leptin resistance there is too much leptin circulating in the blood and it is unable to enter the brain at the proper rate. This causes a person to eat more fat than is needed to feel satisfied. Proper brain leptin levels protect dopamine nerve cells against damage.

Adequate Brain Histamine depress NPY

Carnosine is a primary antioxidant in the brain. It stabilizes right brain chemistry and prevents "brain friction." When carnosine levels are low, carbohydrate cravings increase.

Proper brain carnosine levels protect serotonin nerve cells from damage.

(Antihistamine medication depresses brain histamine causing elevated NPY and food cravings).

High Agouti boosts NPY and increases appetite

A lack of calcium causes agouti to be elevated, increasing NPY and slowing down metabolism.

meat, and high-calorie Mexican food, are foods that individuals may turn to so that the dopamine-reward system in the brain feels satisfied. Individuals who crave high-fat proteins generally crave energy.

Such a craving may be based on an actual need, as in the case of an active person who is maintaining proper body weight. It may also be based on a faulty "need," as in the case of a leptin-resistant individual who seemingly must eat this type of food to feel satisfied. In this latter case, it is converted to an expanding waistline. A person with leptin resistance eats more fat than is needed in order to get the satisfied feeling. This leads to eating too many calories.

SEROTONIN AND NEUROPEPTIDE Y

The parasympathetic side of the nervous system is fueled by the neurotransmitter serotonin. This side of the nervous system has no direct connection to leptin at all.[239] It relies on tryptophan, an amino acid, and higher carbohydrate intake in order to increase the serotonin production.

A higher serotonin level also depresses NPY. This results in a satisfied feeling. While there is no direct connection between leptin and serotonin in terms of regulating each other, they share a common effect on NPY.

The most famous serotonin-raising food is chocolate. Individuals who crave carbohydrates generally try to improve their mood, especially to create a relaxed feeling.[240]

On a subconscious basis, the right brain tries to avoid pain. Therefore, as serotonin levels drop, a person craves carbohydrates in an effort to turn off unpleasant emotional feelings.

Depressed individuals crave more carbohydrates in an effort to raise their low serotonin levels.[241] A far better choice would be moderate aerobic exercise, such as walking. Mood fluctuations prior to the menstrual cycle can cause powerful carbohydrate cravings for the same reason – depressed serotonin.[242]

The last thing people need when they are in a good eating pattern is too much stress that induces cravings for food to satisfy energy or mood needs. Eating to make one's head feel better may work in the short run, but it is a fast path to frequent eating and overeating, behavior that is sure to induce leptin resistance and weight gain.

If individuals know that they will have a demanding day, it is better to eat a large breakfast or lunch, as opposed to having their energy crash and getting into craving patterns. Once leptin resistance sets in, hunger signals are more likely to be incorrect, leading to an inability to lose weight and a tendency to progressively gain weight.

HISTAMINE AND NEUROPEPTIDE Y

There is a new wave of information relating to brain histamine and food cravings. Higher neuronal histamine in the hypothalamus gland of the brain depresses appetite.[243] The action of brain histamine is synergistic with the action of leptin to depress appetite.[244] The working hypothesis in this emerging research is that higher histamine depresses NPY.[245] This also explains why antihistamine medication and antipsychotic medication with antihistamine effects cause weight gain.

Ongoing brain histamine research over the last fifteen years has demonstrated that a proper amount of brain histamine not only helps control excess appetite, it is essential for the brain to feel properly awake.[246]

The nutritional supplement carnosine is a naturally occurring histidine peptide, highly concentrated in the brain, muscles, and heart. New research shows that carnosine is a primary antioxidant in the brain.[247,248] It offers considerable protection from changes in brain structure that lead to dementia,[249] and it is being considered as a novel way to stop changes in the brain that lead to Alzheimer's disease.[250]

Carnosine is a major part of the foundation of the relaxed reserves in the brain.[251] When carnosine levels are proper, the brain can tolerate stress and stimulation. When carnosine levels are lacking, stress induces damage to brain cells and leaves the nerves in an excess adrenaline state. This contributes to high blood pressure, due to a lack of ability to tolerate stress.

In a groundbreaking study, carnosine stopped the effects of excess adrenaline on the kidneys, leading researchers to conclude that carnosine may offset the obesity-associated high blood pressure problems associated with leptin resistance.[252]

Carnosine levels in the brain are directly associated with protecting the brain from damage. Carnosine also helps appetite control, generates a relaxed and awake feeling, and has an ability to reduce adrenaline and leptin resistance.

LOW CALCIUM CAUSES FOOD CRAVINGS

The issue of calcium and weight loss is another emerging finding related to genes and fat cells. Calcium has a direct influence on a brain signal called agouti. Agouti is a best friend of NPY, acting to stimulate food intake while slowing down metabolism.[253] In fact, it is known that this combination of high NPY and agouti block thyroid function, even though common thyroid lab tests appear normal.[254]

Agouti is one of many brain signals involved with promoting appetite. In our genetic evolution it was common not to have enough food. Thus, as we evolved, we developed numerous signals to help the ingestion of food, and very few signals to turn off appetite. This may have been handy many years ago, but it is extra genetic baggage that we do not have a great deal of use for now.

Agouti is a gene signal that amplifies the production of leptin from fat cells, and it blocks the ability of the hypothalamus gland to sense leptin in the brain, thus helping to promote the leptin resistance problem.[255] The net result of this problem is to increase fat storage and inhibit fat breakdown.[256] The agouti gene is regulated by calcium intake.[257] Extra calcium intake can cool off this agouti gene and thereby remove a stressor that enhances the production of excessive leptin and reinforces higher levels of NPY that cause food cravings.

Further, too much agouti causes people to gain weight while eating the same amount of food they could previously eat. This is because it slows down metabolism.[258] A higher level of calcium intake improves thyroid function and metabolism by lowering agouti.

Higher calcium levels also help to settle down excess production of adrenaline. It does this by relaxing the smooth muscles of the circulatory system, thereby helping to bring down high blood pressure. The calcium imbalance that contributes to high blood pressure is the same type of calcium imbalance that leads to obesity.[259] This imbalance is made worse with excess salt consumption and a lack of water.

To help weight loss, calcium is only going to work during times when a person is not overeating. If excess calories are being consumed, the body is simply forced to store them as fat. The combination of appropriate dietary restriction and increased calcium intake has the best weight-loss effects.[260]

SUNSHINE REDUCES CRAVINGS

Americans are constantly being told to stay out of the sun. This results in a reduction of vitamin D, a fat-soluble nutrient. A recent scientific study shows that vitamin D is a powerful inhibitor of leptin secretion from white adipose tissue.[261] When one does not get enough sun, there is a higher risk of leptin excess, leading to leptin resistance.

This takes its toll every winter in the northern states, where shorter and colder days mean less sun exposure. This is not helpful with the tendency to overeat, especially at the holidays, locking in a leptin-resistant pattern the rest of the winter.

Additionally, vitamin D is an important cofactor in calcium absorption. Thus, not only does the lack of vitamin D improperly increase leptin, it also decreases calcium uptake, which predisposes a person to a higher than normal level of agouti. This in turn causes higher levels of neuropeptide Y and food cravings.

EATING TOO MUCH BECAUSE
YOU ARE NOT EATING ENOUGH?

All this information tells us is that feeling satisfied from food is a complex issue. If we have strict rules that prevent eating fat or carbohydrates, we could easily get into a situation of elevated neuropeptide Y that does not shut off.

For example, people attempting to eat a high-fat and high-protein diet who need to raise serotonin will end up overeating fat, because they cannot tell when they are full. Such diets are touted as a way to help prevent insulin resistance, because insulin is secreted primarily based on the amount of carbohydrates in a meal. However, when fat is eaten, it stimulates the intestinal tract to release a compound called gastric inhibitory peptide that causes insulin to rise higher.[262]

While insufficient gastric inhibitory peptide can be a problem in making insulin, it has been found that excess stimulation of gastric inhibitory peptide due to high-fat consumption can induce insulin resistance.[263] This means that high-fat diets which are not supposed to cause insulin resistance are just as capable of inducing the same problem through a different mechanism. As mentioned earlier, when a person cannot metabolize higher fat in the diet, then that fat is deposited in the pancreas and liver, clogging their function and inducing insulin resistance.

Conversely, people on low-fat diets can easily eat too many carbohydrates because the dopamine reward system is not satisfied. These people feel like they have no sustainable energy or ability to focus.

In both cases, the individuals become overweight or stay overweight because they are eating too much, even though they think they are avoiding the "evils" of saturated fat or too many carbohydrates. If they had learned to eat an appropriate amount of saturated fat or carbohydrates, their cravings would turn off, their metabolism would run more efficiently, and they would not overeat in an effort to feel satisfied.

A simplistic guideline about how much fat or carbohydrates individuals should eat so they do not crave food is not possible, because these amounts are different for every person. Issues such as personality type, physical demands, emotional demands, sleep status, and many other factors influence what is correct for any individual. However, people who do not learn this information and how it applies to themselves can easily overeat simply because they are trying not to eat a particular type of food.

DO YOU HAVE A MISGUIDED SWEET TOOTH?

Interestingly, it has been proven that leptin influences the taste system. Properly functioning leptin enables a person to not crave sweets. There are leptin receptors on taste buds. When leptin communicates to taste buds, then the craving for sweet tastes is reduced.[264] If a person has leptin resistance, then the taste buds do not get the leptin message, and overconsumption of carbohydrates and sweets becomes likely.

People without eating problems can induce them by trying to follow dietary advice that makes them feel unsatisfied. A few pieces of cheese can make the leptin-dopamine system feel good, preventing excess carbohydrate consumption. A few bites of chocolate can make the serotonin-satiety center feel good, preventing someone from continually eating other food.

Generally, for more serious eating problems, an entire program needs to be implemented. This includes exercise, stress management, lifestyle modification, and appropriate use of nutritional supplementation. This heads a person toward the goal of being able to eat in a normal rhythm and pattern and to be satisfied on a moderate amount of food.

Even healthy people should be wary of a diet that is too low in fat or too low in carbohydrates. These diets can induce overeating because they fail to produce proper feelings of satiety following a meal.

SUMMARY

The bottom line for any meal is that a person must feel satisfied, or he or she keeps eating. Feeling satisfied is a more complex event than one might imagine. It is especially hard to feel satisfied when there is a major problem with leptin resistance.

As one follows the *Five Rules*, leptin resistance decreases and it is easier to feel satisfied on a moderate amount of food, especially less sweet food. Also, as physical fitness improves, food cravings decrease. Therefore, individuals are able to use their willpower for a few days and follow our eating guidelines, they begin to get leptin resistance under control, and it is easier to not crave meals that are high in carbohydrates and fat.

Stress is the wild card that magnifies any weakness in a person's brain chemistry. If the weakness is on the dopamine side, cravings are for calorie-laden and salty foods. The subconscious goal here is to have an energetic feeling of metabolic drive. If the weakness is on the serotonin side, cravings are for carbohydrates. The subconscious goal in this instance is to have a relaxed state or a more pleasant mood.

Extra nutritional support can be used to help turn off food cravings and turn on metabolism. This type of support is especially helpful for individuals who have so many cravings that they can not get on track, for individuals who do not lose weight even when they are eating in a good pattern, or for any individual who simply wants to make weight loss easier.

When overall natural balance in a person's life is not good, then there is much less tolerance for stress. A person is likely to experience food cravings based on brain chemistry imbalance. This triggers stress eating, in turn causing a disruption in fuel utilization. This leads to leptin resistance, insulin resistance, and adrenaline resistance, a path of increased fatigue and bad moods, no matter what is eaten.

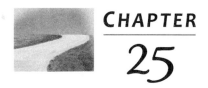

CHAPTER

25

Ghrelin, the Stomach's Cry for Food

THE GASTROINTESTINAL TRACT (GI TRACT) produces a variety of hormonal signals that communicate to the hypothalamus gland in the brain and affect hunger. These signals are part of normal appetite. When the body is out of balance, these signals cause inappropriate food cravings.

We have already shown how that the hypothalamus gland of the brain must be able to correctly perceive the true amount of leptin in order to regulate metabolism correctly. If there is leptin resistance, the hypothalamus gland does not sense the correct amount of leptin, and appetite stays higher than normal, even though a person may be quite overweight.

Scientists have shown that there are many diverse metabolic signals coming to bear on the hypothalamus gland, most of them seeking to stimulate appetite for one reason or another. It is believed that leptin acts as a "brain toner" to enable the brain to properly respond and regulate these diverse signals.[265]

In addition to the hunger signals discussed in the previous chapter, many other appetite-related signals come from the GI tract itself. In this chapter, we will focus on a primary hunger signal coming from the stomach, called ghrelin.

WHAT IS GHRELIN?

Ghrelin is a hormone produced in the stomach that says it is time to eat. The ghrelin hormone signal has a short-term effect lasting up to an hour. If a person does not eat when the hormone signal presents itself, then it goes away and appetite disappears. If there is too much ghrelin, then a person will overeat.

NPY and agouti stimulate the production of ghrelin, and ghrelin tells the pituitary gland how to influence metabolism.[266] This is rather amazing information. It means that the stomach is a major player in human behavior and metabolic rate, and that the brain must coordinate the stomach's input in order for there to be a harmonious situation.

This science reinforces the fact that solving stress eating is only minimally a psychological issue; it is primarily an issue of achieving natural balance so that subconscious signals get along with each other. People can look endlessly for the psychological reasons for overeating and beat themselves up for having feeble willpower; however, this path is likely to have minimal value.

Any person who chooses to view weight and obesity issues from a psychological perspective may find this hard to believe, but eating issues are primarily issues of hormone imbalance. The solutions that work are ones that help establish natural balance. To this end, managing stress more effectively is helpful. However, root causes are programmed into genetic survival information and controlled by subconscious signals. Unless natural balance is returned to the subconscious system, craving patterns and eating problems will simply persist.

GHRELIN, INSULIN, AND LEPTIN

Ghrelin levels rise when the blood levels of leptin and glucose fall. High-fat diets that cause a rise in leptin, depress ghrelin levels. Conversely, diets high in carbohydrates increase the production of ghrelin.[267] Ghrelin directly communicates to the brain to increase the production of NPY, the brain's main hunger signal.

In normal function, once the ghrelin signal is released, it will turn off for one of two reasons:

1) No food is eaten. The hormone can last up to an hour; after

this time it goes away.

2) Food is eaten. The food itself, not insulin, turns off the production of ghrelin.[268]

Very significantly, a normal amount of ghrelin is essential for gastric motility – the forward movement of food through the digestive system – and the correct release of stomach acid to digest protein.[269] A proper amount of ghrelin is essential for emptying food from the stomach into the small intestine.[270] In addition to primary ghrelin production in the stomach, it is also produced in the small intestine,[271] pancreas,[272] and thyroid.[273]

In a normal-weight individual, ghrelin rises before meals to signal hunger. Between meals, in individuals with healthy metabolism, ghrelin and leptin rise together in the bloodstream throughout the day. They create a normal fitness tone, playing off each other to help maintain appetite drive.[274]

Inside the brain, leptin and ghrelin act as metabolic opposites. Ghrelin helps NPY go up, thus stimulating the brain's desire to eat. Leptin makes NPY go down, thus allowing the brain to feel that there is no longer any need to eat.[275]

GHRELIN IN OVERWEIGHT INDIVIDUALS

The levels of ghrelin in normal-weight individuals as compared to the levels in overweight individuals is quite interesting. In overweight individuals, the amount of ghrelin before eating is usually lower than normal.[276]

In normal-weight individuals, ghrelin levels drop when food is ingested. In overweight individuals, ghrelin levels stay elevated after food is eaten, leading to excess consumption of food.[277] Overweight individuals have a blunted response to ghrelin working as it should.

Once again, it is an issue of efficiency. Ghrelin loses its normal rhythmic function in overweight individuals; it is an out-of-balance stomach hormone that adversely affects eating and behavior. Why does it do this? Leptin is too high. As soon as high leptin levels come down, ghrelin goes back into natural balance, and normal appetite patterns of ghrelin reappear.[278]

The issue of leptin resistance causes higher-than-normal blood levels of leptin. This, in turn, causes ghrelin to be released for an abnormally extended period of time during the meal, stimulating excess eating in order for the individual to feel full. This especially causes excess eating of carbohydrates. Following the *Five Rules* is fundamental to lowering leptin and normalizing ghrelin.

A recent animal study shows that taking melatonin can decrease ghrelin levels by enhancing normal rhythmic function of leptin.[279] Melatonin levels drop in individuals as they age; also in the winter when days are shorter and there is less sunlight. And, leptin levels generally rise as an individual ages. Now we know that this combination sets the stage for improper ghrelin timing, a key hormonal signal that fuels the subconscious overeating drive.

SUMMARY

Eating some carbohydrates is essential for normal ghrelin activity and production. The importance of this is further explained in chapter 34 on growth hormone. Here, it is important to understand that carbohydrate cravings and eating excess carbohydrates are associated with ghrelin being released at the wrong time in relation to eating.

In overweight people there is not enough ghrelin before the meal and too much ghrelin after the individual starts eating, causing an improper signal that says keep eating. This is a major reason why overweight people overeat; once they get started, they cannot stop until they have eaten too much food in relation to their true energy need.

Further, natural ghrelin release is essential for normal gastrointestinal flow and digestion. Thus, ghrelin problems cause the GI tract to become sluggish, resulting in indigestion and heartburn. As a person solves this problem by bringing leptin down, then ghrelin timing normalizes, excess carbohydrate cravings stop, and digestion improves.

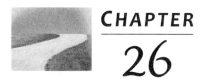

Dangerous Weight Loss

IN 1997, it became obvious that the widely used weight-loss drug fen-fluramine caused cardiovascular toxicity and heart-valve damage. The lesson to be learned from this catastrophe is that even though a drug can suppress appetite by manipulating the brain signals which control hunger, the consequence to the rest of the body can be quite damaging. The drug disrupted natural balance. Yes, it forced down the brain's level of NPY, but it did so at considerable expense.

The drug was removed from the market because of cardiovascular issues, but a closer look shows that it also caused four times the amount of serious episodes of major depression when it was used.[280,281] This is because the drug disrupted natural balance in the brain.

This book is about restoring natural balance everywhere in the body so that metabolism can work correctly. This skill is the hallmark of the competent *Health Asset Manager*. If this lesson is not learned now, the unwitting public will be subjected to the next wave of weight-loss drugs, all attempting to regulate leptin and NPY in some way and throwing the body out of balance in the process.

RATIONALIZING THE MEDICAL ROUTE

Health-care costs relating to obesity are skyrocketing. Disease in our society as a result of obesity is at epidemic levels. Society turns to the medical profession for a quick-fix answer.

Currently, the two medications approved for long-term weight loss are rather tame by comparison to fenfluramine and to what is waiting in the wings.

Orlistat is a fat-absorption reducing medication. The primary side effect is disruption of the GI tract. The GI tract must run smoothly and without symptoms in order for natural balance to be obtained; thus, the drug works against a primary goal of long-term weight management.

Three years of data on Orlistat has shown that the drug gives only minor assistance to weight loss.[282] It has failed to demonstrate that it can reduce diabetes or heart disease. All people have to do is get in to some reasonable condition of natural balance and they will eat less fat. This result can be obtained without upsetting the GI tract and further disrupting natural balance.

The other current weight-loss drug is called sibutramine, a serotonin and norepinephrine transporter blocker. It works by interfering with the normal flow of neurotransmitters in the brain. It attempts to prop them up and have the side effect of depressing NPY. It does not act on NPY or any of the core signals or molecules in the subconscious brain that are under current intense research for the next weight-loss "miracle."

Whenever brain chemistry is manipulated, there are side effects. Medications that target appetite suppression by modulating NPY are likely to have adverse stimulant side effects. This means that adrenaline is extra hyped up and the heart bears the burden, as in an anxiety-prone nervous system.[283]

The most commonly reported side effects of sibutramine are dry mouth, constipation, insomnia, and an increase in heart rate and blood pressure that persist for as long as treatment is continued.[284] Those promoting these drugs rationalize that these disruptions of natural balance are not as bad as being overweight.

That view is likely to change as the cardiovascular-distress picture becomes clearer with ongoing use. In November 2002, researchers from Germany quietly pleaded with the scientific community to more fully understand the adverse consequences of this medication to the cardiovascular system: "Our findings strongly suggest that current concepts regarding the action of sibutramine on the sympathetic nervous system should be reconsidered."[285]

Medications that affect the brain show side effects in areas other than cardiovascular risk. Researchers at Vanderbilt University proved that when women used diet pills before pregnancy or during pregnancy, it significantly increased the risk of leukemia in their children.[286] The risk was even greater if both parents took such stimulants.

The leukemia risk also included the use of antihistamines and allergy medication during pregnancy. This finding is not surprising; we pointed out the importance of brain histamine in maintaining natural balance in the nervous system in chapter 24. Although this major side effect was recently discovered, rest assured that it will not be discussed with patients before putting them on stimulant diet pills. How long will it take health authorities to warn pregnant mothers or women who may become pregnant of increased risk for leukemia in their offspring if they take antihistamines or allergy medication while pregnant? Meanwhile, the quick-fix-oriented public is continuing to pop sibutramine pills.

GASTRIC BYPASS INSANITY

A basic rule of natural balance is to keep all body parts whenever possible. If a body part is altered, then natural balance will be forever altered.

Gastric bypass surgery was once reserved for the morbidly obese. It is being promoted as a glamorous way to lose weight, with various celebrities on covers of magazines and in the media. The frenzy is backed by a medical profession that is too eager to make money by removing body parts. In fact, not only do they want part of the stomach, they want to take the gallbladder for "preventive purposes."[287]

Gastric bypass surgery is complicated and requires considerable skill. The most alarming adverse side effect is a higher level of death, due mainly to blood clots in the lungs, which occur even when precautions are taken prior to surgery to prevent them.[288]

If a person makes it past this initial risk factor, there is a 9.5 percent chance of developing a serious complication that requires more surgery.[289] These are not the annoying GI tract disturbances that are also common; they are major ones.

Nevertheless, a certain number of individuals are willing to take these risks in an effort to be thinner and reduce other types of risks.

Unfortunately, this is a situation where the long-term risks of doing the surgery are just as bad as the health risks of being overweight – they are just different.

It is coming to light that individuals with gastric bypass surgery need to contend with the risk that they are likely to develop serious metabolic bone disease as they grow older. This is a well-documented side effect of this surgery.[290] In the past, it was thought that this side effect was due to malabsorption of food, or eating too little, or both.

New science shows a different cause; the surgery is ruining the body's metabolism. How is this possible?

The surgery reduces the quantity of functional stomach. As we discussed in the previous chapter, the stomach makes a hormone called ghrelin, a key hormone that stimulates hunger and leads to overeating in overweight individuals.

As it turns out, gastric bypass dramatically lowers the levels of ghrelin because there are fewer stomach cells that can make it. This is permanent. A person might think that this is a good thing because they will not be hungry as often.

However, once the surgery is completed there is no normal ghrelin response to food.[291] This is quite different than a normal-weight person's correct and healthy ghrelin function. Gastric bypass surgery permanently destroys normal ghrelin function and rhythm.

This one finding is enough to call a halt to such surgeries. Why? Because ghrelin is the key signal in the body that enables the proper release of growth hormone.[292] Ghrelin is a major discovery in the growth hormone field. Without proper ghrelin function, numerous parameters of aging worsen because the body cannot correctly repair itself. One side effect that has already been noticed is the bone-disease issue. This finding has been confirmed by animal studies showing that low ghrelin suppresses bone mineralization.[293]

SUMMARY

There are no quick fixes for weight loss. Due to the severity of this problem in our society, there is considerable research money being poured into finding drugs or surgeries to help individuals lose weight.

Since there will be adverse effects from such drugs and surgeries, the companies and health professionals involved use the age-old marketing ploy that the benefits outweigh the risks. Once the government agrees, then frustrated dieters jump on board. Years later, the adverse effects accumulate.

The widespread promotion of gastric bypass surgery is a new low. The economic forces behind it use a marketing campaign appealing to thinner America. They promote its "safety," downplaying its serious risks and problems.

There is only one safe and healthy way to lose weight and maintain quality of health. That is a comprehensive approach to achieving and maintaining natural balance. All quick-fix weight-loss solutions are detrimental to natural balance.

The health risks associated with obesity are serious. Taking proactive steps on a consistent basis is essential. There are no shortcuts. There are healthy solutions.

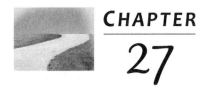

Reviewing Key Food and Fat-Burning Points

THIS CHAPTER highlights important points an individual needs to keep in mind for weight loss. Consistency over the long haul is what will produce results. When an individual gets off track, it is important to learn from the experience. It is also important not to get too far off track, becoming a casualty of the yo-yo diet syndrome. This chapter is the first one an individual should turn for a quick refresher on key points.

WHY FAD DIETS DO NOT WORK

There are many diets on the market. There are two primary mistakes made by virtually every popular diet.

1) Beginning a plan with a highly restrictive introduction phase. This type of diet induces the low-leptin starvation response. It plays on the fact that, for a period of time, a person's metabolism is generally set to burn the higher amount of calories that he or she has been eating. Significant food restriction burns off stagnant calories and dumps water weight. After a week or two, metabolism slows down to match the lower calorie intake. Unfortunately this approach locks in the low-leptin starvation response. As soon as a person's willpower is compromised in this new diet plan, even if it is a good diet plan, weight is headed back to fat storage under the influence of leptin.

2) Allowing snacking between meals. It does not matter how many calories a person snacks on. Snacking disrupts leptin and throws it out of balance, shutting off fat-burning time. In turn, this makes a person want to eat more food at the next meal, which then flares up leptin resistance. Following the diet plan is now a struggle, at which point more food is eaten and all the weight is gained back. The reason diet authors do not understand this point is because none of them understands leptin. If they did, they would not allow snacking.

The Leptin Diet avoids both of these problems, because it advocates eating in a way that maximizes the efficient function of leptin. Doing so increases the rate at which fat can be metabolized in a safe manner. This eating pattern avoids the starvation response and avoids the snacking-induced improper rises in leptin that are the eventual downfall of all popular diets.

WHAT KIND OF MEALS SHOULD A PERSON EAT?

With the exception of Atkins meal plans, many popular diets offer excellent meal suggestions based on a mixture of low glycemic carbohydrates, lean protein, fruit, and vegetables. Any such meal may be incorporated into *The Leptin Diet*. Our diet emphasizes a good protein serving at breakfast to help promote leptin stability the rest of the day. Protein amounts at lunch or dinner may vary significantly; however, at least one of the other two meals of the day should contain a noticeable protein serving.

The Atkins diet is the worst popular diet on the market today. It seeks to solve insulin resistance by eliminating or drastically reducing carbohydrates. This type of calorie manipulation can work for a period of time; however, it turns individuals into carbohydrate cripples. When a person breaks down and eats carbohydrates, leptin problems come back in spades. The diet is doomed to eventual failure for the majority of people who attempt it.

The Atkins diet has an even worse side to it. Overweight people are already stuck in leptin resistance. The new science demonstrates that the UCP3 control system in muscle cells is seriously compromised by the existing leptin problem. It is this UCP3 system that enables cells to dispose of an overload of saturated fat. We now understand that an important function of leptin is to help cells dispose of extra fat. This is so the fat does not become deposited in cells, tissues, and organs, thereby causing disease.

If a person is losing weight on an Atkins diet, then this potential problem is not occurring. However, a high-saturated-fat diet tends toward excess calorie consumption at a given meal, making weight loss stop or weight gain occur. When people are not losing weight or are gaining weight on Atkins' type meals, they run a high risk for depositing fat in their liver, arteries, heart, pancreas, and other places. This directly induces diabetes and heart disease by clogging healthy function with fat deposits.

It is completely fine to have an amount of saturated fat in the diet. That is quite different than high saturated fat and low complex carbohydrates, a risky proposition for the majority – especially over the long haul.

Conversely, low-saturated-fat diets have never produced long term healthy results in the majority of people following them. Government health officials and dieticians have conditioned our society to think that all saturated fat is bad. Eggs take a lot of abuse; but eggs are an excellent food. Almost anyone can eat eggs regularly if they like them and are not allergic to them. They do not raise cholesterol significantly, if at all, and they do not cause heart disease.[294,295,296]

In reality, eggs are a heart-friendly food. They contain the highest amount of choline of any commonly eaten food. Choline acts like a fat solvent in the blood, helping to keep fat from sticking together and clogging vital organs. Further, choline makes betaine in metabolism, which helps protect against cholesterol forming plaque in the arteries. Betaine helps clear homocysteine, a known risk factor for hardening of the arteries.[297]

Milk also has a bad name. True enough, some people are allergic to milk or have lactose intolerance, or they just do not like milk. However, many more people have switched to skim milk because they think the saturated fat in milk will clog their arteries and cause heart disease. Guess what? A new study finds that milk fat intake is inversely correlated with heart disease and the risk for a first heart attack. In this study, insulin levels and leptin levels were lower in relationship to the percentage of milk fat in the diet.[298]

The current milk and egg studies do not support the idea that a low-saturated-fat or low-cholesterol diet is essential or even important for reducing heart disease risk. There is also plenty of data to show that a high-saturated-fat diet is very problematic towards increasing heart disease risk, especially when eaten as part of a general pattern of calorie excess. It is an issue of moderate intake, of balance. Some saturated fat intake in the context of a balanced diet and good eating patterns is completely fine for the great majority of individuals.

MAKING GOOD DECISIONS

It is incredibly difficult for leptin-resistant individuals to make consistently good meal decisions over the course of an entire month. Even when individuals are in a good pattern for a week or two and making progress, temptation lurks.

This temptation typically flares up when individuals get out of their highly controlled personal environment. Eating out and social events are the common downfall times during many well-intentioned weight-loss attempts.

Being good for so many days in a row tends to kick up the subconscious idea that a reward is in order. This will manifest as a desire for something sweet or something higher in fat. The desire for sweets is driven by elevated NPY; fat cravings are driven by dopamine-related stimulus-response reward behavior. Both are quite powerful, capable of overwhelming willpower, if given the chance.

This means people must have a predetermined focus about what they will eat and how they will eat before showing up at a social event. For example, at a restaurant, the people with a dopamine-driven impulse think a steak or filet sounds like a great idea – some type of heavy and high-calorie meal. Those with NPY-driven impulses want to start out with bread and wine, and are likely to feel a need for dessert in order to be satisfied. Foods heavy in meat are not generally appealing. Dopamine-driven people also want dessert, simply because not doing so indicates a lack of reward and unjust deprivation of pleasure, not because they actually need a sweet taste to feel satisfied – they probably got a full signal halfway through dinner.

If the dopamine drive wins out and a steak is ordered, weight loss is going to come to a stop. Such an individual must use willpower to order the tastiest looking fish entrée on the menu. There are no options. Skip all bread and desserts. Eat slower and eat only the entree. Hopefully, the entrée has a variety of tasty vegetables included with the fish. There is usually a moderate carbohydrate. Drink a lot of water with the meal. If leptin resistance is improving, oddly enough this meal will be very satisfying even though it did not seem to be when it was ordered. Next-day bonus – the individual has survived eating out without losing progress on a weight-loss program, rather than being two to four pounds heavier the next morning following the steak.

To satisfy NPY and prevent excess sugar consumption, flavor is the key. By all means, have a glass of wine if you desire it. Pick something that sounds like it will have a lot of flavors you enjoy. Enjoyable flavor stimulation during the course of the meal is vital to overcome that unstoppable feeling of needing something sweet in order to feel satisfied. Oddly, skipping dessert will then not feel like deprivation, and the scale will reward these efforts the next morning.

Anyone attending a buffet or a social situation where there is access to unrestricted food is really putting subconscious impulses to the test. Drink plenty of water just before going. Once there, focus on vegetables and salads, with minimal dressing or dip, until a good base of these is in your digestive system. Keep drinking water. This strategy provides a base of fiber that will buffer the rate of calorie absorption from whatever else is eaten, thus lowering insulin and leptin response to food that is not likely to be a good choice.

If you eat enough veggies and drink enough water, you may not want anything else at all – a sign of improvement. Once the fiber and water base is in place, then make selections that look to be the most flavorful, with the least amount of fat or sugar. Try to avoid the dessert selections or the meat and cheese choices, if possible. The key: once you start eating these foods, eat slowly and finish eating them in fifteen to twenty minutes. Then eat no more food at all the rest of the night. The next morning the scale will indicate that you've survived, with little or no weight gain.

SUMMARIZING GOOD FOODS

It is always dangerous to spell out a list of foods that are acceptable to eat. Invariably, someone will figure out how to eat too much of something on the list, negating its value as a useful food. This list is not a meal plan; it is a guideline of foods that can be eaten on *The Leptin Diet*.

Primary proteins: lean meat, eggs, chicken, turkey, fish, seafood, whey protein powder, cottage cheese, pork, veal, and lamb.

Occasional protein/fat sources, generally used as a condiment: cheese, cream cheese, peanut butter, nut butters, nuts, seeds, avocado, hamburgers, and steak. Only lean cuts of meat should be eaten when you are trying to lose weight. If you are overweight or trying to lose weight, do not eat any of these as an entrée or main feature of a meal.

Two fruit servings per day are fine. Avoid all fruit juice if you are overweight. Have fruit with meals or blended into whey protein drinks (use milk, rice milk, or almond milk as a base for the protein drink). Do not snack on fruit. Do not snack on anything!

Vegetables and salad may be eaten in unlimited amounts at meals, with the exception of carrots, corn, peas, and pumpkin. Their carbohydrate content makes them part of the carbohydrate content of a meal, and this must be taken into account. Go easy on salad dressing and avoid any salad dressing made with partially hydrogenated vegetable oils.

Primary carbohydrates: any whole-grain wheat product, pasta, oats, yogurt, milk, tomato soup, chicken noodle soup, sweet potato, butternut or acorn squash, beans, carrots, tomato-based vegetable juice (not carrot juice).

Occasional carbohydrates (eat a small or moderate portion): rice, low-sugar cereals, lentils, peas, corn, and potatoes.

Condiment sweeteners: chocolate, honey, maple syrup, white sugar. For optimal progress, a person serious about weight loss will completely avoid all these sweeteners. An occasional thumb-size portion is acceptable. More than that amount is likely to slow or stop progress significantly. When a goal weight has been reached, occasional intake is okay, especially if you have planned exercise that day or the next. If you get to the end of a meal and want a little something sweet to finish it off, it is a good idea to fill a glass with water and squeeze some lemon or lime in it. Drink this instead. Or just get busy doing something else, and the desire to eat more will soon pass.

Learn to use herbs to enhance the flavor of food. Our society is conditioned for fat, salt, and sugar intake, leading to cravings for junk. Herbs can introduce flavor back into the picture, a key to help control cravings.

Avoid completely high-sugar cereals, candy, cookies, cake, bakery goods, and foods or beverages sweetened with high fructose corn syrup. Also eliminate all MSG and all artificial sweeteners. High salt and high-fat junk food should be completely avoided. Avoid ice cream. When you eat something sweet and realize that you really do not like it or could have done without, you are making progress.

Saturated fat naturally occurring in the protein foods mentioned above is fine. Butter may be used as a condiment. Cream may be added to coffee, though it is part of the meal's calorie total. Olive oil is highly recommended as a fat source. It is very important to get some high quality omega 3 oils (DHA/EPA) into the diet, as well as GLA. These oils are best taken as supplements, since they are generally lacking in the food supply. Salmon and tuna have the highest amount of omega 3 oils of any readily available food. Avoid trans-fatty acids (partially hydrogenated oils) like the plague. Minimize your intake of any fried foods. Avoid potato chips, corn chips, and French fries.

If you are stuck in a fast food situation, eat the leanest protein sandwich on the menu or a salad with a low-calorie dressing. Eat no side orders or desserts. Drink water.

It is vital to keep the bowels moving every day, or weight loss will come to a halt from backed-up toxins. The above food choices offer a variety of fiber in the form of whole grains, vegetables, and fruit. Supplemental fibers may be helpful for some, if needed. No bowel movement equals no progress.

Drink six to eight glasses of clean water per day – avoid tap water. Clean water is the primary beverage to consume between meals, and it may be consumed with meals. Teas that do not have any sweetener are acceptable in moderation, as long as they do not upset the stomach or induce food cravings. Organic green tea is preferred. Carbonated water may disturb digestion and induce cravings. Some is acceptable as long as it does not cause problems.

A general level of activity can be well maintained on *The Leptin Diet* with total calorie intake in the 1200 to 1800 range for women and 1500 to 2100 calorie range for men. The calorie range for each sex relates to body height. Average American intake of calories is currently between 2500 and 3500 – just too much food. These suggestions are in keeping with the very first human study that shows keeping calories below 1950 can significantly reduce all parameters of heart disease.[299]

Higher physical demands may require a slightly higher intake of calories. *The Leptin Diet* makes it possible to more efficiently extract energy from less food, making lower calorie intake feasible. This is far different than a low-fat eating disorder induced though starvation, wherein the body is locked into a high state of inflammation.

FAT BURNING

Food is needed to sustain energy. The goal of *The Leptin Diet* is not to dwell on food choices; it is to focus on fat-burning times and how to maximize them. There are two prime fat-burning times:

1) When moderate aerobic activity of one to two hours' duration is performed between meals or on an empty stomach. This fat-burn-

ing time can be enhanced by taking antioxidants prior to exercise, especially co-enzyme Q10.

2) During the night while a person is sleeping. This is most effective when no food has been eaten after dinner and no snacking occurred during the day. This fat-burning time can be enhanced by a short-duration strength exercise before bed, like push-ups, and by any type of vitamin support that helps a person sleep better, if needed. Common examples are calcium and magnesium.

Not snacking between meals and not eating after dinner are keys that open the door for prime fat burning.

When a person is in a good fat-burning mode, that individual can expect to have a good energy level, clear head, fewer body aches or pains, and no cravings for foods that are known to promote weight gain.

The whole purpose of the *Five Rules* is to maximize the use of food to facilitate healthy fat burning. This applies to overweight individuals and normal-weight individuals.

ADJUSTING MEAL TIMING

In our hectic world of ever-changing demands, even the best intentions for following a consistent pattern may get thrown off. It is a very unfortunate situation to get home late and be ravenously hungry. A little planning can save a lot of leptin resistance.

If your schedule is such that the next meal is only four hours away, then eat a smaller meal at the meal prior. This creates a smaller rise in insulin and leptin and preserves the rhythm of fat burning.

If dinner is later at night, then lunch needs to be a larger meal and dinner should be a small meal. Even a small dinner should be finished three hours before bed. For a larger dinner you need five to six hours before bed.

The afternoon is a typical weak spot for many people. This is especially true if your schedule has six to eight hours between lunch and dinner. Whenever you go six to eight hours between meals, a larger meal is indicated at lunch, one that has some saturated fat in it. This prevents the afternoon crash.

Some individuals notice they get tired shortly after eating a larger meal. This indicates insulin resistance and leptin resistance, instead of an efficient response to the meal. Yet, if these individuals do not eat enough, they will not have any energy in four to five hours. In this situation the response to a larger meal may be helped with caffeinated coffee or tea. Caffeine in response to a meal is known to reduce the rise in insulin and leptin. It also reduces fat deposition in the liver and acts as a stimulant to the liver, helping the liver factory to more efficiently process the larger-sized meal. Caffeine is a tool, not a requirement. Individuals who do not get tired from a slightly larger meal and have good energy over the next six to eight hours do not need it, as their bodies are working in a more efficient manner.

The weekend poses another typical problem with meal timing. What should people do when they catch up on sleep and wake up two to three hours later than normal? The best solution is two meals that day, both a bit larger. Enjoy a larger breakfast, followed by dinner six to seven hours later. Plan some physical activity for the middle of the day. Do not eat dinner too late.

In reality, there is no technical reason why a person needs to eat three meals a day to master leptin. Three meals a day is the maximum number in order not to upset leptin. Two meals a day may work better for many people, and it certainly works better on a weekend day when an individual has slept in.

Individuals in metabolically weak condition may have trouble going five to six hours between meals, regardless of what they eat. This weakness manifests as low blood sugar symptoms between meals. It is reflective of a congested or inflamed liver, similar to flabby, out-of-shape, or hurting muscles. Just as exercise needs to be improved gradually to help the muscles, eating patterns and time between meals may need gradual improvement. Eating four smaller meals a day, four hours apart, with about ten hours between dinner and breakfast, helps get people into better liver fitness. Eventually they will notice they can eat the three meals a day and feel good energy all day.

THE SCALE

Many people hate scales, a general symptom of weight-loss frustration. A person who has induced low-leptin starvation metabolism finds standing on the scale to be a very unrewarding practice. However, a good digital scale is an essential training tool for individuals to understand their specific body in relation to food choices, energy level, internal body function, mental energy, the demands of life, and weight loss.

Weighing oneself each morning is acceptable. Weighing oneself morning and night is more informative. In ideal fat-burning mode, the scale is seldom ever higher at night than it is in the morning. A true goal of daytime energy management is to have the scale no higher at night than it was in the morning.

It will become immediately obvious that many other factors besides diet come into play. A lack of sleep brings weight loss to a halt. Fighting an infection brings weight loss to a halt. Backed-up toxins bring weight loss to a halt. Too much stress brings weight loss to a halt. And, unfortunately for many, a little bit of sugar or high-fat food choice brings weight loss to a halt. Monitoring the scale on a daily basis is the best way to compare what body weight is doing in comparison to diet and life issues.

All these factors that slow weight loss relate to some type of stress which increases wear and tear and thus inflammation in the body. When a person has a clear head and vibrant energy while following the exercise guidelines and *Five Rules* of *The Leptin Diet*, progress will be made.

However, it is important to realize when some life issue or internal body stress is slowing down weight loss and stopping fat-burning mode. In this situation, along with the head not feeling clear and energy not being good, the scale will be moving up slightly instead of staying the same or lowering. Modern digital scales offer a precise way of monitoring this, even throughout the course of a day if a person cares to check.

When a person has a slight weight gain when following a diet pattern which usually induces weight loss, it means that some form of stress is generating enough inflammation to provoke fluid retention. Sometimes a person may need to get through the stress before the scale starts moving down again. Examples include the friction and fluid retention of the menstrual cycle or fighting an illness. Other times a person can rearrange his or her life so that there is more sleep or exercise time. Stress management life skills are vital.

The ability to lose weight and keep it off is directly related to a personal ability to perceive and correct small changes in metabolism causing it to head in the wrong direction. This skill far exceeds basic information about what to eat. Violations of the *Five Rules* invariably cause problems; there are also many other potential issues.

A huge mistake is to assume that *The Leptin Diet* is not working and head off track. Frustration that leads to eating too much, especially in response to cravings induced by the stress, is a fast track in the wrong direction.

Individuals who are doing everything they can with exercise, diet, sleep, and stress management have numerous nutritional supplement options available to help with issues as to why the scale creeps up during the day. Individuals can gradually increase nutrient support, targeted at their metabolic weak spots, until they are able to maintain a more efficient fat-burning mode.

SUMMARY

There are no shortcuts or quick fixes to attain optimal health and proper body weight. *The Leptin Diet* is not a set of rules to be followed for a few months and then discarded. These are the core rules for building stable natural rhythms in the human body which help a person efficiently burn calories and make energy.

Individuals following the *Five Rules* do not feel like they are on a diet. They do not feel deprived. A significantly improved energy is obvious. It is also obvious when they revert to old ways and get too far off track. The fatigue, cravings, and other health issues are reminders of the wrong way of doing things.

It is incredibly important for individuals to establish proper dietary habits for themselves. The *Five Rules* offer a blueprint on how to do this. They are not set in concrete; they are functional rules that have scientific basis.

Proper eating patterns and consequent energy production from food set the tone for other rhythms in the body. This gives an individual much greater potential to deal with any type of stress or demand and not get worn down.

The *Five Rules* are the secret to maximizing the energy that can be extracted from food. When this ability declines, food easily turns to stored fat instead of energy.

Some individuals struggle with this issue their whole lives. Others have a turning point, such as the start of puberty, going off to college, or having children. These turning points tend to aggravate problems that may not have previously been significant. Maybe a person can violate the *Five Rules* and seem to get away with it. This only means that his or her metabolism is strong enough to tolerate the abuse. Sooner or later, it will catch up.

Individuals entering their forties know that their body just does not respond the way it did when they were younger. Now the *Five Rules* are mandatory. Violating them leads to slow and progressive weight gain and a whole host of other issues associated with aging.

In order to stay on track with the *Five Rules*, individuals must understand cravings and what they mean. They must understand how to get back on track if they get off track. Problems with metabolism tend to lead to obesity.

The *Five Rules* of *The Leptin Diet* are the foundation for attaining and maintaining optimum body weight. Implementing them in one's life requires skill. The reward of doing so is an improved ongoing quality of health.

PART THREE

Preventing Disease

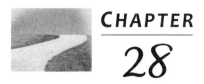

Timing, Inflammation and Aging

TIMING IS EVERYTHING. Our bodies are regulated either by a harmonic symphony, a heavy-metal tune, or something in between. Biological rhythms are the guiding force of human metabolism and natural balance. They are the essence underlying communication in the body. A person either feels in sync or out of balance.

Whenever extra demands are placed upon a person, they could potentially push the individual out of rhythm. A fundamental principle of the human body is that no matter what type of demand is placed on it, it tries to compensate and maintain natural balance.

Hormones are important communication signals in the body that seek to coordinate the body's ability to stay in sync and meet the extra demands or pressures. As a person begins to have problems, the body is thrown out of sync and timing is off.

Poorly timed communication occurs in hormonal systems. This sets in motion a path of wear and tear. This out-of-rhythm situation generates friction; cellular function no longer clicks along in the proper way. Such friction causes excessive and inappropriate inflammation. This is not just an ache or a pain. This is inflammation happening at a cellular level throughout the body.

This cellular friction or inflammation is the primary cause of heart disease, both in terms of the progressive deterioration of the circulatory system over time and as a causative factor in a heart attack.[300,301,302,303]

The problems of inflammation and cardiovascular risk are significantly elevated in insulin-resistant and leptin-resistant individuals.[304] The problems of inflammation extend to many aspects of disease risk, a fact that is being announced loud and clear to the American public.[305]

Slowing the aging process is related to having a good rhythmic base of natural balance and an ability to bounce back and manage stress.

KEEPING TIME AND ESTABLISHING ENERGY

The central biological clock that governs rhythms is called the suprachiasmatic nucleus (SCN). It is found in the hypothalamus gland of the brain. It is the primary timekeeper for all of the rhythms in the human body, much like the conductor of an orchestra. It seeks to synchronize the body through various internal functions, such as hormonal patterns and body heat. It adapts regulation to external cues, such as light. It may change the musical composition at a moment's notice, based on some type of stress or demand. Each orchestra member – those being a body part or a cell – must also keep time and play on cue.

The hypothalamus gland sends out the rhythmic signal that sets the twenty-four-hour leptin pattern, thus permitting energy to be used by other hormonal systems and body organs. When leptin works correctly, the twenty-four-hour rhythm follows, like an orchestra member following the conductor. There is an improper degree of tiredness or fatigue when leptin and the hypothalamus are out of sync. Such a lack of energy is frequently the first symptom of a problem.

The conductor must figure out what musical composition can be played based, on the energy required to perform the composition. In order to figure this out, the conductor must perceive the level of leptin which indicates the amount of fuel on hand. Once this is determined, the conductor will set the pace and energy expenditure of the orchestra as a whole. At the most fundamental level, leptin has a powerful influence on metabolic rate and the feeling of good energy at the most fundamental level.

AGING AFFECTS RHYTHMS

As a person ages, the biological-clock system begins to lose its ability to keep time, resulting in a direct deterioration in the quality of health. There are several changes that occur. All changes result in a lowered quality of communication taking place in the body; and there is a concurrent increase in inflammation, due to the friction caused by the inefficiency.

One change is that the rhythms lose their ability to hit a peak, like the singer who can no longer hit the high notes. This causes the rhythm to "flatten out," resulting in the inability to get the job done with the same quality. The singer can still sing – it just does not sound as good as before.

Another change is in overall timing. The conductor of the orchestra sends signals prematurely, so that instruments are played at the wrong time. It does not sound good, and it does not feel in sync. The general trend of aging is that the timing moves inappropriately forward. This is evident in wake/sleep patterns, in which a person goes to bed earlier and wakes up earlier – especially waking up too soon for a full night's sleep, a sign that the body is losing proper timing.

In this case the peak sleep depth is not hit (like the singer who can't hit the high note), resulting in lessened quality of sleep. This interferes with the ability to repair and maintain the health and well-being of the body.

These issues of timing and quality apply to all hormonal systems and body rhythms, not just to sleep patterns.

Another problem with rhythms is that the members of the orchestra do not follow the conductor well. The conductor may be furiously signaling a whole section of the orchestra to play – like the liver section or the immune section – and the section simply does not respond well. It has become resistant to the conductor's directions. The problem is not entirely in the central clock in the brain; it also occurs in areas of the body that receive the messages.

All this is complicated by the fact that various body organs do not communicate well with each other. There is a breakdown in messages occurring between the pancreas and liver. This makes the job of conducting even more frustrating, as group members are not working together.

A TRIAD OF PROBLEMS

These breakdowns in communication are the essence of leptin resistance, insulin resistance, and adrenaline resistance. Such miscommunication causes internal friction and wear and tear, leading to inflammation and accelerated aging.

Leptin resistance, insulin resistance, and adrenaline resistance are the key problems that lock in hormone imbalance. The "glue" that keeps hormonal imbalance locked in is found in the pro-inflammatory signals: TNFa (tumor necrosis factor alpha) and IL-6 (interleukin 6). These are the primary immune signals that no longer work properly when a person is in a wear-and-tear trend. They become the primary source for generating the inflammation that leads to poor health and disease.

Insulin stimulates white adipose tissue to make TNFa.[306] As higher levels of insulin occur during insulin resistance, higher levels of pro-inflammatory TNFa tend to match the exaggerated insulin level.[307] TNFa can directly induce insulin resistance.[308]

TNFa also sends disturbing e-mails to the adrenaline receptors inside fat cells, telling them not to work, thus inducing the white adipose tissue resistance to adrenaline.[309] TNFa sends e-mails to its pro-inflammatory friend, IL-6, telling it to get into high gear.[310] IL-6 gets the liver all worked up, and then C reactive protein levels increase, a key measure of cardiovascular risk.[311]

IL-6 also tells the digestive system not to move,[312] thus causing heartburn and indigestion. This is why many individuals in a wear-and-tear trend have heartburn, reflux problems, and/or sluggish bowels.

Furthermore, platelets in the blood, the cells that stick together in order to form a clot, have leptin receptors on them. The effect of high leptin on platelets is to induce them to stick together too much. This dramatically increases the risk for excessive clot formation[313] and resulting occlusion in the circulation that can cause a heart attack or stroke.

A common theme in part three is to show how excess inflammation becomes the cause of a variety of health problems. We explain how this issue relates to every major hormone and to numerous diseases. Once a person understands this information, it is no longer a mystery why there is disease; it is only an issue of how to solve the problem.

BASIC RHYTHM MANAGEMENT IS PART OF THE SOLUTION

By keeping our bodies in better biological rhythm, we have more tolerance for stress. Having some level of consistency in our daily behavior and routines can help. This is a form of anti-aging exercise for body rhythms. Scientists have proven that regular behavioral rhythms are conducive to good health and well-being.[314] Establishing routine eating times, sleep times, exercise times, and other life-related timing under our control can have a powerful influence on health.

Many of the hormones work in harmony or disharmony with one another. It is not possible to isolate one from the others; they are all members of the orchestra. They either sound good and make beautiful music, or they do not.

In the context of metabolism and food, eating a meal causes insulin to rise. This is the short-term response to the food. There is also an underlying health issue in the insulin system, one that is part of the overall health trend of the body. This is a longer-term pattern. It reflects the function of insulin in relation to other hormones and body organs on a week-in and week-out basis, independent of a single meal.[315]

Insulin resistance is an issue of this long-term pattern, as too much food over a period of time eventually takes its toll. This is involved with progressive leptin resistance and adrenaline resistance.

Hormones are powerful controlling signals in the body. When they work in harmony, they play like a well-rehearsed orchestra. Everything goes according to plan; timing is perfect; harmony and natural balance are the result.

SUMMARY

Good patterns for eating, exercising, and sleeping form the basis for consistency that sets healthy biological rhythms. These are steps we can take to directly affect how our own hormones work toward the goal of keeping everything in natural balance.

The tendency of the aging process is losing quality and timing in hormonal communication systems. Once this happens, an inflammatory path of wear and tear sets in. If it is not resolved, this path leads to increased risk of disease and accelerated aging.

Leptin is the most powerful hormone in the human body. When it works properly, it smoothly interacts with other hormones. When there are health issues, there is friction and disharmony between leptin and other hormones. Timing is off. Rhythms are erratic. Resistance to hearing the hormonal phone call is common. An individual simply feels out of sync.

In the first two parts of our book, we have focused on the hormones leptin, insulin, glucagon, and adrenaline. We have discussed dietary steps an individual can take to reduce stress and friction in hormonal systems.

In part three, we explain how leptin relates to other hormones, including cortisol, growth hormone, thyroid hormone, and sex hormones.

Once there is a comprehensive picture of how hormones work in relationship to each person on an individual basis, then one can take steps to effectively manage them so that they work together in sync.

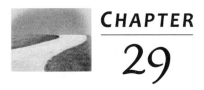

CHAPTER
29

Stress and a Fat Stomach

HOW MUCH STRESS can a person handle on a day-to-day basis before it takes its toll on health? Every person has a different ability to tolerate, adapt to, and manage stress. At the point where stress throws the body out of rhythm, it sets the stage for problems with metabolism, food, weight gain, and poor health.

On an emotional level, such a level of stress feels out of control and uncomfortable. On a physical level, there is wear and tear. The first sign of this wear and tear is fatigue beyond what is normal. The individual no longer pops out of bed in the morning. It is harder to get going or keep going. There is less tolerance for stress because the brain does not have the same energy to deal with stressful issues. As time goes along, one of the undeniable physical issues accompanying this inflammatory wear and tear is weight gain around the middle.

Stress complicates the whole picture of fuel utilization, biological rhythms, and hormones. Stress implies that there is an increased pressure or burden and, therefore, an increased need for fuel. Stress can come from external pressures. These include emotional and physical demands, as well as insufficient sleep or poor-quality sleep. It also comes from internal demands, such as the energy needed to run a menstrual cycle or to fight an infection. Many times there is a combination of external and internal stressors.

Many individuals are already out of sync from wear and tear in their lives. What happens when they get under additional stress? The already inefficient and inflamed body may get overworked and overloaded. If it is unable to meet the demands of the extra burden, a major health turning point occurs.

Sometimes this happens as progressive wear and tear catches up with a person over the years. Other times, there is a major event or series of events that trigger the stress overload. Once this happens, it is the same as a major thunderstorm that knocks out power and downs power lines. This magnifies the degree of communication problems in the body, because the structural integrity of the nervous system and hormonal systems are not functionally up to par.

ADAPTING TO STRESS

If life never had any variables and clicked along at a predictable and monotonous pace, there would be no such thing as stress. Life would also be quite boring. In fact, a great deal of human evolution involved adapting to or overcoming significant threats to survival.

The key hormone that orchestrates the ability to respond to stress is cortisol, produced by the adrenal cortex. In terms of general nonstressed function, cortisol is highest in the morning. It functions as a cellular activator to "turn on the light switches" in all cells so that they wake up and get going for the day.

Morning fatigue or taking a long time to feel energized are common signs that cortisol is in a poor condition. For example, we know that leptin levels must be low for proper cortisol release in the morning. Thus, if leptin-resistant individuals overeat at night, their leptin level stays higher during sleep. It will also be too high in the morning, thus interfering with the proper time for the release of cortisol.[316] This makes a person feel tired and out of balance in the morning.

In fact, once leptin resistance takes hold, the problem gets worse: the normal twenty-four-hour rhythm of leptin is chronically blunted, leading to a four to eight hour delay in proper leptin timing and insulin function. This leptin problem forces normal daily cortisol release to take place at the improper time, thus resulting in fatigue and throwing the entire body out of natural rhythm.[317] This is why a person with leptin resistance has some abnormal level of fatigue, tiredness, or stress intolerance.

Cortisol is secreted in higher amounts under stress. This helps the liver get into action to synthesize blood glucose at a higher rate to meet the need. It is part of the adaptive system of the human body. Think of it as a rubber band stretching. After the stress is over, the rubber band returns to its normal position. This indicates good stress tolerance.

Under the wear and tear of stress, the rubber band does not bounce back properly. A person feels this in an energy level that includes increasing periods of fatigue. There is a feeling of physical wear and tear. Moods are noticeably affected; there is a short temper and ongoing negative feelings such as agitation, sadness, apathy, or even depression. This type of wear and tear causes the body to lose biological rhythms associated with stress tolerance and fuel regulation. A common consequence of this problem is gaining fat around the middle.

LEPTIN AND THE STRESS RESPONSE

We have mentioned that leptin is essential for survival. One of its key operations is managing the body during periods of low food supply and helping the body replenish itself once the period of food deprivation is over.

Leptin also is involved with the short-term energy needs relating to stress. However, leptin is an integral part of the stress response and is purposely released when inflammation occurs.[318] The body must initiate a change of normal operation in order to deal with the stressful irritant. Leptin is a key part of this healthy reaction.

Leptin initiates a wide variety of changes:

1) Leptin enables blood vessels to enter tissue that does not normally contain them, thus enabling a temporary communication and transport system to an area of the body that has been irritated or injured.

2) Leptin stimulates the production of red blood cells. This is es-

sential if there is a wound that causes blood loss.

3) Leptin stimulates the production of white blood cells so that an immune response can be effectively mounted against any pathogens that have entered your body.

4) Leptin stimulates macrophages, which are immune cells that help clean up debris. Leptin also turns up the signals in macrophages, including highly pro-inflammatory signals such as TNFa and IL-6, to help orchestrate the inflammatory response to stress. This is the normal and appropriate use of these inflammatory signals to help deal with an acute challenge.

The net result of this activity is the proper healing of a wound or healing stressful trauma in the body, wherever it may be. This is essential for survival. It is part of the body's perfect defense system. Several scientific papers explain the role of leptin in this capacity.[319,320]

Why would the body utilize a hormone secreted by fat cells in order to help regulate the inflammatory response to stress? So that the body will have enough energy to deal with stress without having to digest food.

Digesting food requires a tremendous amount of energy. If energy is needed for an emergency, then consuming food forces energy to be used for the purpose of digestion. This is why people lose their appetite when they get sick. It is why animals do not eat when they are stressed. It is why some humans lose their appetite when they are stressed. Those who eat in response to stress have serious leptin resistance.

There must be a supply of energy to deal with stress. The body already has a hormonal signal that it uses to manage the longer-term available fuel supply; it is called leptin. Therefore, when there is plenty of fat in storage, leptin levels are higher and signal the brain not to eat anymore. This is what leptin does, unless a person has leptin resistance.

When stress causes an inflammatory emergency, the rise in leptin tells the body not to eat. This is essential for a proper immune response to the emergency.[321] If the stress is dealt with in a shorter period of time, that is great. If not, the body uses the energy in fat cells to fuel the stress response until the problem is brought under control.[322]

If a person is at a normal body weight and in good natural rhythm, then leptin works as designed. Leptin will be a friend in the process of creating a perfectly working stress response.

LEPTIN RESISTANCE AND INFLAMMATION

Leptin resistance is the situation of having too much leptin already in the blood. It is the most common issue in any person who is overweight. There are two situations where leptin is higher. One is a natural response to stressful inflammation, and the other is leptin resistance. Are they the same? No.

Leptin levels rise during stressful inflammation, but there is a 50-50 ratio of free leptin to bound leptin. Half the leptin is biologically active (free). In leptin resistance, only ten percent of the leptin is biologically active.[323]

It has recently been proposed that obesity is an inflammatory condition. Overweight children and adults have elevated levels of C reactive protein, IL-6, and TNFa, all markers of inflammation.[324] Normally, these signals rise when the body mounts a stress response for a given purpose.

In overweight individuals, these markers are stuck at higher levels. This is due to the generation of these immune signals on a chronic basis, from the extra pounds of fat. Remember, thirty percent of cells in white adipose tissue are immune cells. Overweight individuals have more than a normal amount of TNFa because of the amount of fat they have on hand.[325] The rise in TNFa is the actual cause of signals that generate excess inflammation for the rest of the body.[326]

Scientists are just beginning to comprehend the dramatic and far-reaching nature of this information. For example, the inflammation generated by TNFa is understood to be a cause of diabetic retinopathy, which the scientific report calls a "newly recognized inflammatory disease."[327]

CORTISOL AND LEPTIN

Cortisol and leptin generally communicate in a reciprocal manner – as one rises the other tends to fall. In nonstressed situations, both cortisol and leptin follow a twenty-four-hour rhythm. The peak level of leptin is between midnight and two in the morning.

Leptin is mostly an anabolic hormone (one that helps build and repair); correct and properly communicating leptin levels during sleep are essential for repair of the human body. The peak cortisol level is six in the morning; it is the primary get-up-and-go hormone. In a healthy individual, the two hormones have a "communication tone" between each other that is fundamental to natural balance, enabling an individual to respond to stress, deal with stress, and recover from stress.

We know that cortisol is not in control of leptin. Mice that have had their adrenal glands removed still have a normal twenty-four-hour leptin pattern. However, under stress cortisol can influence leptin. Cortisol acts to turn up the volume of leptin activity in fat cells.[328] This is a genetic response in which the body needs more energy to deal with stress. It needs the help of leptin to orchestrate the healing response to stress, including the appropriate inflammatory changes that must take place so that healing can occur.

When this normal reaction to stress becomes imbalanced and natural rhythm is lost, then the same hormones that are needed to combat stress begin to miscommunicate. Cortisol still stimulates leptin production, but the condition of leptin resistance develops. For example, in Cushing's syndrome and other metabolic conditions like Cushing's, there is a chronic overproduction of cortisol. Such patients have markedly elevated levels of leptin, yet the leptin activity inside of fat cells is blunted.[329]

The combination of excess cortisol from stress and leptin resistance blunts the metabolic activity of abdominal fat cells.[330] This is a serious issue: not just one of unpleasant fat. Abdominal obesity is a primary indicator that there are disruptions among cortisol, leptin, and neuropeptide Y. Remember that elevated NPY causes a person to be hungry all the time. Scientists have proven that these hormone imbalances are the actual cause of diseases and mortality associated with the extra abdominal fat.[331]

THE TRUE CAUSE OF STRESS EATING

Yes, a person can seek to manage psychological factors that relate to stress. Anything people can do as a life strategy to feel more in control will help them release less cortisol in response to their personal perception of stress.

However, stress eating is not a psychological issue; it is an issue of disrupted natural balance. It is a key sign that the body is out of rhythm and unable to properly tolerate the perceived demands. It does not matter if the stress is a current issue or a past trauma.

Stress induces overeating only when stress is followed by excessive cortisol release. When this issue is ongoing, there is excess cortisol, leptin resistance, and weight gain around the middle.[332] As mentioned above, this is combined with elevated NPY. Thus, the person has a constant hunger signal locked in place.

ELIMINATE ABDOMINAL FAT TO STOP DISEASE

Scientists have proven in animals that when this extra abdominal fat is removed, insulin resistance, diabetes risk, and the diseases related to these hormone imbalances are significantly reduced or eliminated.[333] How to do this is discussed in the next chapter.

SUMMARY

Good health and proper weight management establish and maintain healthy rhythms. As a matter of lifestyle it is important to have a core rhythmic pattern in place, especially so there is more ability to tolerate a stressful demand when it happens. This pattern prevents excess cortisol from stress.

If a person does not have a good rhythmic base, then stress can throw the entire system out of whack in a matter of days, leading to vicious patterns of weight gain, poor energy, and many other potential health issues. This sets up a problem of internal friction and ongoing excess inflammation, in turn setting the stage for disease risk.

People do not need elaborate testing in order to realize when stress will lead to increased risk of serious health problems. Emotionally, it feels like too much is out of control. The longer individuals feel this way, the more likely they are to be in a state of excess cortisol production.

Physically, it feels like accelerated wear and tear and a poor energy level. This is because cortisol acts by breaking down body tissue to make energy. When there has been too much cortisol secretion, over time it becomes physically wearing. A person with this cortisol excess problem is prone to stress eating, a behavior that is driven by out-of-balance hormones.

Eventually, these emotional and physical trends result in weight gain around the midsection. Over time, the metabolic strain of stress results in a true physical problem, one that reflects a much higher risk for disease.

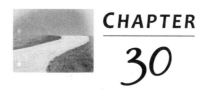

CHAPTER
30

Solving Weight Gain
Around the Midsection

THE KEY to understanding weight loss is getting leptin to work properly. Properly working leptin permits fat burning to occur. It is the hormone that controls the rate of fat burning in the liver, muscles, pancreas, and heart.[334]

Normal metabolism of fat and carbohydrates must be restored in order for weight to be lost correctly. In leptin resistance, there is a slowdown of fat metabolism in the liver. This leads to an accumulation of stored fat, since the fat cannot be burned as fuel. Normal-weight individuals do not have this problem.[335]

Further, once fat utilization is disturbed, carbohydrates also turn into fat. This means that insulin resistance is a consequence of leptin resistance.[336] As long as leptin resistance is present, carbohydrates are likely to turn into fat because of the body's inability to burn fat.

Overweight people have factors working against them that normal-weight individuals do not have. The calories contained in the same exact food are metabolized differently in an overweight person than they are in a normal-weight person. The unfortunate tendency is for the overweight person to convert the food into stored fat.

This is an area where extra nutritional support can balance the playing field, giving the overweight person a significant boost in the ability to metabolize fat.

NUTRIENTS TO SUPPORT OPTIMUM HEALTH

This brings up an important issue about what we seek to accomplish with nutrition. We try to restore healthy structure and function to the body. We work to restore communication in the body, so that it has the ability to establish and maintain proper biological rhythms. We may also need to implement a plan to offset the stressful demands in our lives.

Our government's Daily Values for vitamins and minerals, formerly referred to as Minimum Daily Requirements, evolved because it was discovered that a lack of essential nutrients caused nutritional deficiency diseases. A lack of vitamin C causes scurvy, a lack of vitamin D causes rickets, a lack of B12, or iron, causes anemia, and so on. These stone-age concepts of nutrient needs serve a purpose, but they are woefully deficient when it comes to the general health needs of individuals.

For example, an individual may have one hundred percent of the nutrients that the government thinks are needed for health and still have a raging case of leptin resistance. Excess cortisol from stress makes the problem worse, and the individual gains weight around the middle. What the government thinks an individual needs to prevent the old-time nutritional diseases has nothing to do with how a person tolerates stress and utilizes calories.

Let us define need in a relevant way. If we agree that leptin resistance, insulin resistance, adrenaline resistance, and cortisol excess are not good for health, then a main goal is to eliminate problems with these issues. Whatever a person must do to accomplish this becomes a minimum daily need.

One indicator that such a need is met is that the individuals have a better tolerance for stress, and their midsection shrinks or stays flat while their muscle energy and motivation is good. If nutrients are moving you in this direction and you have improved energy then you are on the right track.

There are shades of gray, wherein people slip into a pattern of wear and tear or they may be gradually improving. It is important to look at the weekly and monthly trend to tell how well a person is doing over time.

A person can take more nutrients than are minimally needed just to be on the safe side or for prevention, but that is a matter of personal choice. The true need is to resolve issues with leptin resistance, insulin resistance, adrenaline resistance, and cortisol excess. This not only helps one attain and maintain proper body weight, it reduces the risk for the diseases of aging.

EVERY PERSON IS DIFFERENT

There are many factors that come to bear on this issue of natural balance besides vitamins and minerals. Food, stress, and sleep are of major importance. If people eat well, exercise, effectively manage stress, get adequate sleep, and have no signs of leptin resistance, insulin resistance, or adrenaline resistance, then they have achieved the goal. They are in excellent natural balance.

The great majority of people, especially those over the age of thirty, have a difficult time getting in a state of natural balance simply by eating well, exercising, and making an effort to get adequate sleep. Certainly, improvement is experienced by making positive changes in these areas, but the goal of being in balance may be difficult to attain or maintain.

There are varying states of difficulty. There can be a moderate case where an individual is five to ten pounds overweight and feeling more sluggish than normal. A person can be stuck in a more significant problem of progressive weight gain, yo-yo dieting, or the inability to lose significant extra weight. Individuals need help to get back on track and to stay on track.

Extra nutrient support can help make this possible by getting the person out of a health rut. This is a relevant use of nutritional support. If the person uses extra support and gets on track, there is a positive outcome for healthy function and structure. In our way of thinking, this is the true minimum daily requirement.

Once individuals are back on track and doing well, they may not need as much nutrient support to stay that way. Thus, two issues arise:

1) What do people have to do to get on track and back in rhythm?

2) What do people have to do to stay on track once they are in a stable pattern?

Do not expect the government to issue guidelines to help people understand nutritional needs in this context. The government has a history of being ten to twenty years behind the times.

For many years, the major medical journals have been anti-vitamin. Now, faced with overwhelming evidence of the health benefits of nutritional supplement support, they are changing their tune.

A rather astounding article published in the *Journal of the American Medical Association* stating, "It appears prudent for all adults to take vitamin supplements."[337] The surprising aspect of this article is that this is mainstream medicine telling the world that even basic vitamins and antioxidants can prevent serious disease.

Leptin-resistance issues are clear; people either have them or they do not. Individuals with leptin-resistance issues age faster, and their health deteriorates quicker than necessary. Something can be done and should be done while there is time. These are factors that help define minimum daily nutritional needs for any individual.

ESSENTIAL FATTY ACIDS AND LEPTIN RESISTANCE

White adipose tissue contains immune cells that in overweight people crank out inflammatory signals, TNFa and IL-6, twenty-four hours a day, seven days a week. This is a somewhat relentless form of stress. Not only do overweight individuals have to deal with the stress of life, they have to deal with the stress of highly inflammatory immune signals being generated by the extra pounds of fat they carry.

Changing the type of fat in the diet can change these inflammatory signals and help stop leptin resistance.

Long-chain omega 3 oils, such as fish oil, can reduce the output of TNFa and IL-6 from white adipose tissue.[338,339] Individuals in inflammatory states such as arthritis can reduce their inflammation signals, including TNFa, by as much as ninety percent using fish oils.[340] By helping to reduce these pro-inflammatory signals, the stranglehold that leptin resistance has on a person can be changed and willpower can start to take charge.

Fish oils are also proven to reduce insulin resistance.[341] Fish oil has a direct bearing on enhancing glucose utilization,[342] including the ability of muscles to use and store glucose.[343] In order to get rid of leptin resistance, glucose metabolism must work properly. This is why extremely low and no-carbohydrate diets do not work in the long run.

It is essential to restore glucose utilization in order to stop excess leptin production.[344] Therefore, fish oils, with their ability to enhance glucose utilization, are one of the many unique nutritional supplements that can have a significant impact on returning natural and normal energy balance to a person who is otherwise stuck in an extremely bad rut.

In a recent study, fish oil and an oil called GLA demonstrated the ability to reduce pro-inflammatory immune-cell activity by up to sixty-five percent within four weeks.[345]

Three to nine grams of these oils added to the diet modify the excessive inflammatory problems generated by the extra pounds of fat. This is a form of stress management for fat cells. It helps to cool them off so they stop generating aches and pains for the rest of the body, as well as locking in conditions of hormone imbalance.

Omega 3 oils were found in much higher amounts in our diets when animals ranged freely and grazed on grass. This caused their fat to have much higher levels of omega 3 oils. Today, other than by eating deep-sea fish such as salmon or tuna, it is difficult to obtain the needed amount of omega 3 oil in the diet. We end up eating too many pro-inflammatory fats without a natural amount of anti-inflammatory fat to keep things in natural balance. This tilts the scale toward inflammation and leptin resistance.

In overweight individuals, extra amounts of these oils become a minimum daily requirement to offset the extra pro-inflammatory immune signals coming from the extra pounds of fat. This serves as a basic example of an increased daily requirement for nutrient intake. The minimum daily requirement relates specifically to how many pounds of extra fat the body has on hand.

PANTETHINE: THE METABOLIZER OF EXTRA FATS

Pantethine is a special form of vitamin B5, pantothenic acid. It is a coenzyme form of the vitamin, meaning that it is exactly the form naturally used in metabolism. It is extremely biologically active, much more so than plain vitamin B5. If we think of fats in the body as a long train, pantethine acts like the locomotive, hauling and transporting fat into metabolic action. No other nutrient is as effective as pantethine.

Pantethine can lower LDL cholesterol,[346,347] raise HDL cholesterol,[348,349] lower triglycerides,[350,351] and make blood less sticky.[352] Unlike drugs, the cardiovascular risk-reducing features of pantethine are accomplished by restoring normal metabolism of fat without any adverse side effects. This includes naturally stimulating the breakdown of stored fat in white adipose tissue.[353]

In a recent study with sixteen individuals who had fatty-liver disease and high triglycerides, each was given 600 milligrams of pantethine a day for six months or longer. At the end of the study, nine of them no longer had fatty-liver disease. Further, CT scans of their abdominal areas showed significantly reduced visceral fat (abdominal fat), the type of fat around important body organs that is the largest concern for fat-associated serious disease.[354]

This study is important because it proves this nutrient helps metabolize abdominal fat which is the type most associated with the onset of disease. It changes the problem of excess cortisol and leptin resistance.

A twenty-year scientific track record of the safe use of pantethine, even in patients with diabetes and kidney failure, demonstrates the power of this natural way to improve fat metabolism. A case can be made – from the viewpoint of healthy function and for the safe and natural reduction of abdominal fat – that this nutrient is essential in higher amounts (600 to 900 milligrams a day); amounts that far exceed what an individual could get from the diet.

CALCIUM: A NEW SOLUTION FOR STOMACH FAT

In chapter 24, we mentioned the importance of calcium in controlling agouti, a gene signal in the brain that helps bolster neuropeptide Y. NPY makes a person hungry, while at the same time blocking the brain's perception of leptin; thus it locks in leptin resistance. In the previous chapter, we pointed out how excess cortisol, leptin resistance, and elevated NPY are locked into a metabolic pattern in stressed-out, overweight individuals, placing them at high risk for stress eating.

As it turns out, agouti and NPY gang up on the body to cause excess food cravings and eating. Excess agouti is directly related to the accumulation of excess abdominal fat.[355] The more overweight a person is, the higher the agouti will be.

It is easy to cool off the agouti gene. To do this, a person needs to take enough high-quality calcium. This may require calcium intake ranging from 2,000 to 3,000 milligrams a day. When the right amount is reached, many cravings for food stop, energy is noticeably improved, and there is weight loss around the midsection.

In our clinical experience, we have had the best results using calcium AEP and coral calcium to accomplish this result.

SUMMARY

Freeing the body of extra abdominal fat is essential to reducing the risk for disease and slowing the rate of aging. When a person gains weight around the middle, it signifies that many issues relating to hormones are going in the wrong direction and that natural balance is disrupted.

If a person is able to eat better and exercise, thereby losing weight, then that is all that is needed to return the body to natural balance.

This issue becomes progressively more difficult to solve when ongoing stress and poor eating habits have set up problems with cortisol, leptin, insulin, NPY, and agouti. These problems tend to lock each other into place and get progressively worse as time goes by.

It is proven that various nutrient supplements can help the body regain better control of fat metabolism and reduce the inflammation coming from fat cells. At the forefront of nutrients in this category are essential fatty acids, pantethine, and calcium.

The science is overwhelmingly clear that these nutrients are safe and effective to help restore natural balance in fat metabolism. From a functional point of view, for many overweight individuals this type of nutrient support is essential to overall health and well-being.

For many others, this support helps make weight loss easier or prevents weight gain from stress. It can be used as part of a health maintenance and anti-aging approach to help metabolism run more efficiently.

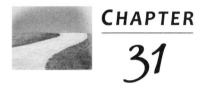

Resolving Eating Disorders

WE ARE CONSTANTLY BOMBARDED by advertising images that tell us ultra-thin is desirable. In an effort to achieve this thin state, one attempted solution is to eat very little food.

Frequently, this involves younger women who try to attain or maintain their idea of a proper body image. Their fear of food is reinforced by their observation that when they eat more they gain weight. Quite often, they look at their overweight parents and do not want to turn out that way.

Individuals heading down this path can easily get into a metabolic pattern they cannot get out of, resulting in a clinically definable eating disorder. The essence of this disorder is that starvation metabolism becomes locked into place, and the individual cannot get out of the problem.

MILLIONS OF BORDERLINE EATING DISORDERS

Millions of Americans who think they do not have eating disorders are headed down this path. This is partly because the public-health officials in charge of dietary advice have been preaching low-calorie and low-saturated fat diets to the general public for years.

The public has become brainwashed into thinking that this type of diet is beneficial for heart health as well as the best way to lose weight. Since it is a recommendation made to the general public, many women who try to be healthy and stay slim employ this method of eating in order to watch their weight. This is a quick way to enter starvation metabolism.

Starvation metabolism comes in degrees of severity. Those most likely to encounter this low-leptin problem are:

1) People who significantly reduce calories on a diet.
2) Young women trying to be thin.
3) Middle-aged women trying to stop progressive weight gain or maintain a too-thin body.
4) Athletes with demanding energy output. Female gymnasts are particularly at risk.
5) People with stress-induced lack of appetite, which causes fatigue, muscle wasting, and weight loss.
6) Elderly individuals whose appetite and health are sliding.
7) Individuals suffering from chronic or serious illness.

THE SIGNS OF EATING DISORDERS

There are many shades of gray between optimum health and a clinically definable eating disorder. A clinical disorder is characterized by the pervasiveness of the starvation metabolism. In some cases, this is caused by a disease process such as cancer or the wasting away associated with advanced aging. In other cases, it is by choice, in an effort to lose weight or stay slim.

The hallmark of the starvation metabolism is a low-leptin situation. Since leptin permits a healthy metabolic rate to take place, a low-leptin starvation metabolism forces the body to run slowly, as if in a hibernation mode.

Forcing a hibernation metabolic rate onto oneself can have devastating metabolic effects. For example, young female gymnasts are known to have a low-leptin problem. This has a profound effect on their estrogen levels, normal female development, hormonal function, and bones. By comparison, elite male gymnasts do not have the same type of problems.[356] Having enough leptin is important to women.

In less obvious low-leptin situations, it is still fairly easy to observe whether there is a problem: there is not enough energy for the body to work properly. Body functions that are energy intense, such as the monthly hormonal pattern or the immune system, do not work properly.

Many young women are naturally thin because they have an efficient and highly functional metabolism. How does one tell the difference between such an individual and one heading down the path of an eating disorder?

This is relatively easy. There should be a normal appetite. Onset of menstruation should be at a normal age, and the menstrual cycle should run each month in a timely manner without symptoms. Individuals should not catch colds easily and should get over bugs readily, if they do get ill. Mood should be good, with no tendency to irritability and depression. Posture should be excellent, with no slumping shoulders or evidence of scoliosis. If a young woman is trim and has none of these issues mentioned in this paragraph, then she is generally eating enough.

Problems in this area range from slight malnutrition to full-fledged anorexia. Excessive exercise, whether done to keep ultra trim or as a result of competitive athletics, aggravates any issue in this category. This is because extra activity requires extra fuel. If a person does not eat enough, the body breaks down protein, fat, and bone to sustain energy needs. This can develop into a full-scale stress response and a serious malnutrition syndrome.[357]

Many athletes fall into this problem by not eating enough fat to sustain their energy. They think that saturated fat will cause them to have too much body fat. However, the failure to take in adequate food results in adverse effects on performance, directly related to a lack of leptin.[358]

Underweight individuals tend to be in low-leptin metabolic patterns, especially if they have any type of ongoing health issue. However, a person who is on a low-fat diet, in an effort to maintain a given weight or in an effort to lose weight, may also enter into a low-leptin metabolic condition.

Many middle-aged women gain weight and then employ starvation-metabolism diet strategies in an effort to prevent gaining any more weight. This induces problems with fatigue, menstruation, hormones, and the immune system. These problems are obvious. Women who follow such diets normally blame their problems on the stress of raising children, working, and so on. These stress factors do indeed raise cortisol, which helps send them down the wrong health path. However, the diet strategy itself makes their health worse and locks in excess cortisol.

Such women are not anorexic by clinical definition; they are anorexic-like in their metabolism because they live in a starvation metabolism. They can also be in this metabolic pattern if they are overweight or their general trend is to continue to gain weight. This can seriously speed wear and tear and accelerate aging, the exact opposite of what they were hoping to accomplish with their low-calorie diet.

We also have the middle-aged women who try to maintain a super-thin appearance because they think it looks good. These individuals frequently run on stimulants such as diet soda, excess caffeine, and/or cigarettes. While these individuals may be thin, they are often in an unhealthy wasting pattern. Such individuals invariably have a variety of health complaints that are difficult to resolve because they do not have a normal metabolic energy capable of fixing their health problems. By the time they are in their fifties, they are likely to have serious bone-loss issues.

It is easy to observe by looking at the skin that there is accelerated catabolic wasting (meaning too much tissue breakdown) in such individuals. This is because the normal fat layer under the skin has been weakened or has broken down. This causes the skin to wrinkle much faster than normal. Many such individuals have already been to the plastic surgeon for face-lifts to help correct their sagging skin structure. However, the neck and the hands are two areas that can easily reflect this problem.

This catabolic breakdown of fat also causes cellulite. This is a main reason why a thin person or a person who is five to ten pounds overweight has cellulite.

If a woman does not want to wrinkle or develop cellulite any faster than she needs to, it is best to maintain a functional level of leptin that is proper for correct metabolic rate. This will not cause a breakdown in the fat layer under the skin at an accelerated rate. While a person too low in leptin may look thin, it is not a healthy look.

There are a number of unmistakable symptoms of the "middle-age" eating disorder. Individual try, and possibly succeed, in using incredible willpower not to eat; especially not to eat foods that they have been conditioned to think of as bad. If they are not governed by some fear of food or rule about fats in food, they will gladly indulge.

This is accompanied by abnormal fatigue and a feeling of wear and tear. Of course, if such individuals have a stressful life, then all factors of fatigue and wear and tear are made worse.

Such individuals do not have the energy to exercise; or, when they force themselves to exercise, they do not feel good. They may get through the exercise feeling all right, but their response to exercise is not as good as it was before they entered the wear-and-tear condition.

Sex hormones, whether in men or women with this type of eating disorder, are not in normal balance and function; and symptoms of one type or another arise – especially lack of sex drive. Women with this problem are prone to infertility and miscarriages. In this metabolic condition, a person is more prone to get sick, be constipated, or have sluggish bowels.

To a greater or lesser degree, every factor mentioned in these paragraphs is present in any individual heading down the path of starvation-metabolism eating disorders. Remember, there are a thousand shades of gray. However, the metabolic trend and picture are clear; there is no hiding these symptoms.[359]

LEPTIN REGULATES HEALTHY METABOLIC RATE

People with symptoms of the anorexic-like starvation metabolism have one thing in common – leptin levels that are too low. Adequate leptin tells the brain there is adequate fuel on hand; thus, metabolic activity in the body can function at an active metabolic rate. This is healthy, a condition in which natural balance can occur.

Too little leptin tells the body it is starving; therefore, the brain turns down metabolic rate and function. The longer and more sustained the anorexic eating metabolism becomes, the greater the chance for chronically induced low-leptin levels. When a person gets stuck in low leptin over a period of time, it locks in a serious eating disorder with serious health consequences.[360]

Many problems of not enough leptin are similar to those of too much leptin. This is because leptin resistance means the leptin message does not get through to the brain. In leptin resistance, there is low leptin in the brain, high leptin in the circulation, and leptin resistance in the pancreas causing metabolic syndrome X. Excess cortisol combines with high circulating leptin to make a person fat in the stomach. This results in a condition of fatigue and increased risk of disease.

On the flip side of this picture, the clinical anorexic has low levels of leptin in the brain and low levels of leptin in the circulation. There is excess cortisol, a catabolic hormone, combined with low leptin. This combination forces body wasting to occur. There is also fatigue and increased risk of disease.

In between these two is the leptin-resistant individual who keeps trying to employ the low-calorie diet to lose ten pounds and who cannot do it. The dieting itself makes the person have anorexic-like wear and tear, yet the five to ten pounds on the tummy will not budge.

The leptin-resistant state and the low-leptin anorexic state share these common features: low leptin in the brain, high cortisol in circulation, fatigue, increased risk of disease, and accelerated rate of aging.

Many individuals flip-flop between leptin resistance and low-leptin issues, the essence of yo-yo dieting. Many dieters hit a starvation-metabolism brick wall long before they get to their goal weight. The longer they stay in this dangerous condition, the more body muscle and bone they lose – not fat.

Thus, we have the starvation dieters who have the metabolic profile and faulty immune response of anorexics. This includes low-leptin induced depression,[361,362] muscle weakness that has been diagnosed as fibromyalgia, and loss of bone density, [363,364] yet they may be fifty to one hundred pounds overweight!

Additionally, animals that lack leptin demonstrate that the immune cells in their livers become overactive, generating inflammation that damages other healthy liver cells and leads to liver disease.[365]

Women who get stuck in the anorexic metabolic pattern begin to lose function of their hormonal cycle. This may show up as scanty or skipped cycles.[366] If the low-leptin problem is left unchecked, it can develop into infertility or a higher risk for miscarriage if there is a pregnancy.[367] This is a primary health issue for the person in low-leptin anorexic metabolism, and it is present as the hallmark of this situation, regardless of the person's body weight. This is a serious health issue. These problems also occur in the leptin-resistant individual.

WHAT IS CACHEXIA?

Cachexia is a term given by the medical community to a disease process, such as cancer, that forces the body into an anorexic metabolism. Common anorexia is frequently encountered due to high stress, fears regarding food, or misconceptions about how to lose weight. Cachexia is the same physical problem as anorexia; it is simply caused by a different source, a disease that makes the body waste away.

Overcoming the cachexia problem is crucial to surviving cancer. High leptin sets the stage for cancer risk. Initially, high leptin may fan the flames of cancer and make it grow and spread. However, as the cancer takes root, courtesy of chronically elevated NF-kappaB, it attacks body structure and destroys protein structures, as well as white adipose tissue. As the white adipose tissue is destroyed by cancer, the leptin levels will drop quite low.

This problem of cachexia is responsible for thirty percent of the deaths in cancer situations.[368] It is fascinating to note that men with advanced prostate cancer seldom have cachexia. This is because they are treated with testosterone-blocking drugs, which have the net effect of increasing their leptin.[369] This same issue of wasting away and low-leptin has also been documented in patients with chronic obstructive pulmonary disease.[370] The main point here is that too little leptin during cancer or other chronic illness causes the body to accelerate the wasting-away problem, leading to life-threatening malnutrition.

IMMUNITY ISSUES, A SIGN OF MALNUTRITION

There is no simple way to think about leptin. Leptin is essential for survival. Too much leptin or too little leptin causes major health problems. Individuals must obtain a good understanding of natural balance and how to eat in relation to the amount of energy they expend. Doing so will help maintain the right amount of leptin and optimum body weight, and help avoid major health issues. Low-fat diets are just as dangerous as high-fat diets. The healthy balance is somewhere in the middle.

Immune function is an important marker that helps define the right amount of food for an individual. People who are overweight frequently have impaired immune function.[371] Such problems may involve leptin resistance or may be due to a variety of other issues. Some overweight people have no problem with immune function.

The great majority of individuals with the anorexic-like starvation metabolism have a problem with immune function. A proper amount of leptin is essential to mount an efficient immune response. If the efficient immune response is not there, then the person is more prone to catching bugs and taking longer to recover. Such a person is also prone to a flare-up of dormant viral infections, such as mouth sores.

Leptin is an essential part of a proper response to inflammation and infection, key parts of the body's natural defense system.[372] Recent research proves that low leptin handicaps the immune response.[373,374,375] This issue is not open to interpretation. If a person is on the thin side, or is attempting to restrict calories too much and is prone to catch bugs, struggles to get over a bug, or gets a breakout of mouth sores, leptin levels are too low and not enough food is being consumed.

Low leptin causes the thymus gland to shrink resulting in serious immune depression.[376] There is always the release of pro-inflammatory signals associated with inflammation and infection. Unlike most of America, there are populations around the world who still struggle with a lack of food that induces serious malnutrition and consequent poor immune function.

AUTOIMMUNE DISEASE

Americans are prone to overeating. As we have pointed out, this leads to excess production of TNFa and IL-6 from the resulting extra pounds of fat. In terms of immune status, the resting metabolic situation is already inappropriately hyper. Researchers have identified that excess leptin due to excess food consumption is a key factor behind the increase in autoimmune problems in affluent countries.[377]

This information sheds light on why some children may experience a debilitating response to immunizations. A recent animal study shows that autoimmune nerve inflammation occurs as a result of immunizations given in the presence of excess leptin.[378] Baby girls have higher leptin than baby boys, placing them at higher risk. Any child who is overfed, overweight, or born to leptin-resistant parents is at a greater risk for such immunologic complications from immunizations.

This information also applies to leptin-resistant adults who are given flu shots. Once again, we find that public-health officials do not keep up with the current science or act on it in a proactive manner. Their focus seems to be on immunizing everyone, not on proving that immunizations are safe or figuring out who might be at risk for serious nerve damage from immunizations.

We learned in chapter 8 that when there is low leptin in the brain, due either to generally low leptin or to leptin resistance, the brain is much more likely to experience nerve damage. In leptin resistance, the low leptin in the brain is combined with high leptin in the circulation. This overheats the immune system, causing a high level of risk for autoimmune disease. This creates a metabolic risk profile of an overly hyped-up immune system in the body, and a brain more susceptible to damage. The fact that so many people are leptin resistant calls into question the safety of any broad-based immunization campaign.

SOLUTIONS FOR EATING DISORDERS

If we are to solve eating disorders, we must understand that eating correctly does not promote excess weight gain. Understanding leptin explains why this is the case.

It is vital to get the individual with an eating disorder to consume more food. With eating, the problem is likely to be improved. Getting young women with anorexia to eat restores their leptin levels and changes their bone metabolism, so that they gain bone mass instead of losing it.[379]

In milder cases of eating disorders, whether in young women or adult dieters, it is simply a matter of explaining to them why diet-induced starvation metabolism does not work. This applies to underweight, normal weight, and overweight individuals.

In more serious situations of metabolic wasting, there are physical reasons why people cannot eat. They are locked in a metabolic pattern where they have no appetite. They are nauseous, or when they eat they become nauseous. Even if they make themselves eat, they may not gain weight or energy.

This state of affairs is usually induced by major stress that has resulted in unhealthy weight loss, purposely not eating and then getting stuck in the problem, or fighting cancer or some other chronic wasting disease.

When such individuals agree that they should eat, the next issue is to get them to have an appetite so that they can eat and benefit from the food. This is not a psychological issue; it is a physical issue.

In our previous chapter, we pointed out how essential fatty acids, such as fish oil, borage oil, and flax oil, reduce excess leptin production by reducing the pro-inflammatory signals such as TNFa and IL-6. This causes a reduction in inflammatory immune signals coming from fat cells that lock in leptin-resistant overeating.

It is interesting to see that the same solution can work for individuals with low leptin, thus helping to solve eating disorders! In low-leptin states, the body is in a stressful wasting condition. There is excess cortisol fueling the wasting away of the body. This state of physical breakdown involves the excess production of TNFa and IL-6. However, this time, these highly inflammatory immune signals do not come from the excess fat, they come from the cortisol and/or disease-fueled wasting process. They cause the loss of appetite.

A study was recently conducted with pancreatic cancer patients who were in a state of cachexia. Such problems are resistant to basic dietary therapy. The individuals are told to eat more food; however, in most cases, they do not have any appetite. Even if they do eat more, they do not gain weight. In this study, patients were given two grams of fish oil per day. Within three weeks, they had stopped wasting away and started gaining weight![380]

The researchers documented that the fish oils lowered inflammatory markers, such as IL-6, that fueled the catabolic process. This enabled the body to get out of high cortisol and highly inflammatory immune situations, thereby returning the body to a better state of natural balance. Once this is accomplished, the individual can eat food and gain weight.

Understanding this information, we began testing this principle on a variety of underweight individuals. Some had no appetite; others had stress-induced weight loss. It generally required a dose of six grams of essential fatty acids to solve the problem. On this dose, appetite returned, body wasting stopped, and healthy weight gain occurred.

Another important nutrient in the recovery of the anorexic metabolic problem is zinc. A lack of zinc predisposes a person to anorexia in the first place.[381] A recent review of literature regarding zinc showed its extreme importance in helping people recover from anorexia.[382] It is proven that zinc supplementation is essential for the treatment of anorexia.[383]

Zinc is essential for hormone function of all types and also for hormone transport in the blood. It helps individuals that are stuck in an anorexic metabolic pattern. In can be helpful for moderate cases of anorexic metabolism, in terms of helping the body to run normally when more food is eaten. We recommend 25 to 75 milligrams of zinc per day to assist in restoring natural balance in any person prone to the metabolic problems of anorexic-like metabolism.

The other major issue for people recovering from an eating disorder is that they fear they will gain too much weight once they start eating again. There is an element of truth in this concern, as leptin begins to rise as more food is eaten. This is normal and essential in order to replenish the malnourished condition.

If individuals eat according to the *Five Rules* and moderately exercises as they regain weight, the leptin signal tends to become accurate; weight gain stops when they are properly nourished, and excess weight is not gained.

These are relatively simple solutions to what can otherwise be a very devastating issue.

In the case of people who are ten pounds overweight and losing energy on a low-calorie diet, they will tend to lose weight and cellulite by eating more and following the *Five Rules*. This is because they improve the efficiency of their body to use calories as well as prevent the catabolic wasting of anorexic-like starvation metabolism.

SUMMARY

Not having enough leptin can pose just as many health problems as having too much leptin. Bouncing around between high-leptin and low-leptin levels, as in yo-yo dieting, is incredibly stressful to the body.

In order to avoid problems of leptin excess and leptin insufficiency, a person needs to adopt consistent eating and exercise patterns over the course of their lifetime; helping them to live in a state of leptin efficiency. This is a true commitment to healthy living, an important skill of the *Health Asset Manager*.

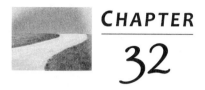

CHAPTER

32

Exercise to Solve Leptin Problems

IT IS WELL KNOWN that exercise is an important part of any weight-loss program. This fact will not change. A lifestyle that places regular exercise as a priority is imperative. Hormones in the body, especially leptin, do not work efficiently over time if there is no exercise.

Exercise conditions the fuel-regulation systems in the body to work more efficiently. The better these fuel systems function, the less likely there are to be problems with weight.

EXERCISE, INSULIN RESISTANCE, AND LEPTIN

Exercise improves insulin resistance.[384] Exercise significantly enhances the ability of insulin to transport glucose into muscles so that the calories can be used for energy.[385] When muscles are depleted of fuel there is a demand to replenish the diminished supply.

The short-term positive effects of exercise on fuel utilization can last up to forty-eight hours. Minimally, a person needs to exercise three to four times a week. This allows for more optimal utilization of the foods that are consumed.

During the first fifteen to twenty minutes of exercise, stored sugar in the muscles, called glycogen, is the primary fuel that is used. Even this small amount of exercise helps with insulin resistance, as the depletion of glycogen causes muscles to demand more fuel. It has been conclusively proven that exercise helps lower insulin resistance.[386]

As exercise progresses beyond twenty minutes, glucose and free-fatty acids from the blood become the primary fuel. This helps clear stagnant calories out of circulating blood. During this time, the adrenal glands begin secreting higher levels of hormones, working with the liver to sustain energy for the exercise.

Individuals who are fatigued and have adrenal wear and tear cannot exercise longer than fifteen to twenty minutes without experiencing unpleasant symptoms. It is important to improve the adrenal reserves and improve liver fitness so that exercise can last at least thirty to forty minutes and produce a pleasant relaxed feeling. This is an important step in strengthening the fuel-regulation system. A positive response to exercise lasting thirty to forty minutes has the beneficial effect of lowering insulin resistance and fatty buildup in the blood.[387]

After forty minutes of exercise, fuel comes from a combination of stored liver glycogen and the breakdown of fatty acids from stored fat. As long as the exercise is refreshing and not stressful to the cardiovascular system or physically exhausting, the longer the exercise time the more stored fat is broken down and burned.

When a person has insulin resistance, the liver does not efficiently store glucose as glycogen. This makes it difficult to exercise for longer than forty minutes. This is because to the fact that fatty acids are most cleanly burned for fuel when some carbohydrates are present. If the liver cannot secrete glucose from its store of glycogen as it tries to burn fatty acids, excess numbers of ketones will form. Ketones are acid byproducts of incompletely burned fats. This inefficiency in burning fatty acids causes hypoglycemia, a lack of energy, irritability, fatigue, and other issues.

People recovering from wear and tear need to find a balance in their exercise, seeking a refreshed response as a priority. Many times this means going at a slower pace than they formerly would, until overall health and energy reserves are built back up.

Exercise is necessary to repair fuel-regulation problems. As adrenal reserves and liver function improve, exercise will be possible for longer periods of time. A refreshing response to longer periods of exercise is important for solving insulin resistance, leptin resistance, and fuel-regulation issues. It may take some time for an individual to build up to this level of fitness; however, it is essential in order to achieve ideal body weight and to keep off the weight, once it is lost.

Fortunately, as we have mentioned, even fifteen minutes of exercise begins to improve insulin resistance. As it gradually improves over time and the adrenals and liver get in better shape, then longer periods of refreshing exercise become possible.

In addition to the immediate benefits of aerobic exercise, it also lowers leptin when done consistently.[388] A consistent exercise program can improve leptin resistance and insulin resistance over time.[389] This fixes the long-term trend and rhythm, a true solution to insulin and leptin problems.

The problems of insulin resistance and leptin resistance are significantly improved when a person can exercise at a moderate pace for at least one hour, three times a week, and have a refreshing response to that exercise.

Such exercise is important for those with a problematic weight history. Even if an individual begins with only five minutes of exercise, it is essential to get started and stay with it.

THE RELAXATION RESERVES

In every person's nervous system there is a natural balance between activation and relaxation. Activation is guided by the sympathetic nervous system. It leads to more assertive behavior and guides the basic stress response (fight or flight). Relaxation is controlled by the parasympathetic nervous system. It leads to a more easygoing and adaptive behavior. It acts as a savings account, or "relaxation reserve," to help balance and tolerate the pressures of life without generating too much friction or internal wear and tear.

Leptin resistance disturbs natural balance in the nerves. This leads to excess sympathetic nerve activity with a loss of parasympathetic nerve tone. Leptin resistance, as well as an unbalanced lifestyle, uses up relaxation reserves. This causes the nerves to "run hot."

This frayed feeling in the nervous system generally accompanies leptin resistance. Eventually, this feeling turns into nerve pain that affects the muscles, a problem referred to as fibromyalgia.

As relaxation reserves run low, too much adrenaline is constantly active in the sympathetic nerves. Normally, white adipose tissue is metabolically stimulated by adrenaline. In this situation of excess adrenaline, the white-adipose-tissue fat cells become deaf to the adrenaline signal, causing weight gain around the midsection. However, the heart and kidneys are irritated by this excess adrenaline.

Once this problem locks in, even on a generally nonstressed day, a person with leptin resistance produces excess adrenaline at night. This is because adrenaline rises excessively with leptin resistance, peaking as bedtime approaches. This extra adrenaline is superactivated by eating at night or by a stressful event at night. It can also be active at night simply due to the overall stress of the day.

It is quite common for people with leptin resistance to be prone to a racing, erratic, or unstable heart rate at night, especially when they lie down to go to bed. This may cause an excessive surge in blood pressure in the evening, disrupting sleep.

Most people understand how stress affects them on an emotional or relationship basis, because they are consciously aware of their feelings. If they have had a stressful day, the heart symptoms mentioned above may be worse, especially at night. However, with leptin resistance, a person is prone to troubling heart rhythms, regardless of how stressful the day may have been. This is due to the excess irritating adrenaline that is in the circulation.

Rhythm disturbances in the heart can lead to ventricular fibrillation, the leading cause of unexpected cardiac death in industrialized nations. Many medications to control heart rhythms have simply failed to be of any value, causing increased cardiac mortality.[390]

Drugging the sympathetic nervous system into less aggressive function does little to restore sympathetic and parasympathetic natural balance. This should come as no surprise, since drugs frequently do little to restore normal function. The risk for a cardiac event is proportionate to excess adrenaline, which in turn is relative to a loss of parasympathetic tone or balance.[391]

EXERCISE TO THE RESCUE

Aerobic exercise is the single best option for anyone who would like to reduce the risk of dying from sudden cardiac death due to heart-rate instability.[392]

Consistent aerobic exercise is the number-one physical act a person can perform to correct leptin resistance. There is no shortcut. The biggest factor is consistency, rather than intensity. How fit one is must be taken into account in terms of how much exercise is done. One must get a relaxed response to the exercise, not exhaustion. It is important to do an amount of aerobic exercise that will enhance the tone of the parasympathetic nervous system.

Even mild exercise, along with watching the diet, improves parasympathetic tone and to reduce the effects of excess adrenaline.[393] In a study with mildly obese women who did not have high blood pressure, all the women improved their heart-rate stability with exercise. At the same time, they lost weight, lowered cholesterol, lowered triglycerides, and improved insulin-resistance issues. They improved the factors relating to leptin resistance, simply with consistent, moderate exercise and mild calorie restriction. The control group who did not exercise showed no improvement.

The reserves of parasympathetic nerve function act like oil in the engine of a car, keeping it from overheating. This parasympathetic tone is the key aspect of natural balance in the nervous system, enabling the body to bounce back from stress and offset the potential wear of adrenaline output.[394] Without this natural balance, a person gets too wound up and too stressed. The degree to which an individual has this problem is related to the risk of dying from a heart attack.[395]

There is simply no question that exercise opens the door to recovery from leptin resistance by restoring parasympathetic tone to normal.[396] No drug can do this. For individuals who are not in good shape, the encouraging part is that it is just a matter of starting and being consistent for there to be improvement.

Even mild or low-grade aerobics, such as walking, enhances para-sympathetic tone in overweight individuals.[397] Walking ten thousand steps a day in the course of your activities can do this; plus it can reduce high blood pressure in hypertensive patients.[398] Study after study shows that mild aerobic exercise improves parasympathetic tone, thereby reducing excess adrenaline.[399,400,401]

GETTING ON TRACK

The better physically fit a person is, the easier it is to get back on track and recover from leptin resistance. People who are fit enough to go out for a thirty-minute jog can boost the parasympathetic tone in a hurry. This can stop the binge eating and cravings of leptin resistance in one day. However, the program needs to be consistent, such as running at least three times a week, in order to maintain tone and build up the reserves in the nervous system.

People who are not in this type of condition should not be discouraged. It just takes a bit longer to work your way back to a level of acceptable fitness – it can be done! As there is improvement, an individual can begin to do more, if it is within physical capabilities. The goal is to obtain a relaxed and refreshing response to exercise, in order to replenish the parasympathetic tone in the nervous system. Doing too much too soon, or exercising too vigorously, will not be of any benefit.

A TRICK TO STAYING ON TRACK

It is quite common for the leptin-resistant urge to eat to attack at night. It may come about even when one is fairly consistent and more or less on a good track. That overwhelming desire to eat starts. At first, it is ignored. Then it starts to take over. What can be done?

If you have enough willpower to overcome this urge to eat at night, congratulations. If not, the best thing to do is to get blood to flow to the head. Overweight individuals with food cravings have an exaggerated lack of blood in their conscious brain and an excess amount of blood overheating their subconscious brain fueling the drive to eat.

Instead of eating, vigorously exercise for a few minutes. Do some jumping jacks or push-ups, or do weight-bearing exercises. Walk up and down the stairs ten times while taking deep breaths. Do something to stimulate circulation. Even go for a walk. If you get blood to flow to your head you will mechanically change the balance of power so that willpower is back in control; the craving will stop. Do not get in a wrestling match with the subconscious mind; it will most likely win.

Intense physical exercise can depress leptin on a short-term basis because it creates an increased demand for fuel. This reaction is felt over a period of hours, meaning that a good workout in the afternoon or evening can help prevent the nighttime desire to overeat. This lowering of leptin in response to resistance strength-training exercise has been demonstrated in athletes,[402] as well as in diabetics.[403] Short-duration intense exercise is a fantastic tool to bring leptin cravings under control.

BUILDING MUSCLE

As a person gains body fat, the internal appearance of muscle becomes more like a slice of bacon than a piece of lean beef. This accumulation of fat inside the muscle is counterproductive to healthy function of insulin and leptin. As we mentioned above, there is a short-term improvement in leptin status from intense exercise. This response is different than a resistance-training program, which converts muscle that looks like bacon back to a leaner and stronger appearance.

Recent scientific evidence shows that resistance training lowers body fat and leptin. This reduction of body fat and leptin enables insulin to function correctly, so that there is no insulin resistance in the muscles.[404]

A combination of aerobic exercise and resistance training in premenopausal women lowered their leptin and TNFa, in turn leading to a loss of all types of body fat.[405] These studies are important because they show that building strength over time helps restore leptin to normal levels, resulting in resolution of insulin-resistance problems.

Strength training also creates a demand for fatty acids to be used by the muscles. This is because muscle tissue breaks down as a result of the exercise. This causes a higher demand for protein to repair the muscle, and for fat to fuel energy supplies in the muscle.

When a person goes five to six hours without eating, the body begins breaking down triglycerides to use for fuel. Triglycerides are a combination of one glycerol, or sugar, and three fatty acids. As these fatty acids are liberated into the circulation, they must go somewhere useful. The muscles are the primary body tissue that uses fatty acids for fuel. The muscle breakdown that occurs during strength training may last forty-eight hours or longer, meaning that strength exercise three times a week keeps up a constant demand for fatty acids to flow to the muscles.

If there is no muscle need for the fatty acids, the next time a person eats and insulin goes up, the fatty acids are packaged back up into tri-glycerides and sent back to storage. Thus, a person who eats properly but does not exercise may not get anywhere in terms of weight loss.

BODY HEAT AND EXERCISE

When cells throughout the body breathe correctly, energy is produced in an efficient manner. As glucose or fat are burned for fuel, energy is made (ATP) and heat is produced. Normal metabolism produces sixty-five percent energy and thirty-five percent heat. A person with the starvation-metabolism problem conserves energy and does not produce adequate heat.

Body temperature is as important as light to help the body set bio-logical rhythms. Scientists have demonstrated that proper body tempera-ture is needed to activate certain parts of the brain which cause alertness during the day; and as bedtime approaches, heat signals other parts of the brain that promote sleep.[406] A shift in heat from the internal part of the body to the periphery signals the start of the sleep process.[407]

Further, even middle-aged adults have already started moving this temperature rhythm earlier in time, indicating the onset of loss of temperature rhythm.[408] Body heat is now recognized as an important factor in proper sleep patterns and, therefore, in all other biological patterns.

This places new importance on exercise. Aerobic exercise increases body temperature; strength-training exercise increases muscle mass, which in turn increases body temperature, even when your body is at rest. Proper production of heat can wake up the head, another benefit for individuals who make the wise choice to exercise regularly.

SUMMARY

There are six critically important reasons to exercise:

1) To improve the natural rhythm and pattern of fuel utilization in the body.
2) To increase the parasympathetic tone of the nervous system, building up the relaxed reserves.
3) To keep leptin food cravings and out-of-control eating behavior in check.
4) To enhance strength in order to more permanently stabilize leptin and insulin function.
5) To improve the muscle use of fatty acids, so that weight loss is easier or optimum weight is more readily maintained.
6) To ensure adequate body heat, an important foundation for body rhythms and patterns.

The most important principles guiding exercise are consistency and achieving a refreshed feeling from the activity. As fitness improves, the duration and intensity of exercise can be increased, as long as consistency and the refreshed feeling are not sacrificed. As a person gains strength over time and can perform aerobics for longer periods, there is a consistent enhancement in leptin function. Exercising is a powerful tool for solving leptin issues.

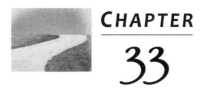

CHAPTER

33

Proper Sleep – Key for Repair

QUALITY OF SLEEP is another issue that must be well managed in order to solve problems with leptin. For there to be good quality of sleep, it is vital to maintain a steady supply of blood sugar during sleep. This enables one to dip into the reserves of fat while sleeping, an essential requirement for healthy weight loss. Sleep is prime fat-burning time, especially when one has not eaten after dinner.

Sleep enables the body to clean house and perform needed repairs. It is essential for recovery from wear and tear. The better the job one does of managing energy resources during the day, the better the quality of sleep at night. This is partly because there is less wear and tear to repair and partly because the body is in overall better rhythm.

The fastest way to disrupt sleep is to eat after dinner, eat too large a dinner, or eat dinner too late. This forces the body to digest food when it should be performing other functions such as fat burning and body repair. Also, as leptin resistance sets in, it causes higher amounts of adrenaline during sleep hours. This causes insomnia, light sleep, restless sleep, sleep apnea, and a general feeling of unrest.

There is no making up for a lack of sleep. A lack of sleep causes energy systems in the body to give out too easily. Even a person with little stress who does not sleep enough finds it almost impossible to go five to six hours without eating. A person who is sleep deprived does not have tolerance for stress, leading to exaggerated hyperglycemic and eventual hypoglycemic responses to stress. Sleep-deprived individuals are irritable.

For people with more demands in their life, it is imperative to keep exercise, eating, and sleep rhythms in a good pattern. A failure to do so results in a steady decline in the quality of sleep and daytime energy. Eventually this can lead to the problem called fibromyalgia, wherein sleep can be so poor that hardly any energy is possible the next day.

SLEEP AND FAT BURNING

Sleep is the most important time for burning fat. If the *Five Rules* are followed, eleven to twelve hours should elapse between finishing the last meal of the day and eating breakfast. As the night progresses, more calories from fat are burned.

Ideally, one should be slightly hungry and tired as approaching sleep. Avoid emotional stress before bed; this is the worst time to rev up the system with excess adrenaline. There should be an absence of hyperglycemic symptoms or hypoglycemic symptoms; otherwise, sleep will not be refreshing.

It requires a level of fitness, in terms of fuel regulation, to successfully go eleven to twelve hours without eating. The liver, pancreas, adrenal glands, and muscles must all be in relatively good working order to get a good night's sleep, one which results in proper fat burning. If at first you cannot do this, follow the information in this book to improve overall fitness and work toward the ideal we describe in this chapter.

BLOOD SUGAR LEVELS AND SLEEP

Hyperglycemic symptoms prior to bed generally feel like the body or mind is working too fast. These symptoms occur even though the person is tired or even exhausted. One can experience an uncomfortable racing feeling that prevents sleep. The heart can feel jittery, skipping a beat or pounding as the person lies down to go to sleep. It is not a normal feeling of energy; it is an uncomfortable feeling of energy. This feeling can come about simply from a lack of fitness because a person is not eating properly and not getting enough relaxing exercise. This racing feeling is easily magnified by stress.

Hyperglycemic-prone individuals often process the details of their life stressors before they go to bed. Their mind can be busy trying to figure everything out and have a plan ready for the next day. In essence, they generate a stress response, releasing adrenaline and cortisol before bed. This fuels the hyperglycemic reaction. Having an argument before bed automatically puts a person in a hyperglycemic mode.

Hyperglycemic states before bed are driven by emotional stress, physical wear and tear, and/or leptin resistance. Because stress hormones are frequently involved, they interfere with falling to sleep, staying asleep, and sleeping deeply. They make an individual prone to going to the bathroom frequently during the night. Hyperglycemic issues cause a person to have problems with fuel regulation the next day, thereby setting up a vicious circle.

Hyperglycemic individuals tend to burn fat inefficiently while they are sleeping. This causes an excess amount of ketones to form at night, which may cause nightmares. Such individuals in the middle of the night or in the morning may wake up with nausea, heartburn, or a queasy feeling.

When people wake up nauseated or with heartburn, they typically find that if they eat a few crackers they can go back to sleep. This is because the rise in insulin from the carbohydrates turns off the hyperglycemic problem and stops the ketones from forming, which are the cause of the digestive distress. While this works as a temporary solution, it does not help weight loss.

Some hyperglycemic individuals may become hypoglycemic during the night. This is because:

1) The liver's reserve of glycogen is not adequate; thus, the person does not have a stable supply of blood sugar, which is important for the proper burning of fatty acids.

2) There is excessively high insulin from insulin resistance and leptin resistance, which suppresses the proper release of glucagon; thus, the liver does not get in gear to make energy before blood sugar drops.

3) The high cortisol level at bed blunts leptin function and disrupts sleep. By the time leptin gets going, it blunts cortisol in the morning. The chaotic rhythms cause energy fluctuations that are abnormal, including hypoglycemia.

This may lead to waking up with extreme hunger, nightmares, excess sweating, and/or headaches during sleep or upon waking up in the morning.

Most individuals who go to sleep hyperglycemic wake up hypoglycemic. This causes them to feel heavy in the head, and their mood is irritable when blood sugar is low. What we have, then, is the morning grouch.

When individuals wake up hyperglycemic, meaning blood sugar numbers are high, then either:

A) the pancreas fails to sense the rise in morning cortisol, or

B) leptin resistance has blunted the morning rise in cortisol, or

C) the liver is stuck in an excess sugar-production mode

Individuals who are hyperglycemic before bed generally find that if they have a small carbohydrate snack before bed, their uncomfortable racing feeling will calm down and they will be able to go to sleep. This is better than not getting a good night's sleep, but it does not promote weight loss and does not address the source of their problem.

Such individuals should avoid a high-protein/low-carbohydrate dinner, since the extra metabolic drive of such a dinner can push them into a hyperglycemic pattern as protein stimulates glucagon release. Individuals prone to hyperglycemia at bed tend to do best on a dinner that is higher in carbohydrate and somewhat lower in protein. Such individuals usually do better on higher protein earlier in the day.

A less common issue is the person who is hypoglycemic before bed. Such individuals feel dull in the head; they cannot remember things easily, and their brain feels foggy and disconnected. These symptoms occur because blood sugar is not adequate to keep the brain in a normal range of function. It is a different feeling than normal tiredness. It is more common for individuals to wake up hypoglycemic in the middle of the night or in the morning than to start out that way before bed.

This type of individual ends up eating too much before bed in an effort to solve the hypoglycemic feeling. This also interferes with optimum fat burning. In many cases, this problem can be resolved by eating a high-protein dinner with moderate carbohydrates. This dinner recommendation is the opposite of that for the person who is prone to hyperglycemia at bed.

Taking any kind of medication to help sleep is undesirable over the long run, as these drugs deaden nerves and pose problems to the liver. Correcting problems of leptin resistance, insulin resistance, hyperglycemia, and hypoglycemia solve most sleep problems. Many sleep medications are functionally addictive, meaning that once they are started, sleep problems become magnified when they are discontinued.

Hyperglycemic and hypoglycemic problems at bedtime, during sleep, or upon waking are key signs that overall fuel regulation is out of balance. Because nighttime is generally the longest period to go without food, it serves as an excellent metabolic test of the health of this system, especially overall liver fitness. It is essential to get it in good working order to properly lose weight. A good sign that this issue is improving is the ability to pop out of bed in the morning and get going with a good energy level, without the need for caffeine or some other stimulant.

When a person is out of balance or if there has been an unusually stressful day or period of days, it is common for there to be difficulty with fuel regulation and sleep quality. Steps need to be taken to get this issue on track as quickly as possible, as well as to improve the overall situation so that sleep is better. Disrupted sleep, whether due to fuel-regulation issues, stress, or inadequate time for sleep, is a fast track to poor health. Over the years, there is no greater form of wear and tear than a lack of refreshing sleep.

MELATONIN, SLEEP, LEPTIN, AND THE FAT STOMACH

When there is good sleep, meaning that energy levels are stable through the night, other hormones have the potential to work properly because the body is in natural balance. When fuel balance does not work well, it shuts off the proper function of these hormones and causes a poor quality of sleep.

Melatonin is an important hormone that is released during sleep. It must peak at the proper time in order to ensure adequate deep sleep. Melatonin levels decline with age. Melatonin released correctly during the night is essential for proper leptin rhythm during the day.

Proper melatonin release helps establish proper leptin rhythm. When melatonin is released incorrectly, leptin is thrown out of rhythm.[409] It has been shown that supplementing melatonin can restore normal leptin rhythm.[410]

An animal study showed that melatonin prevents the accumulation of stomach fat and lowers leptin, independent of the diet.[411] Melatonin improves diabetes in animal studies by eliminating insulin resistance.[412]

It is interesting to note that scientists are demonstrating that low leptin levels in the brain, whether due to leptin resistance or the starvation metabolic pattern, are the actual cause of most hypothyroid problems. We will discuss this in detail in chapter 39.

Too little leptin, the hallmark of the anorexic-like starvation metabolic pattern, causes a drop in serotonin function which leads to depression and other more serious mental disorders.[413,414] We know that individuals with anorexia have low serotonin, making them more prone to depression. The low-leptin, hypothyroid, and low-serotonin picture prevents the proper formation of melatonin, which is normally made from serotonin.[415] Therefore, one of the fastest ways for an individual to become depressed and to have disrupted sleep is to eat too little fat for there to be normal leptin in circulation.

In addition to the importance of melatonin in facilitating proper biological rhythms, this hormone exerts a positive influence on the source of inflammation. It directly lowers TNFa by turning down excess NF-kappaB. This improves the inflammation associated with irritable bowel,[416] as well as helping to lower high blood pressure.[417]

We frequently use one-half milligram melatonin capsules, in dose ranges of one to six per night, to help individuals sleep better. With the proper dose, an individual notices better sleep. A proper dose of melatonin at night can improve leptin function during the day, helping to normalize leptin rhythm and reduce food cravings. This is another tool to help reduce abdominal obesity.

SUMMARY

Too many Americans are sleep deprived. It is difficult to compensate for a lack of sleep. A lack of sleep accelerates wear and tear and pushes the body out of natural balance and rhythm.

In addition to not enough sleep, many individuals have trouble getting quality sleep. It is not possible to separate daytime energy regulation, blood sugar, eating patterns, eating habits, exercise, and stress from sleep issues. Central to sleep problems are fluctuating blood sugar levels, both hyperglycemia and hypoglycemia. At the root of such blood sugar related sleep problems is leptin resistance, insulin resistance, and adrenaline resistance.

For many individuals, a low dose of melatonin can promote more restful sleep and can help restore more normal leptin rhythms.

Quality of sleep is a key metabolic sign that fuel regulation is working well. It is prime fat-burning time. Short-changing sleep time or going to bed stressed not only handicaps repair, it also interferes with the best time for losing those extra pounds.

CHAPTER

34

Increase Growth Hormone, Naturally

GROWTH HORMONE (GH) is one of the most talked about hormones of modern times. Infomercials touting the benefits of human growth hormone saturate the media. It is promoted as the fountain of youth. In the hands of the uninformed, it may just as well be the fountain of death.

There is no question that GH levels decline with age. Also, overweight individuals have seriously handicapped GH function. Lack of GH activity promotes weight gain around the midsection, the worst possible type of weight to gain.[418] As GH levels decline, the cardiovascular-risk picture significantly worsens.[419]

GH can be measured in the blood to establish a lack of the hormone. GH can be given with the intent of replacing the lacking hormone and returning the GH blood test to a normal score. This is how Western medicine likes to operate: when the number on paper improves, it is thought that the body is back to normal.

Unfortunately, in the case of GH replacement, the short-term risk of this therapy is diabetes; in the long term it is increased cancer risk. This serves as an example of the shortcomings of the Western medical approach as it seeks to measure improvement and to monitor the function of the body.

It may seem hard to understand why a hormone that is essential to the body and declines with age can be involved as a primary factor in certain types of cancer.

A general way to understand the issue is to say that when a person takes GH and is already in an out-of-balance situation, GH may stimulate the growth of cancer even though the level of GH looks normal in the blood. Since most individuals who seem to need GH replacement are out of balance, taking GH is very risky. Taking GH does not fix the problem of why GH is low, and, it may in fact cause serious health problems.

The reason GH levels decline with age is that leptin and the inflammatory signals TNFa and IL-6 block the function of GH, causing GH resistance and depressed GH function. GH is depressed in response to these problems; it is not in control of them. The way to enhance GH function in the body is to solve leptin issues and reduce excess inflammation, not take GH drugs.

WHAT IS GROWTH HORMONE?

GH is produced in the pituitary gland of the brain. Its production is activated by growth hormone releasing hormone (GHRH), produced in the hypothalamus gland. GHRH is one of the oldest hormonal signals in human evolution. As the gene encoding GHRH evolved, its "children" became insulin, glucagon, and various other signals that affect reproduction.[420] Thus, the activity of GH is intimately involved with fuel utilization and reproduction, essential features that allow survival of the species.

When GH is released by the pituitary gland, it travels to the liver where it activates a family of hormonal signals that help carry out repair in the body. True to the family tree, these signals look almost identical to insulin. The primary signal made by the liver that reflects GH activity is called insulin-like growth factor 1 (IGF1). IGF1's main role in a healthy person is to facilitate growth, repair, and cell proliferation.[421] It is a driving force behind building up the body and maintaining it, in terms of physical structure.

The recent discovery of ghrelin, the hormone secreted by the stomach that initiates hunger, is a major breakthrough in understanding the function of GH. Ghrelin binds to cells containing GH, initiating the release of GH into the circulation. This finding is of extreme importance, one that is revolutionizing research in the GH field. We discuss it in more depth later in this chapter.

There is a natural ebb and flow in the body between anabolic activity and catabolic activity. Anabolic activity repairs and builds up the body; catabolic activity breaks down body structure to provide energy to meet demands. The ability to sustain natural balance between these two activities is essential for health.

GH and IGF1 are primarily anabolic hormone signals that help the body use protein to build and repair. This is essential for body growth. This is how growth hormone was named in the first place. In adults, GH is essential for body repair. Thus, it is a prime hormone that helps an individual recover from the wear and tear of living.

GH and IGF1 are closely associated with insulin, in terms of both structure and function. When insulin works properly in the body, it transports calories into storage, an anabolic activity. In a healthy person, this means insulin helps deposit calories in body tissue so that the tissue can use them as a fuel source or as a building material. Thus, there is synergistic harmony among GH, IGF1, and insulin when a person is in a state of natural balance.

By comparison, the stress hormone cortisol is a catabolic hormone. Cortisol promotes the breakdown of body fuel supplies, and potentially of body structural tissue, to use for fuel to meet the demands of stress.

GROWTH HORMONE AND CANCER

A person should seek to restore natural GH function by getting the body back into a state of natural balance and rhythm. Unlike taking a GH pill or injection, this is not a quick fix.

When a person develops insulin resistance, then IGF1 levels become resistant to normal repair activity. This resistant condition causes higher levels of circulating insulin and IGF1. A deleterious side effect of this problem is that excess and nonfunctioning IGF1 will cause cancer to grow, especially breast cancer. This is why insulin resistance reflects breast cancer risk, an issue we discuss in chapter 47.

Higher than normal levels of IGF1 are associated with breast, prostate, colorectal, and lung cancer.[422] Numerous scientists are reporting these problems from a variety of research facilities worldwide.

Breast and prostate cancer cells use GH to fuel their own growth.[423] It is well documented that high IGF1 is associated with colorectal cancer and specifically acts to block cell death in colorectal cancer cells, helping them to survive and spread.[424]

GHRH is a primary growth stimulator of endometrial cancer.[425] Blocking GHRH activity suppresses the growth of cancer cells derived from reproductive tissue.[426] It is recognized that GH and IGF1 activity are major determinants of breast cancer.[427] Blocking GHRH activity reduces the spread of cancer cells and induces cell death in MDA231 breast cancer cells.[428]

GHRH activity is prevalent in human prostate-cancer cell activity,[429] which explains why GHRH-blocking drugs reduce prostate cancer activity. Further, GH and IGF1 are both associated with an increased activity of prostate cancer cells.[430]

A review published in 2002, of 1,848 patients treated with human pituitary growth hormone from 1959-1985, showed "significantly raised risks of cancer mortality overall...incidence of colorectal cancer was also greatly raised...and of Hodgkin's disease mortality."[431] In a smaller recent study treating thirty AIDS patients with recombinant human growth hormone (rhGH) in an effort to reduce their stomach fat, four of them developed diabetes and three of them developed cancer.[432]

GROWTH HORMONE AND DIABETES

Problems with GH and IGF1 lead to insulin resistance and diabetes.[433] Remember that GH and insulin come from the same family tree and look almost identical. Scientists found that GH causes insulin resistance because it binds to insulin receptors, clogging their function.[434]

Turner's syndrome is a condition in which an X chromosome is lacking, causing GH impairment. This results in short stature and sexual underdevelopment. Girls with Turner's syndrome are commonly treated with GH therapy. GH treatment helps correct the lack of GH, but the medical therapy has a major adverse side effect: it causes insulin resistance and greater risk for diabetes and heart disease.[435] When long-term GH therapy is discontinued, the insulin resistance of these individuals goes away and their lipid values and cardiovascular risks improve.[436]

The *Journal of the American Medical Association* recently published the results of a twenty-six week double-blind study to test the effects of GH therapy in healthy older adults. It was conducted with fifty-seven women and seventy-four men, ages sixty-five to eighty-eight, to see if GH therapy could help improve strength. As expected, the researchers found a decrease in fat mass in both sexes. However, there was only a marginal strength increase in men and no significant improvement in strength or aerobic fitness in women.

The conclusion of the study is alarming: "Because adverse effects were frequent, importantly, diabetes and glucose intolerance, GH interventions in the elderly should be confined to controlled studies."[437]

GH serves as an excellent teaching lesson for the *Health Asset Manager*. Here we have a hormone that is lacking as a person grows older. It is depressed more readily in overweight individuals, contributing to many of the health risks associated with obesity. Traditional straight-line thinking, the type on which drug dispensing is based, says that when a number is low on paper, prescribe a drug to bring the score back to normal.

When this line of reasoning is followed with GH, the short-term adverse effect is insulin resistance and diabetes; the long-term adverse effect is significantly increased cancer risk.

THE NATURAL BALANCE OF GROWTH HORMONE

In order to get GH to work properly, it is essential to be in a state of natural balance. A lack of GH is a consequence of the entire body being out of balance, with a loss of natural rhythm.

GH drives the body to fix and repair itself. When the hormone is given the opportunity to do its work, then it works in harmony with other hormones. When the body is out of balance and not communicating properly, then GH activity is depressed or malfunctioning.

We have explained how leptin is produced during the day in numerous rhythmic pulses, creating a "leptin tone" in the circulation. Overall leptin rises throughout the day and peaks at about midnight. Proper leptin function allows metabolism and energy to run at a proper level. When there is leptin resistance or not enough leptin, energetic drive is handicapped.

Similarly, GH is released in ten to twenty pulses per day. The pulsing activity of GH secretion reflects its rhythmic tone. As blood levels of GH fall, the hypothalamus gland sends out GHRH to induce a surge of GH production by the pituitary gland. The largest amount of GH in a twenty-four-hour period is released at night, several hours after the leptin peak.

When the GHRH surge is not there, the system loses its tone, GH cells in the liver lose their physical size, and GH production is seriously depressed.[438] GHRH is responsible for the quantity of the surge of GH production.[439]

GH and leptin have "opposing tone." When leptin levels are high, GH levels are correspondingly lower. Thus, leptin and GH have an ebb-and-flow relationship that is an essential part of natural balance. It is a synergy of coexistence. Leptin's main effect on GH is to restrict it.[440]

In terms of a general trend in the body, GH acts to lower leptin activity in fat cells,[441] leading to a reduction in fat mass, particularly abdominal fat.[442] However, GH does not seem to affect leptin genes in overall white adipose tissue,[443] meaning that the effects of GH on leptin seem to be concentrated in the abdominal fat area.

LEPTIN RESISTANCE AND GROWTH HORMONE

Once leptin resistance sets in and there is excess leptin in the circulation, then GH production is depressed. This is the true cause of the low GH problem.

For example, diabetic girls entering puberty have a significant problem with leptin resistance and blunted growth due to interference with GH.[444] This data shows that leptin has dominance over GH.

In overweight individuals, the daily pulsing of GH release is missing, signifying the leptin-resistant and GH-resistant state.[445] Once abdominal obesity and insulin resistance set in, there is disruption in the normal rhythms and relationship among leptin, insulin, and GH.[446] When rats are genetically bred to have low GH levels, they rapidly develop leptin resistance and obesity.[447]

TIMING AND STRESS AFFECT GROWTH HORMONE

Excess cortisol from stress stimulates the formation of excess fat in the abdominal area. Once GH is lacking, there is no metabolic force to help reduce abdominal fat, and it will keep accumulating as part of a leptin-resistant and insulin-resistant picture.[448]

Normal-weight young women with polycystic ovarian syndrome (facial hair growth, acne, disrupted menstruation) have lost their natural GH pulsing rhythm that enables proper ovarian function. Instead, they have higher and more consistent surges of GH, more typical of a male pattern of GH secretion.[449] This is a situation of too much GH at the wrong time.

In women the proper amount of GH must be present at the right time in the right amounts for normal function of the ovaries, sexual development, and sex drive.[450]

During fasting, GH levels rise, but this is not because the brain is stimulating GH production. Rather, in a fasting state, the hunger hormone of the stomach, ghrelin, promotes extra GH production.[451] This is a natural adaptation to stress. Patients who overproduce GH because of genetics or a pituitary tumor, have depressed ghrelin levels and no normal ghrelin response to a meal, indicating a loss of natural rhythm due to excess GH.[452]

THE GHRELIN BREAKTHROUGH

Understanding ghrelin may be the key to the great paradox of GH. Ghrelin acts to stimulate the secretion of GH from cells that contain it; thus, it is called a growth hormone secretagogue (GHS).

In aging individuals, it is not just a case that GH levels decline;

the stimulation of the production of GH in the brain declines (lack of GHRH) and the secretion of available GH does not occur (lack of GHS). GH itself is in a state of resistance, similar to leptin resistance. GH is in a state of stressed-out tension because it has lost its natural rhythm and ability to communicate.

GHS in drug form is being tested. It can help offset the lack of GH production in aging individuals because it helps the body release its own GH. This is the forefront of GH research.[453] Since the long-term safety of drugs for this condition is unknown, it will be years before consumers are tempted with a new quick-fix pill or shot.

However, since drug companies and scientists have figured out that GH replacement is a risky proposition, the focus for drug development turns to GHS. In the meantime, even though the dangers of GH are known, the public continues to be bombarded by the promotion of GH until the next class of drug is ready. The marketing of an unsafe therapy continues until there is a new drug that can financially take the place of the older and less-effective drug, regardless of potential adverse health consequences.

The *Health Asset Manager* must back up and realize that the body already has a natural way to make GHS; it is called ghrelin. Why do we need a drug for something we already have? Let us get what we already have to work properly.

We pointed out in chapter 25 that overweight individuals have lower-than-normal ghrelin before eating.[454]

In normal-weight individuals, ghrelin levels drop when food is ingested. In overweight individuals, ghrelin levels stay elevated after food is eaten, leading to excess consumption of food.[455] Overweight individuals have a blunted response to the correct working of ghrelin.

Once again, it is an issue of efficiency. Ghrelin loses its normal rhythmic function in overweight individuals. It does this because leptin is too high. As soon as high leptin levels come down, ghrelin goes back into natural balance and normal appetite patterns of ghrelin reappear.[456]

This information means that we can restore natural GH function by lowering leptin and getting it back into natural balance and rhythm.

THE INFLAMMATION CONNECTION

Individuals with serious physical trauma, sepsis, or burn develop GH resistance. Even though they have adequate GH, their bodies tend to go into a wasting pattern. The stress of such conditions causes excess amounts of TNFa and IL-6. Researchers have shown that it is these inflammatory markers which bind to GH receptors and turn them off.[457] Inflammation signals have the opposite effect of ghrelin on the secretion of GH.

This information has been confirmed in other studies. TNFa is shown to be elevated in sepsis, causing GH resistance and body wasting.[458] Mice that genetically make too much IL-6 have normal or high levels of GH; yet they have growth retardation, reflecting the problem of growth-hormone resistance. The excess IL-6 production in these mice reduces the GH receptor function of the liver by half.[459]

Patients with fibromyalgia, a painful condition of muscle aching, have a nighttime surge of GH that is only about one-third that of normal.[460]

Patients with cancer and cachexia lose weight and muscle even when they eat, reflecting a condition of GH resistance. Researchers demonstrated that the level of IL-6 predicts the seriousness of the GH resistance and consequent body wasting.[461]

In these serious health conditions, the body is usually in a highly catabolic state, with excess cortisol and low levels of leptin. The TNFa and IL-6 are inflammation signals coming from the disease process itself, causing GH resistance by blocking the activity of GHS. This science allows us to understand why obesity causes a depression of GH function.

As we explained in chapters 6 and 30, extra pounds of fat contain immune cells that generate excessive amounts of TNFa and IL-6. Since excess amounts of these immune messengers cause the disruption of GH, turning them off is part of the key to getting back in balance.

Some of this can be accomplished in the short term. For example, taking fish oils reduces the output of TNFa and IL-6. Nutritional support can be used to help turn down acute inflammatory signals that disrupt GH and natural balance. This opens the door for weight loss, instead of for being stuck in a metabolic trap.

Further, as weight is lost, the actual number of fat cells making pro-inflammatory signals is reduced; this in turn resolves the issue of depressed GH.

THE IMPORTANCE OF SLEEP AND GH

Because the largest surge of GH occurs during the night, getting sleep back into natural balance is of primary importance to restore proper GH function.

If individuals have leptin resistance, their leptin and insulin levels will stay too high for too long, including during sleep time. For example, in individuals with insulin resistance, GH is depressed during the early part of sleep.[471] Since GH controls the rate of nighttime repair, this interferes with the general repair functions of the body. As repair does not happen at the rate it should, the fuel needed to carry out repair is not in demand. The normal rise of insulin and glucose in early sleep is blunted.

As morning approaches, the level of cortisol rises in the blood. The purpose of cortisol is to turn on all the light switches in every cell of the body, to wake it up and get it ready for the day. In a normal-functioning person, as cortisol begins to rise, it signals the pancreas to stop making insulin. This in turn lowers blood glucose and ends the sleep process.

In a person with insulin resistance, the pancreas ignores this signal, causing a person to wake up with higher-than-normal insulin and glucose levels.[472] If, due to insulin resistance, the liver is unable to store and release enough fuel to get through the night, the individual may wake up with low blood sugar. In either case, it means a poor energy level in the morning and being tired and irritable. It is like getting up on the wrong side of the bed. Sleep is not refreshing.

When sleep is out of rhythm, insulin, glucose, leptin, and GH are out of rhythm as well. Insulin and glucose occur in the wrong amounts at the wrong time of the night. The individual wakes up with a poor blood sugar condition, starting the day on the wrong foot. Therefore, waking up tired and in a bad mood are signs that GH is out of balance with the other hormones which influence energy and repair.

When people follow the *Five Rules*, leptin and insulin levels are in better balance when they enter sleep, and they do not suppress the release of GH. This permits GH to be released at the right time with a normal surge, thus promoting a better condition of natural balance.

THE ALC SOLUTION

It was recently discovered that taking the nutrient ALC (Acetyl-L-Carnitine) before bed can help the hypothalamus gland stimulate the production of GH during sleep.[473] ALC enhances the release of GH, as well as prevents hormonal depletion from stress.[474] ALC helps offset the effects of stress that induce sleep problems.

In a landmark study, ALC was found to help clear leptin resistance in the brain.[475] ALC can help the brain correctly sense the true amount of leptin, thus overcoming leptin resistance. This is a major discovery and signifies an unquestionable ability of nutrient support to prevent serious health issues by restoring natural balance.

Much of the early research on ALC addressed cognitive issues, in which ALC consistently showed an ability to improve cognitive function, mood, and behavior in difficult situations, even in Alzheimer's.[476,477,478,479,480,481] It has been proven effective against serious depression, actually restoring normal stress response and stress tolerance patterns. [482,483,484]

Amazingly, ALC can metabolize stuck cholesterol out of brain cells, thereby helping those cells to be more normal and functional.[485,486,487] A new chain of discoveries shows that ALC can normalize glucose utilization in the brain,[488] thus helping to provide the energy for normal nerve transmission.[489,490]

ALC is a nutrient that acts in the nervous system to promote the return of normal communication among hormones. This is a key underlying issue at the center of "resistance," regardless of the hormone we are discussing. This includes enabling the brain to answer phone calls from leptin, meaning that it helps reduce leptin resistance. It also enhances the ability of the brain to make GH at night.

EXERCISE AND GH

We have mentioned in this chapter that GH is released during the day in a pulsing manner. It needs to maintain this "tone of fitness" in order to function properly.

Exercise by itself does not restore GH to youthful levels; however, it is one thing a person can do to help maintain proper daily tone and fitness in the GH system of the body.[491] While any exercise helps, consistent resistance training is the best for promoting healthy GH function.[492,493,494]

SUMMARY

There are no shortcuts, quick fixes, surgeries, or drugs that will ever restore normal and natural balance in the GH system.

Current GH therapy, in an effort to replace the seemingly lacking hormone, significantly increases the risk of diabetes and cancer. It is a classic example of the shortcomings of Western medical evaluation, wherein a lab test shows a bad number on paper and a drug is given to improve the number.

The only way to reverse the trend of declining and ineffective GH is to get the body back into natural balance. Many factors work against GH, including stress and inflammation. A primary factor that blocks GH is excess leptin due to leptin resistance.

By following the *Five Rules*, eating some carbohydrates to ensure ghrelin release, being consistent with strength-building exercise, and sleeping better, a person will improve leptin function and GH function at the same time. Nutrients such as fish oil, melatonin, and ALC can be used to help this process along, if needed.

Even serious and lifelong problems with obesity can be improved by following a consistent path. We have helped countless people who think they have tried everything. Diet drugs and gastric bypass surgery have serious and long-lasting effects on metabolism and overall health.

There is a healthy way to solve these issues. It begins with understanding the body and how it is supposed to be working. It continues with the consistent application of what one has learned. Only in this way can a *Health Asset Manager* solve the problems of leptin.

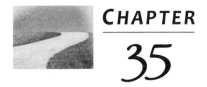

CHAPTER

35

Male Hormone Fitness

TESTOSTERONE is the primary male hormone, the behavioral essence of a man's competitive drive. Estrogen is the primary female hormone. Men and women have both hormones, and it is the balance of these hormones working properly in harmony with other hormones that is essential for health.

Too much leptin puts the breaks on testosterone. A man suffering from leptin resistance has too much leptin in his circulation, forcing down his testosterone. As he gains weight from the problem, especially weight on the lower half of the body, he converts testosterone into estrogen in the accumulating fat cells.

Leptin resistance and depressed testosterone are reflected by weight gain around the midsection. Higher estrogen that is draining testosterone is reflected by weight gain on the buttocks and thighs, the common female places for weight gain. Many men have a combination of both problems.

TESTOSTERONE, LEPTIN, AND AGING

Andropause, the decline of testosterone as aging takes place, is now considered a multi-system disease state.[495] There is nothing "natural" about a lack of testosterone. As testosterone declines, so does masculine motivational drive, sex drive, and sexual-performance ability. Further, declining testosterone is related to increased risk for cardiovascular disease.[496,497,498,499,500,501,502]

The general trend of aging in men, even "healthy" men, is increased body fat and body weight and declining testosterone levels. In this context, the term "healthy" implies "free of abnormal disease," but it is far from optimum health. Men with significant andropause problems lose testosterone faster than what is the agreed-upon "normal" rate. Such men have hypogonadism, excess weight in the midsection, and higher leptin levels than normal.[503]

As body fat accumulates, leptin levels increase and testosterone levels decrease.[504] When there is a lack of testosterone, leptin is inappropriately elevated.[505] There are leptin receptors in the testicles of men, meaning that communication between leptin and the male system is intended. Higher leptin levels tell the male system not to synthesize male hormones.[506] High male hormones suppress leptin levels.[507] Replacing testosterone in men with a lack of that hormone lowers leptin levels.[508]

Leptin communicates to the male hormonal system. Scientists are trying to figure out exactly what it is doing. Some amount of leptin is essential for stimulating the production of male hormones. In men with infertility, too much leptin is present in the seminal fluid.[509]

Leptin controls other hormones. In many situations, the fundamental role of leptin is to permit other hormones to function. Just as the brain senses leptin in order to determine the allowable metabolic rate, many specific body areas require a certain amount of leptin to permit metabolic function.

It is not surprising that leptin is involved with reproduction in both men and women. Reproduction is one of the most energy-intense activities possible. It makes sense that the primary hormone governing the use of energy has an active role in this endeavor.

The idea is not to get rid of leptin – as the proper leptin level allows correct metabolic function, including sex drive and fertility. The idea is to have the right amount of testosterone and leptin in relation to each other.

Throughout this book we have mentioned the triad of problems called insulin resistance, leptin resistance, and adrenaline resistance.

We have discussed how too much cortisol and not enough GH relates to abdominal weight gain. In the case of men, as aging takes place, the issue of low testosterone is consistent in this picture.[510]

There is oftentimes low sexual function in any man with these leptin-related problems, especially as the problems advance with age. Judging by the sales of Viagra, this involves quite a few men.

In fact, the problem of low testosterone and high leptin is passed on genetically by parents who have similar problems, specifically leptin resistance and diabetes. It is proven that first-degree relatives of individuals with diabetes are likely to have the problem of low testosterone and high leptin.

Male children with parents or relatives who are leptin resistant or diabetic are more likely to experience low testosterone and become diabetic.[511] This type of hormone problem is not passed along this way to women, only to men. Further, male hormone replacement prevents the problem from evolving, lowers leptin, prevents insulin resistance, and prevents diabetes.[512]

Andropause is not a pretty picture. Serious cases cause loss of sexual function, hypogonadism, heart disease, diabetes, and increased cancer risk. Milder cases see the male system deteriorate more slowly. The pivotal hormone in this picture is testosterone. It is governed by leptin function.

SOLUTIONS FOR LOW TESTOSTERONE

In addition to improving the efficient function of leptin in order to lose excess weight and enhance testosterone status, another approach is to give nutritional precursors to either help form or help transport testosterone.

Zinc is an important mineral in the formation and transport of testosterone.[513,514] Animal studies show that marginal zinc deficiency can reduce testosterone formation by forty percent, whereas serious zinc deficiency can reduce it by sixty percent. Furthermore, when male animals go through puberty with zinc deficiency, testosterone gene expression is depressed and a significant increase in feminizing characteristics takes the place of the proper male traits.[515]

Tribulus Terristrus is an herb that has been used for centuries in India to treat male sexual problems. Animal and human studies show that it raises luteinizing hormone in the brain, which in turn stimulates testosterone production in the testes. It increases sexual stamina, sex drive, helps get rid of impotence, and increases ejaculatory volume, sperm concentration, and sperm mobility.[516,517,518,519]

DHEA is a testosterone building block. There are numerous studies pointing to the benefits of DHEA. These benefits include weight loss,[520] immune enhancement,[521] and increased energy and sex drive in men.[522] DHEA acts as a major anti-stress hormone, helping the body to adapt to change more efficiently, thereby offsetting wear and tear.

The neurotransmitter dopamine turns out to be a main stimulus to the male sex drive and function.[526] In chapter 24, we explained that leptin is a key to the dopamine drive system and that there needs to be a certain amount of fat in the diet to ensure that there is a normal leptin level. Dopamine production is reinforced by the amino acid tyrosine. This shows that a certain amount of leptin in balance with testosterone is essential for male drive.

In addition to lowering leptin, men can take nutritional support that helps build up testosterone. Men can combine this with strength training for a good fitness program to reduce leptin, build muscle, improve GH, and enhance the function of testosterone. This approach helps improve the amount of testosterone and helps offset the declining trend of aging.

THE ANTI-TESTOSTERONES

It is one thing to build up testosterone; it is quite another to maintain testosterone. There are various factors, both environmental and internal, that create an anti-testosterone situation. Remember that too much leptin is a primary anti-testosterone factor.

There is a natural enzyme in the body called aromatase. It is highly active in white adipose tissue on the lower half of the body. It has an effect on determining the fate of testosterone. In essence, it siphons off testosterone into other activities. Specifically, it converts testosterone into estrogen. This is normal, and a certain amount of this activity is needed for proper male function and drive.

Unfortunately, many men get an excess production of aromatase, a problem that becomes more prevalent as men grow older and gain lower body weight. This tends to make men stay fat and de-energized, contributing to the loss of male function.[527]

It is normal for fat cells to change some testosterone to estrogen; this is a main reason why women have more fat than men.[528] However, progressive increase in body fat in a man tends to lock in an abnormal level of estrogen production, thus keeping testosterone depressed. This is caused by the activity of the aromatase enzyme inside fat cells. As a man gets heavier, more of the aromatase enzyme is active. The extra pounds of fat are the cause of the problem.

Animal studies demonstrate that blocking the aromatase enzyme reduces the conversion of testosterone to estrogen, thereby leaving the testosterone level higher.[529] This helps correct the lack of male drive that is associated with too much estrogen coming from the aromatase enzyme.

It sounds as if every man should just get rid of the aromatase enzyme and suppress it. However, as is the case with virtually everything in the human body, an appropriate amount of aromatase is needed for proper male sexual function.[530] The problem is the out-of-balance situation caused by extra fat on the buttocks and thighs that excessively convert testosterone to estrogen.

Male mice genetically programmed to make excess aromatase develop female breasts. This issue can be reversed by giving them aromatase inhibitors.[531]

When a man gains weight on his buttocks, there is an increase in aromatase conversion of testosterone to estrogen. This is because the amount of aromatase activity in fat cells of the buttocks is ten times that of fat cells of the abdominal area. Thus, a man gains excess midsection weight due to high leptin, insulin resistance, adrenaline resistance, excess cortisol, a lack of GH, and a lack of testosterone. He gains weight on his buttocks and thighs due to excess conversion of testosterone to estrogen by aromatase.[532] Green tea is a powerful inhibitor of the aromatase enzyme.[533]

Atrazine, the most commonly used herbicide in the U.S. and probably the world, decreased testosterone in male frogs tenfold at a dose exposure common to our current environmental levels. It induced demasculinizing effects in the frogs.[534] It does this by increasing the activity of aromatase. This is a serious issue and is the other main reason for increased aromatase activity in men besides extra pounds of fat. Excess environmental chemicals cause a lack of testosterone in men.

CALCIUM FOR MEN

A recent study with old male rats showed that a lack of calcium caused an increase in testicular aromatase activity 2.4 times above normal, resulting in an elevation of estrogen four times normal in their blood.[535]

Thus, calcium is a solution for men with erectile dysfunction. In the brain, a main activator of male sex drive are the melanocortin 4 receptors.[536] When these receptors are activated, erectile activity is dramatic. Anything that gets in the way of these receptors will turn off sexual function.

As it turns out, a primary blocker of these receptors is the agouti gene. Since agouti is easily controlled by adequate calcium intake, getting enough calcium permits the proper nerve signal to flow from the brain and induce an erection. This is good news for men.

Remember that agouti is best friends with neuropeptide Y, the main signal in the brain that makes a person hungry. An excess of NPY directly blocks the function of testosterone.[537]

There are several different pathways in the brain that relate to appetite, especially involving excess consumption of carbohydrates, which block male sexual function. A long-term pattern of excess carbohydrate consumption, reflected by the extra pounds of fat that progressively accumulate and do not go away, takes its toll on male function, sooner or later. Any man who has lost his sex drive and function should lose his sweet tooth and eat fewer carbohydrates.

SUMMARY

Testosterone is an important hormone for proper male function, energetic drive, and cardiovascular health.

Too much leptin depresses testosterone. Not enough leptin causes metabolism to slow down, and this includes male function. Thus, men require a proper amount of leptin. Problems occur when hormones are out of balance. Low testosterone is involved with weight gain around the midsection. Higher-than-normal estrogen causes excess weight on the buttocks and thighs. Many men have both problems.

In addition to balancing hormones and reducing leptin, a man can take steps to build up testosterone and reduce the conversion of testosterone to estrogen. Strength training is the best form of exercise for men to get GH and testosterone to work together in order to stabilize the male energy base. When everything heads in the right direction, weight is progressively reduced and male energy is progressively enhanced.

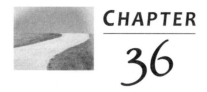

Female Hormone Balance

WOMEN have three times the amount of leptin as men do; this is normal. Even when body fat differences are adjusted, women still have more leptin than men. In fact, it appears that the amount of testosterone in women is the key factor that separates leptin levels in men and women, not body fat.[538]

The comparative lack of testosterone in women enables a permissive relationship between estrogen and leptin, allowing for a combination of higher circulating leptin, estrogen, and body fat. This not only defines a key difference between men and women, it is essential for reproduction and survival of the human race.

Leptin allows for the accumulation of body fat, enabling energy-demanding events to take place, including puberty, pregnancy, and lactation. Extra amounts of leptin are even produced by the placenta during pregnancy.[539] Leptin is essential for survival – not only for preventing starvation, but also for the reproductive function of women.

When a woman is in a state of natural balance and feeling good, then leptin, estrogen, testosterone, and body fat are present in proper amounts and are in harmonious function. Puberty occurs at the proper time, and there is no excess weight gain associated with it. Menstrual cycles run without symptoms and are in a regular pattern. Pregnancy is possible, and healthy pregnancy is typical. Transition is not accompanied by extra weight gain before, during, or afterward. Bone health, heart disease, and breast cancer and other female cancers are not issues.

Too much leptin or too little leptin causes serious problems for women. Leptin resistance means that the brain or ovaries do not respond to the leptin message. This causes serious problems even for women who are not overweight. Leptin efficiency, leptin timing, and the right amount of leptin are important for the female system to work properly.

LEPTIN AND FEMALE PROBLEMS CAN BEGIN EARLY

Girls who start their menstrual cycle early have leptin problems. They typically have higher body fat and are overweight, causing them to have twice the level of leptin than is normal for their age.[540]

This may lead to excess androgen, male hormone production, and polycystic ovarian syndrome in their teens and early twenties.

This leads to at least a forty percent increased risk of breast cancer, simply because there are more estrogenic exposures due to more menstrual cycles in the course of a lifetime.

Girls who begin their menstrual cycles early make estrogen much earlier than they should. However, this problem may quickly shift to low estrogen production in their teens or early twenties.

LEPTIN HELPS REGULATE THE MENSTRUAL CYCLE

In the first half of the menstrual cycle, ovarian follicles are stimulated and an egg is ripened. This happens under the influence of a signal coming from the brain called FSH (follicle stimulating hormone). As the egg ripens, it gives off estrogen. The estrogen enters the general circulation.

When estrogen levels in the blood reach a certain level, the brain knows the egg is ripe. The brain now produces an androgenic signal called LH (luteinizing hormone). New information shows that the rise in estrogen parallels a rise in leptin, and it is the rising leptin that triggers the release of LH.[541] LH stimulates the release of the egg to go down the fallopian tube. The corpus luteum, that was previously holding the egg, now makes progesterone for the second half of the menstrual cycle to help proteins attach to the wall of the uterus, in case there is a pregnancy.

If there is no pregnancy, then progesterone production stops and the wall of the uterus is sheathed off, resulting in menstruation. The process repeats itself, generally in a twenty-eight day pattern.

Returning to the story of the *ob/ob* mouse, which has no leptin; it has great difficulty reproducing. This was the first clue that leptin played a significant role in the menstrual cycle.

We know that there is a normal circle of communication between the brain and the ovaries, which involves leptin. Leptin acts as a primary regulator of proper menstrual rhythm. Problems with leptin resistance or the anorexic-like, low-leptin starvation metabolism disrupt the correct function of the menstrual cycle.

LEPTIN PROBLEMS DISRUPT MENSTRUATION

There are leptin receptors on the ovaries. Just as leptin resistance can occur in the brain, it can also occur in the ovaries. In the first half of the menstrual cycle, estrogen production occurs when a proper amount of leptin binds to the ovaries. When there is leptin resistance in the ovaries, estrogen is produced incorrectly. This causes higher levels of leptin in the follicular fluid surrounding the ovaries, compared to the levels of leptin in the blood.[542]

In this situation, the ovarian follicles are stimulated but may not become fully mature. This means that an egg does not properly ripen or that much more effort than normal is required to ripen an egg. Minimally, this causes excess friction in the female system. In more extreme cases, no egg is ripened at all. These problems significantly affect twenty percent of menstruating women.

Once there is leptin resistance in the ovaries, the brain becomes out of balance and starts to produce excess luteinizing hormone.[543] This leads to excess production of male androgens. This causes acne related to menstruation.

If the problem becomes more significant, there is facial hair growth. The problem can lead to disrupted, irregular, skimpy, or missing menstrual cycles.

Remember that leptin resistance provokes insulin resistance. Insulin resistance aggravates the issue and further magnifies the problem of excess male androgen production.[544]

This is why leptin resistance that triggers early menstruation is such a problem. Excess fat prior to puberty accelerates female development and causes early onset of menstruation. It does this by inappropriately magnifying estrogen production via the aromatase enzyme inside of fat cells. This throws off female hormonal timing in relation to overall lifespan. Since leptin resistance drives this problem, once the menstrual cycle starts, there is a high risk for developing leptin resistance in the ovaries. This may happen right away, or it may develop over a period of a few years.

Women who start menstruation later than normal generally have a low-leptin situation or non-obese leptin resistance. This is due to erratic eating patterns or genetic leptin issues passed down from one or both parents. The result is a lack of leptin-driven stimulation to the ovaries; thus female development may be delayed. An extreme example of the situation of the female gymnast, explained in chapter 31.

POLYCYSTIC OVARIAN SYNDROME (PCOS)

When problems of excess male androgen production are ongoing and significant, there is serious clinical disruption of the menstrual cycle. This is a medical condition known as polycystic ovarian syndrome (PCOS). Leptin problems cause PCOS. There are two types of PCOS, the obese and non-obese versions.

A fascinating study was conducted with young, normal-weight women with PCOS and those who did not have PCOS. Blood was sampled overnight every twenty minutes, in order to monitor the levels of leptin, luteinizing hormone, and androgen levels. Because the women in this study were not overweight, the general leptin issue was not yet developed to the point of obesity. However, the women had PCOS, reflected by their abnormally light or infrequent menstruation and other symptoms.

In both groups of women, leptin levels were about the same. In the healthy women, leptin release lagged behind the release of luteinizing hormone and androgen by about twenty minutes. In the PCOS women, this timing relationship was absent.[545] This inability of proper timing to occur in hormonal rhythms is caused by resistance to the hormonal signals. It means that the ovaries and the brain do not sense leptin correctly, and that leptin resistance takes place in the ovaries and possibly in the brain as well.

Insulin resistance and leptin resistance occur in women with PCOS. These issues coincide with abnormally low ghrelin levels.[546] Low ghrelin reflects abnormal GH activity in relation to the food that is eaten. Additional studies show that women with PCOS have abnormal GH responses to eating food.

Overweight women with PCOS have a blunted GH response to food. Normal-weight women with PCOS have an exaggerated GH response to eating food.[547] In women who do not have PCOS, GH is depressed in response to eating food. The reason it is elevated prior to food consumption is to help induce a normal hunger signal to eat. Once food is eaten, the proper response is to turn off the GH-related signal to eat food. This does not happen in women with PCOS.

Data on GH levels in overweight women with PCOS show that their GH level is reduced by sixty percent, and there is a seventy-five percent loss of pulsing rhythm in GH release.[548] In normal-weight women with PCOS, the GH level is higher than normal in terms of consistent production. However, these women are lacking the pulsing rhythm that is seen in normal-weight women without PCOS. This abnormal GH-release pattern causes excess LH and androstenedione, the precursor to testosterone, to be elevated in direct relation to the improperly timed release of GH.[549]

The overall level of GH is about half that of normal women.[550] Thus, we see the release of a hormone at the wrong time, in an out-of-balance way. Even though the total amount of hormone is only half that of normal women, the improper timing is enough to fuel excessive production of male androgens.

LEPTIN AND PMS

Estrogen and leptin are directly related to one another. Leptin enables there to be a greater amount of body fat. Fat cells, in turn, can increase the metabolic activity of estrogen. When a woman attains natural balance between leptin and estrogen, there is an unmistakable feeling of smoothness and calm. There is also an ability to maintain normal body weight.

Unlike men, who must have a base level of testosterone drive in order to feel normal, women need a rhythmic balance between leptin and estrogen. When women have this working for them, there is a sense of being at emotional ease and in harmony.

Some women go their entire life and do not feel this way, just as some men never have much drive. Instead of being at ease and in harmony, they have an unsettling internal feeling that is magnified in different phases of the menstrual cycle. There may be a certain number of "good days" per month, and then there are the bad days. Even the good days are generally defined as an absence of the uncomfortable feelings, rather than a sense of being at ease and in a state of harmony. Leptin levels are higher in women who experience PMS, reflecting the issue of leptin resistance.[551]

Research shows that leptin levels can be raised in the second half of the menstrual cycle by estrogenic stimulation.[552] Overweight women have elevated leptin levels in the second half of their menstrual cycles, whereas normal-weight women do not.[553] Thus, women who are overweight have more problems with leptin adversely affecting their menstrual cycles in terms of PMS symptoms. The combination of high leptin and low serotonin set up powerful sugar and carbohydrate cravings prior to menstruation.

LEPTIN, PREGNANCY, AND INFERTILITY

A woman entering childbearing years with leptin resistance may have difficulty getting pregnant. If she does get pregnant, she is at higher risk for miscarriage or complications of pregnancy.

Properly communicating leptin is involved with the correct development of the fetus. This happens in part because of its synergistic release of TNFa, which may play a role in fetal growth or development. This is a "good" role of TNFa, in the right amount at the right time, as opposed to excess TNFa causing inflammation and disease.

When there is too much leptin, there is a risk for high blood pressure. Remember the issue of adrenaline resistance discussed earlier. When adrenaline resistance happens during pregnancy, it causes fluid retention and results in a fairly common and potentially serious medical condition called preeclampsia. This condition is associated with excessively high leptin levels.[554] The excessive production of TNFa, due to coexisting high leptin, causes insulin resistance during pregnancy and increases the risk for gestational diabetes.[555]

The reason for high leptin levels in the female system is one of leptin resistance in the actual female organs. For example, fertility specialists have demonstrated that in-vitro fertilization is not likely to work in the presence of high leptin, clearly indicating that leptin resistance may prevent pregnancy from occurring.[556] There is a female-organ leptin resistance that is central to the problem of infertility.[557]

In fact, a certain amount of leptin must exist, along with estrogen, in order for pregnancy to begin. If there is a lack of leptin, then a woman may not get pregnant. If she does, there is a much higher likelihood of a miscarriage.[558]

LEPTIN AND ENDOMETRIOSIS

High leptin due to leptin resistance has a tendency to promote high estrogen, thus causing a relative lack of progesterone in the second half of the menstrual cycle. Warning signs of excess estrogen include heavy blood flow, frequent periods, breast swelling/tenderness, and PMS. This problem may lead to abnormal cell proliferation, such as endometriosis. It can also set the stage for estrogenic-stimulated cancer.

There are leptin receptors on the wall of the female endometrium,[559] meaning that leptin has a direct method of communicating to this tissue.

In a study comparing a group of women with various degrees of endometriosis to a control group, women with endometriosis had significantly higher leptin levels than did women without the condition. Excessive inflammation caused by too much leptin is another factor that fuels endometriosis.[560]

These findings have been confirmed by a more recent study showing that leptin is highly active in endometriosis and is likely a major factor causing it to proliferate.[561] In chapter 47, we discuss the breast-cancer risks associated with high leptin triggering excess TNFa and its companion, NF-kappaB. At this point, it is worth noting that excess NF-kappaB is the key elevated signal that causes endometriosis.[562]

THE POWER OF LEPTIN

The female hormonal system requires a tremendous amount of energy in order to run normally. The week prior to a menstrual cycle, during which time a significant amount of protein is placed on the wall of the uterus in case of pregnancy, is the equivalent of eight hours of construction work per day, on top of whatever else the woman does.

If there is a lack of energy for any reason, it shows up at this time of the month. The primary hormone in the human body that regulates energy use is leptin. Leptin allows the use of energy to go forward in the female hormonal system. Women with leptin resistance have impaired energy regulation.

In the same fashion, women with the anorexic-like starvation metabolism do not have enough leptin to allow normal energy expenditure to run their menstrual cycles.

In addition to allowing a proper energy level and metabolic rate, leptin is involved with governing the female hormonal system. Leptin resistance signifies a breakdown in communication among the brain, ovaries, and other female organs.

SUMMARY AND SOLUTIONS

The health principles in this book – especially the *Five Rules*, consistent and refreshing exercise, and quality of sleep – form the core health program for any woman. This lifestyle is the foundation for solving the numerous female problems discussed in this chapter. It promotes natural rhythm and balance in all hormones in the body, including female hormones.

Any nutrient recommendation given in this book, such as higher essential fatty acids and calcium, is relevant to supporting female health. These recommendations support improved leptin communication and leptin function.

For example, acetyl-l-carnitine (ALC) enhances the correct rhythmic release of growth hormone as well as prevents hormonal depletion from stress.[563] Major female hormonal improvement was noted in women with missing menstrual cycles who took ALC.[564] ALC works by restoring proper communication of leptin, thus helping to resolve leptin resistance.[565]

Anything done to support more natural rhythms and function in any hormonal system – for example, anything that helps to tolerate stress more efficiently – has a synergistic benefit on female hormones.

Trying to manipulate female hormones with drugs is a testament to the lack of skill of the general medical profession. These are common issues, facing well over fifty percent of women.

For example, many physicians prescribe birth-control pills to stop menstrual symptoms. This approach provides a steady stream of external hormones that override natural function. They may spare a woman the turmoil of experiencing how out of balance her menstrual cycle is, but they are far from an actual solution.

Similarly, antidepressants are the "gold standard" for treating PMS.[566] It is easy to see that serotonin levels are low in women with PMS, reflecting a problem of leptin. It is a sad commentary on the skill level of the medical profession when they think they are solving PMS by giving an SSRI medication.

While such symptom suppression may make a woman feel better for a while, SSRI medications frequently have weight gain as a side effect.[567] Another common side effect is sexual dysfunction, hardly a desirable result in correcting female hormone issues.[568] These medications are known to override body rhythms and can induce sleep disorders.[569,570]

If a medication causes weight gain, induces sexual dysfunction, and throws the body out of rhythm, it can hardly be considered a proper solution for the cause of PMS. Short term symptom suppression does not address the cause of the problem, and may in fact make it worse.

Even naturally oriented health-care practitioners may make the mistake of focusing on hormone manipulation of the menstrual cycle. This can involve natural hormone support or various herbs that are known to help hormonal regulation. This strategy may have some value, but if the underlying issue of leptin resistance or lacking leptin is not addressed, it is merely symptom management.

Regardless of whatever strategy a woman uses to help manage her hormonal symptoms, she should have her eye on changing the true cause of the problem. Invariably, hormonal symptoms have some aspect of leptin problems as a primary cause.

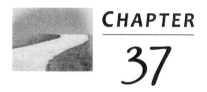

CHAPTER

37

The Estrogen Confusion

The recent development in the medical world of taking women off conjugated estrogens derived from horse urine leaves many women of transition age in a quandary about the subject of estrogen replacement. This type of estrogen drug, in combination with synthetic progesterone, was found to cause more disease than the estrogen drugs were able to prevent.[571]

This problem has been obvious for many years. Western medicine was in denial about the dangers of these medications. In fact, the only reason the problem came to light was because a drug company funded a study to prove these drugs helped heart disease. It was quite a shock to them when the study data came back proving the opposite.

Many women are confused about the subject of estrogen and the appropriate use of it in the context of an overall health program, for women at any age.

THE THREE TYPES OF ESTROGEN
There are three primary types of estrogen:
1) Estradiol (E2): Estrogen made in the ovaries and the primary type produced during the menstrual cycle. It is the type of estrogen that was given in the above-mentioned study as estrogen replacement therapy, the study that demonstrated an increase risk of life-threatening disease.

2) Estrone (E1): Estrogen made mostly in fat cells under the influence of aromatase enzyme. The body can convert estrone to estradiol.

3) Estriol (E3): The protective estrogen. It is made in the ovaries and by conversion of adrenal hormone precursors. The placenta makes significant amounts during pregnancy to protect the developing baby. The body does not convert estradiol or estrone into estriol. The body only slightly makes estriol into estrone or estradiol; it is not a primary or common metabolic path.

The general medical profession considerably misunderstands estriol, calling it a "weak estrogen." It got this name because it has a very slight effect on stimulating the growth of the endometrium. In this regard, estradiol (E2) is eighty times more potent than estriol. Estrone (E1) is seven times more potent than estriol. This perceived potency is more reflective of potential risk, meaning that estradiol or estrone are more likely to cause inappropriate stimulation of estrogen-receptive tissue (breast, cervix, uterus), leading to abnormal growths or cancer.

THE VALUE OF ESTRIOL

There have been several lone voices in the main medical journals over the years pointing out the value of estriol.[572] As far back as 1966, the *Journal of the American Medical Association* published research that showed women with breast cancer had much less estriol than women without breast cancer.[573] New interest in estriol research is fueled by the proven dangers of estradiol and estrone replacement therapy.

Recent discoveries shed light on the essential value of maintaining a proper level of estriol as an important aspect of healthy aging, a topic we discuss more in depth in our next chapter. This new science reshapes the way we think about hormones.

Estriol is the primary estrogen made during pregnancy. Its role during pregnancy is to act as a powerful antioxidant to protect the nervous system of the fetus.[574] A low level of estriol places a woman more at risk for post-partum depression.[575] Other female hormones, such as estradiol or progesterone, were not associated with depression; thus, estriol is a protective hormone in the female system. We pointed out that the condition of high blood pressure during pregnancy is caused by leptin resistance. In severe cases, there is a lack of protective estriol.[576]

Higher levels of estriol protect against MS,[577] whereas higher estradiol may actually promote MS. Treating women who have MS with eight milligrams of estriol per day, a dose similar to pregnancy levels, significantly reduces the problems of MS.[578] Researchers found that brain imaging showed significantly fewer brain lesions in women with MS while they are taking estriol. When estriol was stopped, brain lesions increased. When estriol was resumed, brain lesions went away again. Thus, the lack of estriol is a major finding relating to autoimmune disease. As we mentioned in chapter 31, leptin resistance is also a primary cause of autoimmune disease.

There is a synergistic relationship between the proper amount of leptin and estriol. Both have a protective role in the brain and the female system. During leptin resistance, brain and/or ovarian levels of leptin drop. If estriol levels also drop, there are major problems. If leptin levels and estriol levels reinforce each other in a supportive role, then both the brain and the female organs are offered major protection.

Women who have seizures prior to menstruation have lower levels of estriol, whereas women who have seizures at any time of the month have lower estriol and lower progesterone.[579]

The byproducts of an AIDS infection can be neurotoxic. Not only does estriol protect brain cells from such toxicity, it is the most important form of estrogen in terms of protecting brain cells from calcium displacement (which causes natural balance in the brain cells to be disrupted).[580]

Another interesting study found that estriol was able to stop toxin-induced injury to brain cells, acting as an antioxidant in the brain, almost twice as effectively as estradiol.[581] This study showed that estriol protects dopamine receptors, the same type of receptors that are protected by leptin.

This makes it clear that estriol is the estrogen of choice for protecting the brain; and in this regard, it is much more powerful than estradiol.

In this case, it is the estradiol that has a "weak effect." New science is turning the tables on our previous definition of weak estrogen.

ESTRIOL AND OVARIAN FUNCTION

In an interesting study, it was discovered that estriol maintains a constant level inside of ovarian follicles.[582] This is much different than estradiol, which rises and falls as eggs ripen in the follicles. It has been known since 1993 that estriol protects the ovaries from developing PCOS.[583] As we mentioned in the previous chapter, PCOS, and varying degrees of it, is a major problem for many women. Estriol acts as a protective buffer, so that the female system can run without the symptoms of PCOS.

Thus, any degree of PCOS, such as hormonal-related acne, is a sign that estriol is lacking. Using estriol from days three to fourteen, and possibly longer, in the menstrual cycle, in the dose of two milligrams per day, is helpful in stabilizing this problem.

Using natural micronized progesterone in the second half of the menstrual cycle can help improve symptoms of PMS or estrogen excess.[584,585,586] Medical researchers like to say that the results of using progesterone to improve PMS are statistically significant but not clinically important.[587] They say this so they can justify the use of SSRI medication, which has a higher degree of symptom suppression but numerous adverse side effects that may make the problem worse.

To the contrary, our personal use of micronized progesterone with hundreds of women over a fifteen-year period shows it to be quite helpful much of the time. However, progesterone can easily be converted into stress-fighting hormones, a main reason why it is lacking in the first place. Thus, women get the most benefit from using progesterone in combination with an overall hormone-balancing program.

SUMMARY

Natural balance in the female hormonal system requires an adequate amount of leptin that is communicating efficiently. Not enough leptin or leptin resistance pose major problems to female hormone function.

Estriol and micronized progesterone are useful hormonal support to help balance symptoms in the female system. These are body-identical hormones derived from natural sources. They need to be used in conjunction with proper leptin management to ensure a true resolution of any problem.

Once leptin is properly balanced, especially in younger women, additional hormone support may no longer be needed. This is because the female hormonal system is back in natural balance.

As transition approaches, natural hormonal support can help ease the symptoms of transition. It is especially important to have an effective stress-management and leptin-management program in place; otherwise, no level of natural hormone support may stop out-of-balance transition symptoms.

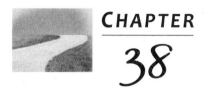

CHAPTER
38

Menopausal Weight Gain

As a woman enters her forties her estrogen levels rise. This is because the brain does not sense when an egg is ripe as efficiently as it did when she was younger. These higher estrogen levels increase leptin production and make a woman more prone to gain weight in her forties, even if she did not have a weight problem before. In mild cases, it is only five to ten pounds, but it does not respond to previous strategies she used to manage her weight.

A recent study comparing fat metabolism in healthy pregnant women, healthy premenopausal women, and healthy postmenopausal women showed that premenopausal and pregnancy were significantly elevated times for fat storage. There was a reduced ability to burn fat as fuel, directly related to the higher estrogen at these times. By comparison, postmenopausal women had an increased ability to burn fat but had higher insulin levels.[588]

This explains why women gain weight before menopause: higher estrogen leading to higher leptin.[589] But why do many women gain weight after menopause? The answer is leptin resistance.

LEPTIN RESISTANCE AND TRANSITION
The drop in estrogen in the female system creates a communication breakdown between leptin and estrogen. The natural rhythm and pattern of estrogen and leptin are disturbed.

Animal experiments show that the drop in estrogen causes leptin resistance in the brain, with an increase in neuropeptide Y.[590] Leptin resistance may develop as a result of a drop in estrogen, a contributing factor to weight gain in postmenopausal women. Since NPY also goes up, hunger is more common and a woman may eat more carbohydrates. During a hot flash, NPY is elevated by thirty-four percent.[591] A high level of calcium is not only helpful for bones, it also helps turn off hot flashes by lowering agouti, which in turn lowers NPY.

In a study comparing premenopausal and postmenopausal women, it was found that postmenopausal women are more likely to gain weight in their abdominal area, as compared to the hips and buttocks, which are the typical estrogen weight-gain areas.[592] The drop in estrogen causes a relative excess of male androgens, even if blood levels of testosterone are low, thereby promoting weight gain around the stomach.

After transition, both leptin and estrogen levels drop.[593] Seemingly, this should help weight loss. However, leptin resistance increases because there is a concurrent increase in insulin resistance. Even though there is less leptin, it does not work as well in the absence of its friend estrogen. The degree of this abdominal weight gain in postmenopausal women reflects the level of leptin and insulin resistance.[594]

IL-6, the inflammatory messenger that disrupts hormone balance, is significantly higher in postmenopausal women.[595] Its partner in crime, TNFa, is also elevated in specific white blood cells. As estrogen drops, these immune cells start to hyper secrete TNFa, posing a specific risk of inflammatory-driven bone loss.[596]

Once again, we see the pattern of leptin resistance, insulin resistance, and inflammatory immune signals fueling the weight-gain problem after transition.[597]

PREPARING FOR TRANSITION

How smoothly a woman handles transition depends on her overall level of physical fitness, her pre-existing body fat when entering her forties, her stress level, and her hormonal history.

In general, estrogen levels rise during her forties and leptin levels go up in response. If she is already leptin resistant and overweight, it is likely there will be a significant struggle with weight during this time. A woman who enters her forties with normal body weight will still struggle with these issues, which typically shows up as a problem with five to fifteen pounds of extra weight.

A woman who takes good care of herself for the ten years prior to transition will have much less trouble before, during, and after transition. The ability to stay fit, eat well, manage stress, and maintain a state of natural rhythm and balance are the cornerstones of health.

SOLUTIONS FOR MENOPAUSAL WEIGHT GAIN

In chapter 30, we discussed the approach to solving weight gain around the midsection. We discussed the importance of essential fatty acids, pantethine, and calcium. In chapter 34, we talked about acetyl-l-carnitine (ALC), another useful nutrient for weight loss. These nutrients are especially helpful in combating weight gain related to transition, which is primarily an increase in abdominal weight.

Because menopause is about changing levels of female hormones, especially a drop in estrogen with a correspondingly higher level of "male" hormones, it is important to know that estriol is a safe and effective way to naturally support estrogen balance. Estriol is much different than the dangerous form of estrogen, estradiol. These differences were explained in the previous chapter.

We have already pointed out in this chapter that leptin resistance is the key problem of postmenopause, with a relative higher level of "male" hormones due to the drop in estrogen. Keep in mind that this issue is not accurately reflected in blood or saliva tests for hormones. Commonly, when postmenopausal women get such test results, they will show low testosterone. However, testosterone will be relatively higher than estrogen, and there will be resistance to the efficient working of the hormones. If a woman takes testosterone to prop up her test scores, she will just grow facial hair and gain more stomach fat, and she may not experience any improvement in energy level, regardless of what lab tests say.

As we also pointed out in the previous chapter, a lack of estriol coexists with problems of leptin resistance. In this chapter we have pointed out that transition-related weight gain is primarily an issue of leptin resistance, which happens as estrogen levels drop. It is logical to conclude that estriol is a supportive estrogen to help maintain proper body weight during and following transition, safely restoring a better harmony between estrogen and testosterone.

There is additional information to support this view. We know that there is greatly increased cardiovascular risk for any person who has leptin resistance. By comparison, estriol was recently proven to reduce atherosclerosis.[598] Furthermore, estriol levels are normal in healthy older women over age eighty-five. Estriol specifically enhances circulation.[599] This indicates that there is a lack of cardiovascular problems in women who have adequate estriol,

Estriol supplementation given to postmenopausal women causes a significant decrease in triglycerides, indicating improved function of insulin and fat transport throughout the body. Since insulin resistance is a key part of the postmenopausal weight gain, estriol helps with this issue as well.

Estriol is proven to prevent a rise in total cholesterol.[600] On the other hand, conjugated drug estrogens that contain estradiol can lower cholesterol but they raise triglycerides, indicating that they make the overall metabolism of fat less efficient.

Only with estriol does scientific data support a favorable relationship in terms of helping to prevent leptin resistance, adrenaline resistance, and insulin resistance. Since the stress of menopause is a drop in estrogen, with a relative increase of androgen, estriol is the estrogen of choice to help keep hormones in balance.

OTHER POSTMENOPAUSAL BENEFITS OF ESTRIOL

There are additional benefits of estriol. It can restore bone density in older women.[601] Estriol can also help relieve urinary incontinence and urinary tract infection.[602,603,604] It can return vaginal flora to normal in postmenopausal women, thus relieving itching and other problems of abnormal discharge.[605,606]

Because estriol binds tightly to vaginal estrogen receptors, it can have a significant impact on correcting vaginal dryness and thinning of the vaginal wall. One study showed a complete resolution of vaginal atrophy in eighty percent of women, within four months of estriol use.[607] Another study demonstrated significant improvement in vaginal dryness and atrophy.[608]

In addition, estriol can significantly help improve the symptoms of transition, including hot flashes.[609]

ESTRIOL SAFETY, CANCER-RISK REDUCTION

A recent study with estriol and 241 postmenopausal women (125 taking estriol, 116 controls) found: "No clinically relevant difference between the endometrium status of postmenopausal women on long-term oral estriol therapy and untreated controls. This trial supports the endometrial safety of maintenance treatment with oral estriol."[610]

In a study comparing the now-infamous estradiol with estriol, breast density was measured by mammography. The estradiol group had a forty percent increase in breast-tissue density, a result that alarmed the researchers. Estriol had only a six percent increase.[611]

In another study with 53 postmenopausal women taking two milligrams of estriol daily for one year, there was a satisfaction rating of eighty-three to ninety-five percent, which was based on reduction of symptoms. The results also showed, "Histological evaluation of the endometrium in all women of Group I and ultrasound assessment of the breasts following 12 months of estriol treatment found normal results in all women. Therefore, estriol appeared to be safe and effective in relieving symptoms of menopausal women."[612]

Estradiol, the dangerous form of estrogen replacement, is shown to magnify the effect of a toxin that promotes ovarian cancer. Estriol, on the other hand, actually reduces the activity of the toxin and prevents cancer.[613] Several animal studies show the ability of estriol to inhibit breast cancer, even when breast tissue is exposed to known carcinogens.[614,615] Estriol binds to estrogen receptors in breast tissue, thus reducing excess amounts of stimulative estrone and estradiol from binding to the same receptors.[616]

In a groundbreaking study, estriol was found to work by down regulating NF-kappaB.[617] Researchers, in this case, were actually looking into why estriol helps multiple sclerosis. This unexpected discovery is of major importance, as excess NF-kappaB is the prime cause of virtually all types of cancer, including female cancers, as we explain in chapter 47. The bottom line is that adequate estriol may be a key component of any woman's cancer risk-reduction plan.

Estrone and estradiol produce estrogen sulfates that in excess cause cancer. This effect of estrogen sulfates can be blocked by progesterone, which is one reason why natural progesterone is also helpful to women.[618] Not only is this therapy effective, it is safe, as demonstrated in a large trial with over nine hundred women.[619]

SUMMARY

The evidence shows that estriol is the core estrogen of immense importance to maintaining health in any woman. Not only is estriol safe and effective for a variety of age-associated female complaints, it appears to be a key hormone that can help prevent leptin resistance and abdominal weight gain in postmenopausal years.

It may also be the case that women who do not have leptin resistance and do not have abdominal weight gain have been able to naturally maintain a higher level of estriol. For those who have not been so fortunate, estriol supplementation is a definite option.

Any support of female hormones works best when other hormones are in a better state of natural balance. Thus, a woman who learns and applies the leptin-managing skills of a *Health Asset Manager* will have an easier time keeping female hormones and health intact as she grows older.

CHAPTER

39

Thyroid Problems Finally Resolved

THE LIVER is the metabolic factory of the human body; it is safe to consider it the brain of the physical body. Metabolic rate is largely determined by the rate of activity of the liver. Thyroid hormone, by comparison, is like a gas pedal on metabolism. The liver is the engine. Leptin is in charge of both of them, because the brain, based on its perception of leptin, tells the liver and thyroid what metabolic rate to employ *(figure 11)*.

Many individuals have the symptoms of hypothyroid function, yet their thyroid lab tests come back normal. When it is understood that leptin is in control of the metabolic rate via the liver, it is logical to assume that thyroid hormones play a secondary role in overall body metabolic rate. We have already explained that if the body thinks it is starving, whether or not this perception is correct, then the metabolic rate slows down for the purpose of survival.

Research relating to thyroid function and leptin shows that thyroid hormones are not in control of leptin levels. It is true that leptin levels are higher in obese, hypothyroid individuals, but the hypothyroid state is not what causes the levels to be higher.[620] These observations are confirmed by multiple studies[621,622] and lead to the conclusion that any thyroid hormone impact on leptin levels is secondary or of minor importance.[623] This data means that thyroid problems do not cause leptin problems. New studies now show that a proper level of leptin in the

Normal Metabolic Rate & Thyroid Function

Figure 11

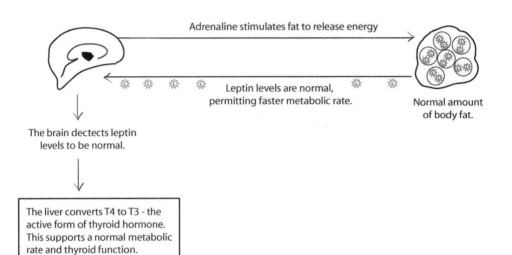

Adrenaline stimulates fat to release energy

Leptin levels are normal, permitting faster metabolic rate.

Normal amount of body fat.

The brain dectects leptin levels to be normal.

The liver converts T4 to T3 - the active form of thyroid hormone. This supports a normal metabolic rate and thyroid function.

brain directly sends out a message to other areas in the brain to simulate the production of thyroid hormone. Leptin controls thyroid. [624,625]

What is evident in these studies of thyroid hormone and leptin is that the percentage of body fat determines the amount of leptin.[626] The combination of insulin resistance and high body fat is the main factor associated with high leptin.[627] Leptin exists as a primary regulator of metabolic rate. When leptin resistance occurs, the body thinks it is starving even though there is plenty of fat on hand. The liver stops converting thyroid hormone into active thyroid hormone because of leptin resistance, the true cause of the seeming thyroid problem *(figure 12)*.

LEPTIN CONTROLS THYROID HORMONE ACTIVATION

T3 is active thyroid hormone. Normally, most T3 is made in the liver, which converts T4, the hormone made by the thyroid gland, to T3, the metabolically active form of the hormone. When the liver is told a starvation situation exists, it slows down metabolism by reducing the production of T3. Researchers have shown an inverse relation between T3 and leptin.[628] This proves that a primary role of the liver is to help leptin control of metabolic rate.

It also means that the huge numbers of individuals suffering from hypothyroid symptoms suffer from leptin resistance and sluggish liver function, a result of instructions from the subconscious brain, which unfortunately perceives the situation incorrectly.

It is interesting to note that the conversion of T4 to T3 works differently in the brain. Whereas the liver handles the major portion of T4 to T3 conversion for the body, the brain is under its own control. Every cell in the brain can convert T4 to T3.

If the individual is in a starvation situation, the liver metabolic rate slows down to save nutrition for the body. However, if the brain slows down too much, the person cannot function. Thus, the brain activates its own thyroid hormone independent of the liver, so that the brain can keep a higher level of metabolic function during times of food deprivation.

This also explains a common, adverse, and now recognizably seri-

Abnormal Metabolic Rate & Poor Thyroid Function   Figure 12

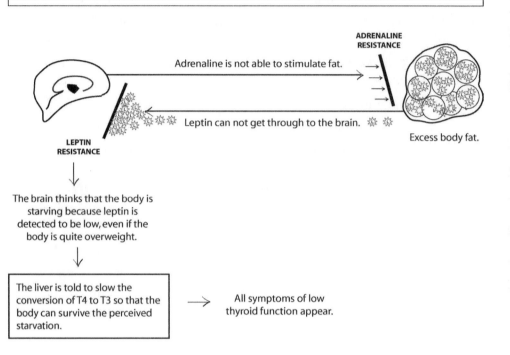

ADRENALINE
RESISTANCE

Adrenaline is not able to stimulate fat.

Leptin can not get through to the brain.

LEPTIN
RESISTANCE

Excess body fat.

The brain thinks that the body is starving because leptin is detected to be low, even if the body is quite overweight.

The liver is told to slow the conversion of T4 to T3 so that the body can survive the perceived starvation.

⟶   All symptoms of low thyroid function appear.

ous problem with thyroid medication. Blood levels of thyroid hormone reflect overall body metabolism and not brain metabolism. Even a person with clinically definable low thyroid is likely to be suffering from primary leptin issues.

If a person takes too much replacement thyroid hormone in an effort to get "blood scores into better range," adverse effects may occur in the brain long before blood scores begin to look normal. If a person takes more hormone than the brain needs, the head feels heavy and out of sync, literally creating a worse hypothyroid problem in the brain.

We bring this up because the common behavior of endocrinologists is to continue raising the dose of thyroid hormone until the numbers look good on paper. The fact is, they are not looking at numbers that mean anything in terms of how one's head feels or how one's actual liver-driven metabolism works. If leptin resistance can be corrected, thyroid problems will likely go away. Leptin is the boss, and thyroid answers to it.

STRESS AND THYROID PROBLEMS

Two other main variables get in the way of metabolic rate; stress and toxic waste.

Stress creates internal friction and inflammation, causing body tissue to become "hot." This is why ice is applied to an injury. However, in the case of stress wear and tear, the heat is all around the body, as multiple tissue areas have "micro injuries" that generate heat. This type of heat comes from inflammation, not as a byproduct of normal metabolic energy production.

In the case of metabolic symptoms, it is like having a sprained metabolism. If metabolism tries to keep up a normal pace, then further overheating and damage occurs. It is like running on a badly sprained ankle.

This is a case of stress overload slowing down metabolism, rather than leptin resistance slowing down metabolism. The conversion of T4 to T3 by the liver is slowed down by high stress.[629,630,631,632] This is a natural defense mechanism against burning up body tissues.

In this situation thyroid lab scores may or may not be low, but the typical symptoms of hypothyroid are present. If individuals take thyroid medication to force their body to go faster, the result can be harmful to health. This problem is recognized in the scientific literature. A recent study warns doctors not to give thyroid hormone to seriously ill patients, even if their thyroid lab scores are low, because significant problems can easily result.[633]

TOXINS AND THYROID PROBLEMS

Another major contributor to poor metabolism is the increase in environmental pollution. It is known that environmental pollution aggravates thyroid problems.[634,635,636,637,638]

Troublesome levels of pollution exist across the United States in groundwater.[639] Rodents eating contaminated fish from the Great Lakes region have significant adverse thyroid problems, even at lower doses of exposure than studied in most toxicology testing.[640]

Nitrates can interfere with thyroid function.[641] Thyroid function is dysregulated by radiation exposure.[642] Infants can have impaired thyroid function from secondhand cigarette smoke from their parents.[643]

The most recent major study in this area, conducted in Canada, confirmed the serious thyroid problem from typical pollutants containing a variety of contaminants and heavy metals.[644] Not only do these pollutants disrupt thyroid function, they have a major impact on disrupting brain function.[645]

This constant burden of excess chemical pollution poses an ongoing metabolic challenge for any person. If the body cannot keep up with elimination of the toxins, then they are sure to overload metabolism and cause metabolism to slow down. It is like pouring sand into the gas tank of a car. It does not matter if the car is old or new, when the engine gets clogged, it will not run correctly. The liver must clear all such chemicals.

When the liver cannot keep up, there is a backlog of toxins in the blood. People feel poisoned, fatigued, irritable, and they have dark circles under their eyes. The lymph system gets backed up, causing stiff upper shoulders, head pressures, excess mucous, and numb arms, especially during sleep. These are plumbing problems, indicating an overload of waste products. Such individuals eventually become sensitive to environmental chemicals and/or have been diagnosed with fibromyalgia.

It has been our consistent clinical experience that individuals with the most severe collection of hypothyroid symptoms also have the most severe symptoms from toxins. This makes weight loss even more complex, because the body frequently tries to get extra toxins out of circulation by stuffing them into fat. Thus, a toxic person has great difficulty losing weight because the body does not want to give up the toxins stored in fat. Doing so will re-expose the person to the chemicals. The liver, lymphatic, and bowel elimination systems must be improved; then, toxins can be more efficiently eliminated, the constraint on metabolism can be removed, and weight loss can occur.

High levels of leptin, like those present in the leptin-resistant situation, induce liver damage.[646] Even more alarming, these high-leptin situations magnify the potential damage that toxins create for the liver.[647]

This is a significant reason why a combination of extra fat and environmental pollution is involved with the diseases associated with obesity. It is a major Catch-22 that must be addressed. While an individual can certainly support detoxification and enhance thyroid function, the primary solution is to master leptin and overcome leptin resistance.

SUMMARY

The symptoms of hypothyroid are common in any person who is overweight and not feeling well. These issues are magnified by stress and chemical environmental pollution.

The primary cause of the problem is leptin resistance, which forces the body into an inappropriate hibernation state. Fixing leptin resistance fixes the source of the problem.

If the problem is not fixed, then health deteriorates because the ability to tolerate emotional or physical stress is reduced, leading to accelerated wear and tear from common stress. Further, the high levels of leptin magnify the damage caused by environmental pollution, and that in itself is another primary burden to thyroid metabolism.

We have found that individuals with the greatest number of hypothyroid symptoms also have the most difficulty with chemical sensitivity and general "toxic symptoms," eventually resulting in fibromyalgia.

Since it is virtually impossible to escape environmental pollution, and it may or may not be possible to reduce stress, the one ticket to health is resolving leptin resistance. Mastering leptin is the key to improving thyroid function, restoring metabolism, and being more able to withstand the stress factors in our lives and in the environment.

Understanding that leptin resistance is the true cause of virtually all hypothyroid symptoms is a major advancement in our understanding of metabolism.

In chapter 41, we give additional information on thyroid hormone function. We will discuss it in the context of weight-loss plateaus and how to get out of a starvation metabolic problem.

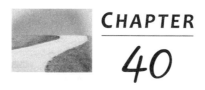

Fibromyalgia: Is Your Metabolism Worn Out or Clogged?

Up to this point, we have discussed the role of various hormones and placed them in the overall context of leptin management. The major reason for understanding any individual hormone is to help it work better. When individual hormones work more efficiently, then all hormones as a group work in improved harmony. This enables an improved condition of natural balance.

There are many shades of gray between optimum health and a diseased state. We have explained how failing to manage leptin results in progressive problems with body weight, insulin resistance, inflammation, and hormone issues, among others. Many levels of less-efficient function exist between optimum fuel regulation and type II diabetes.

Problems with leptin are a key indicator that a person is heading for trouble. These problems include leptin resistance, which leads to obesity, or a lack of leptin, which causes anorexic-like starvation metabolism. Since proper leptin function permits other hormones in the body to work properly, it is fundamental to health.

A person who is overweight is likely to have other hormonal problems, because being overweight reflects of a lack of proper hormone balance, thus setting the stage for progressive decline. However, normal-weight or underweight individuals can easily have trouble with hormones, including inefficient function of leptin.

Fibromyalgia is a serious problem in the hormonal balance system.

In terms of natural balance, significant fibromyalgia reflects of worn-out metabolism. Any person who struggles with any hormone imbalance is more at risk for developing fibromyalgia.

The defining symptom of fibromyalgia is body pain, particularly in the muscles. This leads to disrupted sleep and consequent fatigue.[648] The greater the amount of pain and sleep issues, the more severe the case of fibromyalgia.

Everyone knows how fibromyalgia feels. It is like having a nasty flu bug. The body feels as though it had been run over by a truck. Now, imagine feeling that way without having the flu. There are varying degrees of fibromyalgia. There is always some level of abnormal pain, disrupted sleep, and increased fatigue.

Similarly, individuals with leptin resistance have some level of disrupted sleep and abnormal fatigue. Progression into fibromyalgia simply adds pain to this equation. The best way to avoid getting into the chronic pain of fibromyalgia is to master leptin. The tools of mastering leptin also provide the way out of the fibromyalgia rut.

WESTERN MEDICINE IS OF LIMITED VALUE

The medical approach for fibromyalgia treatment is to modulate pain where possible and hope for improvement in other issues because pain is lessened. Tricyclic antidepressants, such as amitriptyline, and SSRI antidepressants are the common medical treatment specifically for pain.[649] This approach has a degree of workability, since lowering pain improves sleep and lessens fatigue.

This bandage approach of using pain-related medications to improve quality of life has a degree of value, but it does nothing to restore natural balance to the hormonal systems. A person in intense pain and unable to sleep benefits from medication that lowers pain and improves sleep. However, the actual cause of the pain is not addressed. This is reflected by the fact that many patients find the benefits of drugs like amitriptyline wear off after a month.[650]

Fibromyalgia is not an easy problem to solve. In state-of-the-art nursing care in Europe, patients are made to understand that they will never get better: thus they are relieved of the stress of trying to find a solution.[651]

A primary reason why medical people have trouble figuring out the nature of fibromyalgia is that hormone levels in the blood of people with this condition frequently look normal. Medical people have great difficulty understanding a problem if they cannot see it in lab scores on paper. This typically leads them to conclude it must be in the mind of the patient.[652]

However, fibromyalgia is a classic condition of hormonal resistance and improper hormone timing, the hallmarks of an out-of-balance system. Frequently, lab scores on paper look normal enough, yet the proper function of those hormones is far from normal. This is because hormone levels in the blood or saliva do not reflect hormone resistance or improper hormone timing – the actual problems in fibromyalgia.

When lab scores come back normal, yet individuals hurt all over, are fatigued, and do not sleep well, they get a diagnosis of fibromyalgia by default.

The reason modern medical treatment has no solutions for fibromyalgia is that this disease does not have a traditional cause. It is a breakdown in homeostasis, or natural balance. The solution is to fix natural balance. In the case of fibromyalgia, this is not so easy because fibromyalgia is a problem in which the natural balance system has become worn out.

Once people are in this situation, they are handicapped in dealing with various forms of stress. For example, if they get an infection, they have difficulty mounting a proper immune response to get rid of it. If they have an emotional problem in their life, they may have great difficulty dealing with it. If they break a bone, they may have trouble healing it.

Thus, although fibromyalgia is its own problem, it makes other problems more difficult to solve. Under traditional medical care this leads to a longer list of medications, in an effort to manage the body's inability to bounce back on its own. Each time there is a new problem, a new medication is added.

Generally, the medications have adverse consequences to natural balance, making the underlying problem worse. Thus, the increased use of medication places a person between a rock and a hard place. Such individuals feel bad on medication and feel bad off medication; they frequently have to figure out which "bad feeling" they would rather have.

We have helped thousands of people with fibromyalgia. Unraveling these problems takes work, but it can be done. It is easier to prevent fibromyalgia than it is to deal with the condition itself. Thus, we hope that many readers who struggle with leptin but have not yet progressed into fibromyalgia will heed our warnings and learn to master leptin, keeping hormones in a healthy condition of natural balance. Unlike the European nursing profession and general medical community, we offer hope of a true solution for the problem.

THE HORMONE IMBALANCE OF FIBROMYALGIA

Fibromyalgia is a loss of hormonal fitness; it reflects a hormonal system that does not bounce back and recover properly from stress.[653] There is a picture of hormonal tiredness and consequent inefficiency related to the hypothalamus gland in the brain.[654] The command-and-control center is too worn down to do its job.[655]

Fibromyalgia patients have generally lower levels of growth hormone, cortisol (the main stress hormone), and androgens (the main energetic drive hormone for both sexes) compared to normal.[656] However, if people with fibromyalgia have acute stress, they get an exaggerated release of stress hormones, as if desperately trying to solve the stress. Unfortunately, nothing much in their body responds properly to this effort to manage stress.

This reflects their path into fibromyalgia, one in which they have been overloaded by stress. Keep in mind that such stress triggers can be emotional or physical in nature. There is typically a major stress turning point, an event or period of time that acts like the straw that breaks the camel's back.

Thirty percent of patients with fibromyalgia have a definable level of GH deficiency.[657] Patients with fibromyalgia do not release GH in response to exercise, as do normal people. The scientists investigating this issue surmised that the GH regulatory system had lost its "tone"; in other words, it is tired and not working anymore.[658]

Corticotropin-releasing hormone (CRH) is the central hormone in the hypothalamus gland of the brain that initiates the stress response. When this hormone is injected into fibromyalgia patients and healthy individuals, there are different responses. In fibromyalgia patients, the hormone stays elevated in the blood. It commands no appropriate reaction, which reflects general hormone resistance across the board in adapting to stress.[659]

As we have pointed out all along, leptin, adrenaline, NPY, agouti, and numerous other signals are processed in this brain center. Fibromyalgia is a condition of fatigue of the hypothalamus gland. The hormone-regulation system is worn out.

BACKED-UP PLUMBING

The consequence of this problem is physical pain and the accumulation of waste products, due to clogged plumbing in the body. The longer the plumbing stays clogged, the greater the amount of localized tissue damage.[660]

Clogged plumbing in the body is like clogged plumbing in a house: the restrooms need to be used on a regular basis, but the waste products are backed up. This is certainly the case with fibromyalgia, as the backed-up waste products get in the way of hormones and cellular energy production. This magnifies the obstacles that must be overcome for the body to return to natural balance. This is why it is such a difficult problem to solve – there is no drug that does housecleaning; there are no plumbers to call.

WEIGHT LOSS IS MORE DIFFICULT

Leptin-resistant and overweight individuals who have fibromyalgia have an even more difficult time. This is because the body seeks to get toxic waste out of circulation. Since normal plumbing routes are clogged, a secondary place to stuff toxic waste is fat cells. This at least gets toxins out of the circulation and away from key body organs. The formation of fat is enhanced by the condition of fibromyalgia as a natural defense system.

In order to lose weight, such a person must get the plumbing to work better. The toxins in the body, as well as the stored toxins that come out of fat cells as weight is lost, must have someplace to go. The body is reluctant to break down toxic fat if there is no place for the toxins to go.

NERVE PAIN

There are three primary reasons for the pain of fibromyalgia. All three need to be addressed in order to solve this problem. The first one is nerve pain.

Nerve pain is the result of a worn-down nervous system. A normal response to stress involves the release of cortisol, as well as sympathetic nerve stimulants such as adrenaline and dopamine. At the same time, the body releases beta-endorphins to improve pain tolerance and regulate the inflammation involved with stress.

When stress is ongoing, a person enters a phase of excess sympathetic nerve activity or surplus adrenaline. This leads to adrenaline resistance, insulin resistance, and leptin resistance, with a corresponding lack of "relaxation reserves."

At the point where the natural-balance systems run out of energy, fibromyalgia sets in. In this worn-down condition, the nerves hypersecrete inflammatory signals, which come out of nerve endings and bang into muscles, causing pain in muscles.[661] The phone poles and phone wires that make up the nervous system are now in a broken-down condition. Any energy going through them, even too much positive emotion, can induce a flare-up of painful symptoms.

At the same time, the overall analgesic that helps a person normally tolerate pain, beta-endorphin, is exhausted and not available. This is easily seen in the absence of a refreshing response to exercise: the normal rise of beta-endorphin does not occur and, in fact, too much exercise or physical activity in the day overloads the already exhausted system and induces pain that may last for days.

In fact, the ability to get a refreshing response to exercise, to perform more physical activities during the day, and to tolerate positive energy going through the nerves without pain are key signs that a person is solving fibromyalgia.

The antidepressant medications the medical profession prescribes target these nerve-related pain signals and blunt the pain-related communication system. This is potentially helpful when pain is out of control. However, the actual cause of the problem is worn-down nerves.

SOLUTIONS FOR NERVE PAIN

Solving this problem involves restoring nutritional energy to the nervous system while at the same time being consistent with whatever amount of exercise the person can perform.

B vitamins are the most fundamental nutrients for nervous-system function, and in our experience the coenzyme forms of B vitamins are easy for nerves to use and work better to assist nerve health in individuals with fibromyalgia. Minerals are also important for nerves and muscles, especially calcium and magnesium. Magnesium malate helps offset muscle fatigue while soothing nerves, magnesium glycinate is also useful. We like a unique form of calcium called calcium AEP. Calcium is important for nerve function; however, calcium AEP is special. This form of calcium builds up the myelin sheathing of nerves, enabling the nerves to carry more energy, a key problem for those with fibromyalgia.

There are other nutrients that can be used to help nerves, such as acetyl-l-carnitine, phosphatidylserine, DHA, carnosine, and many others. These nutrients may be quite helpful. It is best to start out with basic support and gradually increase nutrients to amounts that support healthy nerve and muscle function. As a person's fitness improves, pain goes down. Nutrients can be very helpful support in this context.

Some people start out with five minutes of walking. As they begin to improve, exercise gradually increases and higher amounts of nutritional support help to strengthen the nerves at a quicker rate.

As nerve-related pain declines, sleep automatically improves. As part of a fibromyalgia program, melatonin can be used to help the sleep process. The dose can range anywhere from 0.5 to 6 milligrams a day, taken before bed.[662]

CLOGGED PLUMBING PAIN

The primary internal plumbing system of the human body revolves around the functioning of the lymphatic system. The lymphatic system is the fluid between all cells of the body. It leads through various channels and glands to its two major thoracic ducts, which drain on both sides of the shoulders back into the veins. Waste then flows to the liver, is processed, and most then flows to the GI tract on its way out of the body.

The lymph system is a one-way pressure system. Thus, when it is clogged, there are unmistakable symptoms. A person may not have every one of these symptoms, but to a greater or lesser degree there is a collection of them. The shoulder area builds up pressure that does not easily go away. This is like having constipation; instead of the bowels, it is the lymph system that is stuck.

Such pressure tends to go backwards when the thoracic ducts are clogged. A person may feel pressure going up the back of the head; it may feel like the top of the head is going to blow off, and/or there may be recurring sinus or ear pressures not necessarily related to infection.

Once the lymph is clogged, the body looks for alternative ways to get rid of waste. This usually involves making extra mucous and trying to excrete it through the sinuses. Thus, clearing the throat, especially after eating, is a sign of lymphatic congestion. This can also cause ear popping, ear ringing, and ear noises, because the fluids in the ear cannot drain properly and there is a backup. In some people, this can be severe, causing pressure on the inner ear and dizziness.

Because the lymph system is most active while people are asleep, individuals wake up with excess congestion, mucous, and body aches. As the lymph swells during sleep, it pushes on nerves that go to the hands or arms; thus, it is common for individuals with lymph congestion to wake up with an arm or hand that is asleep. This can also happen during the day as the wear and tear of the day overloads the lymph system.

Because the lymph system is a pressure system, it responds to environmental pressure changes. Prime examples are flying in an airplane or a change in weather fronts. A secondary example is the full moon or no moon. These environmental influences of pressure change are felt as symptoms of congestion, aches, and backed-up plumbing by a person with a sluggish lymph system.

Once the lymph system is backed up, then lactic acid tends to accumulate more easily in the muscles, aggravating the pain of fibromyalgia. This is especially true in relation to exercise. With serious fibromyalgia, individuals feel like they have run a marathon when all they did was go for a walk. People with fibromyalgia "hit the lactic acid wall" with normal everyday activities.

Medical professionals generally do not understand this problem, do not know how to alleviate it, and frequently make it worse with medications.

SOLVING CLOGGED PLUMBING PAIN

Stagnation is the enemy of the lymph system. Overdoing it is also a problem. In significant fibromyalgia, there is sometimes very little difference between stagnation and overdoing it, an issue that must be resolved in order for a person to get better.

Thus, we seek to get people to do whatever baseline of exercise is possible for them. It is important to be consistent, not intense. As individuals improve, they will consistently be able to do more.

The most effective compound we have found for helping the lymph system move along is arabinogalactan. This unique nutrient wakes up the macrophages in the lymphatic system and puts them back on cleaning duty, as well as facilitates other aspects of immune function.[663] Doses may range from one-half teaspoon to one heaping tablespoon, one to four times a day. Once again, finding a dose that alleviates the symptoms of clogged plumbing is the key. A dose at night is typically quite helpful to improve lymph function during sleep.

We also use magnesium malate to help clear lactic acid from muscles. It is also important to help the liver process its waste. We use a "liver multiple nutrient" for this job, one that has a good base of silymarin and other toxin-clearing nutrients. Of course, if a person is constipated, the bowels must move or waste products back up in the body.

When an individual improves the lymph system and related plumbing, the pain of fibromyalgia can be greatly reduced. Just like the plumbing in a house, this plumbing is always in use. It is not that a person goes through a detoxification and is then free of fibromyalgia. Efficient function of one's plumbing on a daily basis is essential; a backlog has serious repercussions for hormonal balance.

TISSUE-DAMAGE PAIN

Individuals with fibromyalgia have much higher levels of advanced glycation end-product (AGE) modified proteins. The proteins of muscle fibers are cemented together in abnormal structures and no longer work properly. This is a form of tissue damage that causes pain. Unfortunately, this tissue damage activates excess production of NF-kappaB, which contributes to the pain and perpetuates the damage.[664]

This AGE-induced tissue damage occurs once the antioxidant reserves of the muscle are used up. When nerve pain is initially directed at the muscles, the muscles activate their cellular defense mechanisms in an effort to withstand the problem. As the problem continues, the antioxidant defense system is used up. At this point, excess NF-kappaB is activated in an inflammatory manner. This in turn causes a progression of the local tissue damage and resulting pain.

The longer a person stays in the fibromyalgia pain condition, the more likely it is that damage is being done to the muscles.

SOLVING TISSUE-DAMAGE PAIN

The solution for this type of pain is to stop fibromyalgia hormone imbalance in the first place. However, even on a good program this may take some time. In the meantime, we cannot simply stand by as tissue is damaged.

There are various nutritional strategies that can be employed. R-alpha-lipoic acid, a potent antioxidant, has proven to stop AGE-associated damage by turning off the excess production of NF-kappaB.[665] There are numerous studies demonstrating the ability of R-alpha-lipoic acid to turn off the production of excess NF-kappaB.[666,667,668] It is an excellent antioxidant for the nervous system; thus, it is helpful for the nerve pain and nerve inflammation of fibromyalgia.[669,670] It is a primary nutrient to help stop the progression of tissue damage.

There is also hope for repairing tissue damage. We use the enzymes bromelain and papain to help dissolve abnormal tissue protein damage.[671,672] We combine them with quercetin and curcumin to further reduce inflammation and help turn off excess NF-kappaB.[673,674,675]

We may add a nutrient such as hyaluronic acid. Hyaluronic acid signals genes to help synthesize new cells and it acts as a connective tissue raw material itself.[676] Our goal is not only to reduce pain but also to improve the response to exercise. We especially try to find a level of support that will help people do strength-training exercise.

When we can get a people with fibromyalgia onto a strength-training program and get a good response to that program, we can fix their problem. In part, this works by enhancing the release of growth hormone, helping to put the hormone-balance issue back into natural function.[677]

However, in order to get a good response to even mild strength training, a person must be able to repair tissue damage induced by the exercise. Unfortunately, fibromyalgia patients may already be in a condition of tissue damage that they are not able to repair. If they try to do strength training, they may make their overall problem worse, judging by the amount of pain they are in after they work out.

For example, normal individuals who perform exercise they are not conditioned to perform may experience muscle-tissue breakdown and stiff muscles for two to three days. This stiffness goes away or is shortened once individuals are conditioned. People with fibromyalgia may induce the same sort of pain response, but the pain may last one to two weeks! Furthermore, doing the exercise again may result in the same problem, rather than improved conditioning.

Thus, anti-inflammatory and structural nutritional support is important for people with fibromyalgia to improve their muscle fitness and ability to recover from tissue damage. This enables them to begin to get a good response to improved muscle fitness. At the same time, it signifies they have enough nutritional support to prevent excess muscle-tissue damage and to enhance the repair of muscle.

SUMMARY

Fibromyalgia is the problem of a worn-down hormonal system. It especially reflects that the commander-in-chief of the subconscious brain, the hypothalamus gland, is too tired to properly carry out its work. Since its work is primarily the job of ensuring that natural balance takes place, this is a major problem.

Leptin resistance and related issues set the stage for this problem. When these problems exist, the body struggles to maintain natural balance. Fibromyalgia is a progression of these problems into a state of hormonal-regulation exhaustion. There are still hormones in the blood; however, the hormones do not work the way they once did. Quality, timing, and overall efficiency of the hormonal system is lacking – hormone resistance is dominant.

Refreshing response to aerobic exercise and a healthy muscle response to strength-training exercise are important steps on the path to recovery from fibromyalgia. Doing whatever it takes to solve these issues helps alleviate fibromyalgia. Re-energizing the nervous system, improving the plumbing operation, and restoring physical fitness are imperative to solving the problem of fibromyalgia.

By taking it a step further and learning to be a *Health Asset Manager*, a person can prevent sliding back into the problem of fibromyalgia, or ever having the problem in the first place.

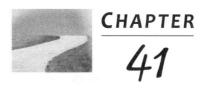

CHAPTER

41

Rapid Weight Gain and Yo-Yo Diets

INDIVIDUALS can rapidly gain weight from eating too much food. Some individuals gain weight from eating a normal amount of food. This is especially true for people who finish dieting and start eating more food. This typically results in gaining back the weight that was lost and frequently five to ten additional pounds. These issues are caused by leptin. In the person who is overeating, leptin resistance fuels the excessive weight gain.

In the case of the person who gains back weight after dieting, the natural response of leptin following a diet is to replenish the supply of fat. It is this survival instinct of leptin that causes dieters to have so much trouble.

The more history individuals have with weight gain and weight loss, the greater the degree of leptin resistance and leptin problems they are likely to have. The body does not trust them anymore. It is all too eager to put extra fat back in place just, to be on the safe side. The body considers the scarcity of food to be an extreme threat to survival. The subconscious brain does not know that when the diet is over, there is food available on every corner.

When individuals lose weight by following the *Five Rules* and a consistent exercise program, the weight loss tends to be permanent. Whenever people try to lose weight by reducing calories, they are prone to gain it back once they start eating more. That is the nature of leptin.

EATING MORE SAFELY

Many individuals keep themselves in anorexic-like starvation metabolism because they want to look thin, and they are afraid that if they eat too much they will gain unwanted weight.

If individuals follow the *Five Rules* and they exercise, they will not gain inappropriate weight as they begin to eat more. Rather, they will gain energy, strength, proper immune function, and improved sex-hormone balance.

Individuals with a history of yo-yo dieting have trained their nervous system and leptin response into a bad habit or routine. While such individuals know they should follow the *Five Rules* and exercise consistently, and may in fact do so, they are more easily thrown into leptin problems resulting in weight gain. For example, they may do fine until they get under stress. All of a sudden they start to eat more. They cannot get out of the pattern; they are sucked back into leptin-resistant weight gain.

Such individuals have a real problem with leptin running their life, as opposed to they themselves managing leptin.

SUMMARY

Yo-yo dieting is very unhealthy. Eating insufficient food in order not to gain weight – essentially staying malnourished – is also unhealthy.

The base for solving these problems is implementing the *Five Rules*, consistent exercise, adequate sleep, and hormone-management skills.

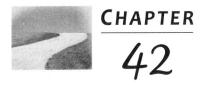

Solving Stubborn Weight Loss

WE HAVE EXTENSIVELY discussed the anorexic-like starvation metabolism. This problem may exist as the dominant metabolic pattern in an individual. Such a person can eat like a bird and still not lose weight.

Anorexic-like starvation metabolism may also be encountered in the dieting process. It causes a person to hit a plateau or be unable to get rid of the last few pounds. When this happens, a person gets stuck at a particular weight and does not progress.

Remember, the subconscious brain does not look in the mirror; it has no clue about how overweight a person may be. The subconscious brain determines where calories head based entirely on one thing, the perception of leptin.

If the subconscious brain does not receive a perception of leptin that permits active metabolism to occur, it enforces starvation metabolism on the person, regardless of how much fat is already in storage. This is the reason an individual cannot get past a certain weight.

VARYING DEGREES OF DIFFICULTY
This perceived state of starvation comes in different levels of severity. Many individuals who follow the *Five Rules*, exercise consistently, and get adequate sleep will be able to solve this problem easily. Remember, these steps are essential for anyone, even those with a more severe problem.

Individuals may practice these basic leptin management skills correctly in terms of eating and exercise, but their weight still will not budge, or they will hit a plateau and have trouble getting past it. This is a more serious problem.

It does not mean that our approach is incorrect; it simply means that the underlying hormonal system is too out of balance to respond to the fundamentals. If these individuals go against the basic leptin-management approach, they will simply get worse. However, they need more help to get their metabolism in gear and out of the perceived state of starvation.

THE GREAT WEIGHT-LOSS MYSTERY

Understanding the problem of perceived starvation is the key to overcoming stubborn weight-loss issues.

Thyroid hormone is blocked during perceived starvation. In perceived starvation, there are elevated levels of reverse T3, the form of T3 that puts the brakes on metabolism. Overweight people who are not in starvation metabolism do not have elevated reverse T3. This occurs in people who are overweight and in perceived starvation.[681]

This is the case even if the basic thyroid lab tests say there is no problem, as most thyroid tests do not look for reverse T3; it can continue to be the case even if a person takes thyroid hormone. A person is either in a perceived state of starvation or not, regardless of what the thyroid lab tests says or whether thyroid medication is being consumed. Thyroid medication is definitely not the answer to this problem.

It should be pointed out that anorexic individuals also have this same problem of elevated reverse T3. In the case of a true malnutrition, starvation, or anorexia, we can understand the increase in reverse T3: the body is trying to slow down metabolism so that it does not waste away. However, why would a person who is fifty pounds overweight become stuck in a perceived state of starvation?

We have stated in chapter 39 that the cause of most thyroid problems is leptin resistance. In difficult metabolic situations, some aspect of the leptin resistance will not budge; in less difficult ones, following the *Five Rules*, exercise, and adequate sleep would have solved the problem.

THE CAUSE OF THE REVERSE T3 PROBLEM

It has been known since 1990 that TNFa causes an increase in reverse T3.[682] It has been known since 1996 that IL-6 causes an increase in reverse T3.[683] We are not saying TNFa and IL-6 simply coexist with the problem of elevated reverse T3; we are saying that science clearly proves TNFa and IL-6 actually cause elevated reverse T3.

In the case of true anorexia, the elevated reverse T3 comes from the inflammatory wasting process.

The great discovery of leptin and consequent scientific exploration into the structure of fat cells shows that fat cells produce IL-6 and TNFa. The more pounds of fat on hand, the greater the likelihood of excess production of these two pro-inflammatory immune signals.

Now we understand why overweight people can get stuck in a perceived state of starvation. It is due to excess production of TNFa and IL-6 coming from the extra pounds of fat on hand, a nasty Catch-22. If they do not lose the extra pounds of fat, the elevated reverse T3 problem does not go away. On the other hand, the elevated reverse T3 prevents them from losing the extra pounds of fat by locking in the leptin resistance and causing perceived starvation.

Before we explain how to solve this problem, it is worthwhile to understand the significance of reverse T3 to overall health.

REVERSE T3 – MORE THAN A WEIGHT-LOSS ISSUE

It is more expensive to determine reverse T3 on a blood test than it is to determine the basic thyroid scores normally evaluated. Testing for reverse T3 is not needed to determine primary hypothyroidism. Because it involves increased cost and is not needed in order to determine if a doctor should give a patient thyroid medication, it is not done as a matter of routine.

As it turns out, testing for reverse T3 may be one of the most useful tests a doctor can order in a routine health check. This fact has been pointed out to doctors in their literature for over twenty years.[684] It is certainly helpful in our understanding of the overweight person who is stuck in perceived starvation.

This lab test demonstrates to what degree a person is stuck at a weight-loss plateau due to perceived starvation. It is valuable for guidance in weight-loss issues, especially for those who have struggled with weight loss. However, it is much more than that.

We know that reverse T3 can be induced by stressful trauma. Being wheeled into an operating room for surgery can activate elevated reverse T3; this is in addition to the surgery itself.[685] Major stress trauma that involves elevated cortisol, including life stress, sets the stage for reverse T3. These are the "health turning points" in one's history.

Reverse T3 status is related to whether or not a person survives a heart attack.[686] The more elevated the reverse T3, the more likely it is that the person does not survive. The level of reverse T3 following a heart attack is related to the amount of cardiac damage.[687]

Another study was conducted with bone marrow transplant patients. These patients, unlike heart attack patients, could be tested for reverse T3 before the surgery as well as after. This information sheds light on the pre-existing nutritional status before stress, as well as the effects of the major stress itself. Researchers found that poor nutritional status prior to the operation, as determined by elevated reverse T3, and the failure of reverse T3 to return to a lower level following the operation, were the determining factors in who lived and who died.[688]

This information is of immense importance to society. It tells us that by managing the problem of elevated reverse T3, we can significantly improve any person's chances of survival. A person who does not have elevated reverse T3 prior to a trauma has a much better chance of surviving, because the energy-regulation systems in the body work more efficiently and have an appropriate energetic response to the emergency.

It is not surprising to find elevated reverse T3 occurring in various inflammatory conditions and issues of poor health during the aging process.[689] It is interesting to note that the anorexia of aging – that is, the deterioration of the body as one grows older – is associated with elevated reverse T3 and lower levels of active T3.

Elderly people on low-fat, low-energy diets are likely to enter self-induced perceived starvation-metabolism with low levels of active T3, increased reverse T3, and poor health.[690]

This is one more scientific fact which tells us that not eating enough calories for energy, including an appropriate amount of saturated fat, is counter-productive for the cardiovascular system. Rather than being a cardiovascular protective measure, it can create a low-energy, low-leptin environment that makes a person less likely to survive a heart attack.

Thus, we have two primary risk groups for cardiovascular disease. One is the over-nourished individual, stuck with leptin resistance, adrenaline resistance, and insulin resistance, otherwise known as metabolic syndrome X.[691] The other is the low-leptin malnourished individual, whose LDL cholesterol may be too low due to malnutrition, and who is in an inflammatory or progressive wasting pattern. This problem also occurs in the dieting person who gets stuck at a plateau and is in the anorexic-like starvation metabolism. A key cardiovascular-risk measurement is elevated reverse T3.

SOLVING PERCEIVED STARVATION

Solving the perceived-starvation problem requires a high degree of skill on the part of the *Health Asset Manager*. There are no shortcuts and there are many variables.

It is important to remember that there are degrees of this problem. The better the overall health and fitness of the person, the easier the problem is to solve. Gradually improving fitness over time is essential.

In addition to the *Five Rules*, consistent exercise, and adequate sleep, there are five important additional issues to work on in order to improve and solve the problem of perceived starvation.

1) Reduce TNFa and IL-6 levels, prime causes of the problem. Since there is no getting away from the extra pounds of fat that generate these signals, nutrients that help turn them off can be of great assistance. Virtually any nutrient that acts as an antioxidant or anti-inflammatory aids this situation (there are many).

2) Provide nutrition to help the stressed-out thyroid gland and to enhance the conversion of T4 to active T3. This includes nutrients such as selenium, manganese, tyrosine, iodine, and calcium.

3) Learn to more effectively manage stress and ensure that there is enough nutritional support to feel on top of stress. Stress is a trigger that sends people down the reverse T3 path. Elevated TNFa and IL-6 lock in this problem over time.

   However, people who are under constant stress, keep tilting their metabolism in the direction of elevated reverse T3, especially if there is a major stress event or an extended period of stress.

   If individuals are losing weight and the weight loss stops, they should look for changes in stress. This can be emotional stress or physical stress, such as an infection. They should also look at any changes in medications. These are common changes that interfere with the progression of weight loss.

   Nutrient support for stress requires extra antioxidants, B-vitamins, calcium, magnesium, zinc, coenzyme Q10, acetyl-l-carnitine, and other possible choices including immune-boosting nutrition. A person needs enough nutritional support to feel on top of stress.

4) Move stagnant calories out of the circulation. Under the influence of reverse T3, especially in overweight individuals, it is common for cholesterol and/or triglycerides to accumulate in the blood. It is like having trucks parked on a highway. These show up on a lab test.

   Rather than trying to suppress the production of cholesterol with a drug that has unpredictable effects on natural balance, we like to take the approach of hauling the stagnant fat into metabolic action.

   The best nutrients for this are pantethine, acetyl-l-carnitine, chromium, vanadium, and tocotrienols. Pantethine acts as an energetic carrier to move fat into action. Acetyl-l-carnitine improves the ability of cells to burn fat for fuel and helps the brain sense leptin more accurately. Chromium and vanadium help calories enter cells to help lower insulin resistance. Gamma tocotrienol helps slow down the excess production of cholesterol, training the liver into a better metabolic pattern and out of the bad habit of making too much cholesterol. Alpha tocotrienol protects the arteries from damage.

The net effect of these nutrients is to help natural metabolism clear the surplus of stagnant energy from the blood. Once this happens, it is a lot easier to get reverse T3 problems solved, as there is not so much "sludge" in the circulation.

5) Effectively manage all symptoms of fibromyalgia. Desired weight loss is not possible if the plumbing system gets backed up and the body is stuck in inflammatory pain. Toxins do not come out of fat if there is no place for them to go. Individuals who have fibromyalgia issues must address these issues as a priority.

Others encounter fibromyalgia-like issues as they try to lose fat that contains toxins. This is reflected in a distinct "poisoned," irritable, and possibly queasy feeling. Dark circles under the eyes appear. Headaches may also occur as part of this process.

Managing toxic symptoms is an important factor involved with weight-loss plateaus and losing the last five to ten pounds. This "core fat" is frequently the most toxic fat and the body has difficulty losing it.

We have provided extensive recommendations for this issue in chapter 40 on fibromyalgia.

A person in perceived starvation metabolism may have problems in any one or all five of these areas. Improving any one of them tends to improve the others. As overall fitness improves, all five areas tend to improve at the same time. Thus, the best that some may hope for is gradual improvement over time, corresponding to gradually improving fitness.

Addressing these areas can speed up weight loss and make weight loss possible for those prone to perceived starvation. How much any person must do is based on the result. Do enough to get into metabolic gear. Once in metabolic fat-burning mode, be thankful, and resist the temptation to get off a plan that is finally working.

SUMMARY

The hallmark of frustration with weight loss is hitting the perceived state of starvation. Some individuals are in this condition before they begin to lose weight. Others encounter it on a weight-loss plateau or when they get down to the last few stubborn pounds that do not want to leave the body.

If individuals get frustrated and throw away their good eating patterns and exercise habits, they will simply gain back excess weight and be miserable. Thus, we need solutions for perceived starvation.

The mystery of this problem has now been identified. It is an issue of elevated reverse T3 fueled by chronically elevated TNFa and IL-6. Stress, toxins, fibromyalgia, and a buildup of stagnant fat in the blood are issues that work against the situation and keep aggravating it.

The *Five Rules*, consistent exercise, and adequate sleep are the cornerstone solutions relating to leptin. In this chapter, we discussed five additional areas of nutritional support that may be needed. Our basic recommendations are capable of breaking a person out of perceived starvation and onto a path of better health.

Solving perceived starvation is a true test of the skills of a *Health Asset Manager*.

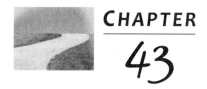

Leptin, NF kappaB,
and the Cause of Cancer

EXCESS LEPTIN is a primary cause of too much inflammation. Excess inflammation disrupts natural balance, or homeostasis, in the body. It can have a domino effect that may lead to virtually any disease; therefore, it is a general health issue of extreme importance. Extra pounds of fat are a pivotal factor in the quality of health.

New information uncovers the true significance of these discoveries. Leptin resistance leads to a situation that promotes major risk for cancer and numerous other diseases.

TNFa CAN BE FRIENDLY AND HELPFUL

So far we have portrayed TNFa as an enemy that generates inflammation. We also pointed out that TNFa is a needed signal in the response to stress. Additionally, we should point out that TNFa, also known as tumor necrosis factor alpha, is a main signal in the body that kills cancer cells. This is how it originally got its name. The word necrosis means death to a cell; thus, tumor necrosis means death to tumor cells. TNFa is a known factor that kills tumor cells. How can that be a bad thing?

The answer to this question goes back to our underlying themes. It is an issue of efficiency. When TNFa works properly, it helps regulate the immune response, the inflammatory response, the healing response, supports healthy pregnancy, and acts to knock out cancer. Timing is everything.

When TNFa is released at the right time for the right set of circumstances, it is part of the body's perfect system of natural balance. When TNFa is released continuously, due to excess fat pounds, the outcome of what it does is unpredictable. Instead of helping to kill cancer, it is unfortunately the case that excess TNFa causes cancer.

HOW TNFa LEADS TO CANCER

What determines if TNFa acts in a good way or in a cancer-causing way? Scientists have been studying this issue rather closely. In conducting experiments on cells that behaved differently in response to TNFa, it became clear that in cells leading to cancer progression, the TNFa activated a substance called granulocyte macrophage colony stimulating factor, GM-CSF.

GM-CSF is a growth factor that facilitates cellular growth, possibly to the point of being resistant to normal death mechanisms. If a cancer can hijack this mechanism in the human body, then it is extremely difficult, if not impossible, to kill. In an effective natural immune response the cancer cells that TNFa was killing do not generate any GM-CSF.[692]

Why does a cell generate excess amounts of GM-CSF that can perpetuate cancer and make it resistant to medical treatment? Answer: excess production of NF-kappaB.

HOW NF-KAPPAB DOES ITS JOB

NF-kappaB is the 911 switchboard of a cell's defense against stress. When a cell clicks along in a normal mode of healthy operation, then NF-kappaB is dormant, much like a 911 operator at the police department who is not getting any calls. NF-kappaB exists in every cell of the human body in this dormant state, when things run as expected.

Under the influence of a stressful irritant, NF-kappaB is activated. We are not talking about a simplistic biological mechanism. We are talking about a 911 activation system that has had millions of years of genetic evolution to deal with a great variety of stress. It can be chemical/pollution stress, infection stress, injury stress, or emotional stress. Literally, there can be a multitude of various stressors confronting a cell.

NF-kappaB goes to the DNA of the cell. It tells the DNA what proteins to make to fight the stress, so that the cell can survive. This is a complex activity, one we are only beginning to understand. For example, if it is a chemical stress, the cell has to figure out how to deactivate or detoxify the chemical before its gets stuck to the DNA and induces mutation. If it is a viral stress, the cell has to figure out how to kill the virus before it kills the cell.

Exactly what the cell should do to defend itself is commanded by NF-kappaB. NF-kappaB contains the genetic intelligence to deal with stress, as well as to adapt to new stress. The survival of any cell, and consequently the survival of the human body, is based on the efficient operation of NF-kappaB.

NF-kappaB also makes the tough decisions about who lives and who dies. Many of the activities of NF-kappaB include survival mechanisms so that a cell can withstand stress. In other words, there may be an emergency need to make cellular components or tissue in order to withstand the type of stress the cell experiences. Thus, GM-CSF can be made to help sustain body structure under duress. Once the duress is over, the need for extra GM-CSF decreases and NF-kappaB stops its production.

On the other hand, the cell may be overwhelmed by the type of stress it is experiencing. If a horribly malfunctioning cell mutates, it is likely to be in a cancerous form. Therefore, NF-kappaB has to decide at what point sustaining the cell life is no longer a good idea. NF-kappaB then initiates death signals that cause the cell to die, a situation known as apoptosis.

Thank goodness there are not a lot of politics involved with these decisions. They are tough life-and-death decisions. They are based on the potential ability of the individual cell to survive, but not at the cost of inducing damage to other cells. It is an incredibly complex and sophisticated defense system. When the body is in a state of natural balance, it works perfectly!

NF-KAPPAB AS THE CAUSE OF CANCER

In March 2002, researchers from the Department of Pharmacology, University of California, published a paper titled, NF-kappaB at the Crossroads of Life and Death.[693] In July 2001, researchers at the Harold Simmons Cancer Center, University of Texas Southwestern Medical Center, published a paper titled, Role of the NF-kappaB Pathway in the Pathogenesis of Human Disease States.[694] These studies show that scientists are aware that excess NF-kappaB is central to serious disease.

Cancer's goal is to survive while it destroys the human body. Cancer that is resistant to treatment has successfully hijacked NF-kappaB and is using the cell's own perfect defense system to perpetuate its own survival and to kill other cells. This is a major breakthrough in our understanding of the nature of cancer.

The issues going on at genetic levels are complex. An easy way to understand this is as follows:

1) There is a normal activation of NF-kappaB to deal with stress.
2) There is an abnormal constant elevation of NF-kappaB that exists in cancer situations, wherein the cancer has hijacked NF-kappaB and uses it to foster its own survival, while the cancer destroys the body.

A key mechanism that causes NF-kappaB to become elevated is the excess production of TNFa. Excess TNFa keeps generating other excess gene signals (Bcl-2, Bcl-x(L)), which then feed the excess production of NF-kappaB for no good reason other than the survival of cancer.[695]

TNFa, the substance that is supposed to help the body kill cancer cells, has turned traitor. It becomes the pivotal signal that causes NF-kappaB to be elevated, as well as the one that causes itself to continue excess production.[696,697]

NF-kappaB, in turn, uses the body's own antioxidant defense system to protect cancer cells from destruction by TNFa.[698] Furthermore, the excess NF-kappaB keeps producing GM-CSF, which makes the cancer resistant to the normal destruction by TNFa. This is completely upside-down and backwards from what should be happening.

Excess NF-kappaB is like a forest fire raging out of control. Once the forest fire is put out – meaning that the excess levels of NF-kappaB can be lowered back to normal – then TNFa starts working again to kill cancer instead of helping perpetuate cancer.[699,700,701]

Pancreatic cancer, a very resistant type of cancer, is an example of this excess NF-kappaB-driven issue.[702] It was recently discovered that suppressing NF-kappaB stops the progression of oral cancer.[703] Further, suppressing NF-kappaB makes cancer cells more susceptible to being killed by chemotherapy. This has recently been demonstrated with lung cancer.[704]

SUMMARY

The important point to understand is that the body's own defense system is being used against itself to perpetuate cancer. The exact mechanisms of how this works in all cancers are yet to be defined, but the overall picture is established.

A person's extra body fat generates excess amounts of TNFa. It is essential, as far as cancer is concerned, to have excess amounts of TNFa in order to generate excess amounts of NF-kappaB. Extra pounds of fat are a primary risk factor for developing cancer. This does not mean that all overweight people develop cancer; it simply means that they have a much higher risk.

A person with normal body weight can get cancer quite easily. For example, a smoker can be at any body weight and have an increased risk for cancer. The constant poisoning of the body with toxins causes excess inflammation and excess NF-kappaB production, leading to cell mutation and risk for any type of cancer. Lung cancer may develop that is resistant to treatment. Any type of excessive inflammatory condition, regardless of the individual's body weight, can increase the risk for cancer by constantly elevating NF-kappaB.

We talk more about leptin, NF-kappaB, and the cancer issue in chapter 46 and 47. This principle is a dominant theme in cancer, especially among those resistant to treatment. Solutions to this problem are key for improving the chances for a positive treatment outcome.

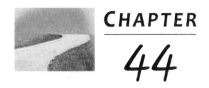

CHAPTER

44

Leptin, NF kappaB, and the Cause of Disease

IN THIS CHAPTER we discuss how leptin, TNFa, and NF-kappaB, when in a condition of excess, contribute to virtually all types of disease associated with the aging process. This is a general and far-reaching principle of health.

LIVER HEALTH

The liver is the metabolic factory of the body. Keeping it in excellent working order is of primary importance. Excess body weight leads to fatty liver issues, meaning the liver is infiltrated by excess amounts of fat that should not be there. These extra amounts of fat increase the production of TNFa.

Too much TNFa induces excess production of NF-kappaB, setting the stage for significant liver injury and liver damage.[705] This issue is further magnified when the body is exposed to pollution. Common pollution, such as air pollution, inducing specific excess production of NF-kappaB in the liver.[706]

The combined issues of extra body fat and exposure to common pollution cause a synergistic negative stress on the liver. With these issues, the rate of liver damage accelerates and the risk for liver cancer increases. Because every person in America is exposed to excess pollution and has no choice about the issue, the primary way to reduce this risk is to reduce body fat.

When a person consumes too much alcohol at any one time, liver cells are infiltrated with alcohol, causing NF-kappaB levels to rise.[707] How much alcohol the liver can tolerate before this happens varies from person to person.

MORE ON CARDIOVASCULAR HEALTH

The usefulness of NF-kappaB to help regulate stress and the problems of excess NF-kappaB in causing disease are definite factors in heart health. Both TNFa and NF-kappaB act to protect the heart from stress, just as they act to protect single cells from stress.[708,709] Therefore, if the body is in natural balance and is exposed to cardiovascular stress, TNFa and NF-kappaB behave in a healthy way and protect the heart from damage.

The endothelial lining is the Achilles' heel of the circulatory system. It is a "skin," or membrane, of cells. It acts as the buffer between what circulates in the blood and the structural walls of arteries, veins, and capillaries. The endothelial cells have a regulatory effect on blood pressure and many other aspects of circulatory function; they are not a passive structure. Damage to the endothelial-cell lining leads to plaque accumulation in the lining of arteries, which eventually leads to cardiovascular disease.

It has been known since 1999 that elevated leptin in your circulation, as in the case of the leptin-resistant individual, induces excess production of free radicals. These damage the endothelial lining of the circulatory system, thereby triggering plaque accumulation and setting the stage for cardiovascular disease. Part of the damaging free-radical process involves the excess production of NF-kappaB.[710]

Around the same time as this discovery, other researchers proved that inflammation leading to plaque formation involved excess production of TNFa and NF-kappaB.[711] Both studies show that these issues can be reversed with antioxidants.

There is no question that excess inflammation is a prime cause of plaque accumulation. There is also no question that leptin resistance tilts the entire body into a more pro-inflammatory condition. Excess

NF-kappaB is at the core of this issue, in terms of how much plaque forms. It is the prime causative mechanism behind the excess clotting that leads to a heart attack or stroke.[712]

Even in medical settings, the value of this new information may soon be put to advantageous use. For example, when an individual has balloon angioplasty, the entire endothelial lining is stripped and damaged. This is an unfortunate side effect of calling in a plumber to clean out a clogged artery. In this emergency medical situation, it is essential to open up the clogged artery so that blood can flow.

The fact that the artery wall is damaged in the process is undesirable, but it is viewed to be not as important as the clogged artery. After the operation, in a relatively short period of time, it is common for the artery to clog again, an issue called restenosis. This happens in large part because of the injury caused by the medical procedure. Animal experiments show that suppressing the production of NF-kappaB can prevent the artery from clogging after surgery.[713]

We are back to our bottom-line issue. NF-kappaB is essential for survival and defending the body against stress. Too much NF-kappaB causes excess inflammation and progression of cardiovascular disease. Extra pounds of fat cause excess TNFa. This in turn stimulates the excess NF-kappaB which led to the problem. Extra body weight is therefore a major cause of cardiovascular disease.

ALZHEIMER'S AND MENTAL DECLINE

NF-kappaB is essential to the healthy function of the human brain. It is involved with the survival of brain cells, especially when brain cells are exposed to some type of stress.[714]

It should come as no surprise that excess production of NF-kappaB is a prime cause of Alzheimer's and mental decline.[715]

An out-of-control inflammatory situation in the brain is at the root of Alzheimer's and cognitive decline. This is confirmed by the evidence that excess amounts of TNFa and other inflammatory markers are all elevated in these conditions, along with the excess amount of NF-kappaB.[716,717,718,719]

These studies show that this is not a trivial side issue which results from Alzheimer's. Rather, this is a causative issue related to the severity and risk of death from Alzheimer's. In centenarians, those who have the most cognitive decline have the highest amount of circulating TNFa.[720]

Further, extra fat in the diet raises the deposition of the brain-plaque forming Apo E, in direct proportion to extra body weight.[721] High levels of Apo E are a primary risk factor for developing Alzheimer's disease.

While being overweight does not necessarily cause Alzheimer's, it certainly tilts body chemistry in the direction of risk for the disease, especially in people with a genetic predisposition to the problem.

A recent study with dogs demonstrated that air pollution activates all the above inflammatory factors and leads to changes in the brain consistent with Alzheimer's disease.[722] Similarly, exposure to aluminum produces the same elevation of NF-kappaB and TNFa, leading to damaged brain cells.[723] Exposure to lead, methyl mercury, and aluminum are known to cause developmental issues in children and brain disease in the elderly.[724]

Alzheimer's is predicted to be a major health epidemic as the baby-boom population ages. The cost to society will be staggering. There will be no easy cure for Alzheimer's. Worldwide pollution must be curtailed as a priority. If this is not accomplished, any person who is overweight and/or genetically at risk is likely to get Alzheimer's or significant cognitive decline as they age.

ARTHRITIS

Excess amounts of leptin increase the amount of immune cells that attack joints, otherwise referred to as rheumatoid arthritis.[725] Excess amounts of TNFa and NF-kappaB are present in rheumatoid arthritis and multiple sclerosis, as causative factors of the problems.[726,727]

Feverfew is an herb that has been used traditionally to help arthritis and migraine headaches. The active component of this herb, parthenolide, is proven to work by lowering NF-kappaB, which reduces inflammation.[728,729,730] The herb is highly effective at getting straight to the gene signal causing the problem.

These findings are spurring other research into parthenolide, including cancer prevention and treatment. Parthenolide can change the way human leukemia cells progress, so that the cells are changed into normal monocytes instead of cancer. This is done by altering the NF-kappaB gene signal.[731]

Parthenolide also helps reduce the activity of breast-cancer cells and makes them more susceptible to be being killed by cancer drugs. Once again, this is due to parthenolide's ability to lower NF-kappaB.[732]

Interestingly, parthenolide is able to differentiate between appropriate cell death, as in helping to kill cancer cells, and inappropriate cell death. It has been shown to turn off inappropriate signaling of NF-kappaB that causes T cells to be killed when they should not be.[733]

VIRAL INFECTIONS

Being sick with the flu is bad enough. Now we have to start looking at the effect of low-grade and chronic viral infections on our health. Everyone in America is exposed to a variety of viral infections; most are cousins and best friends of each other.

Many individuals suffer from low-grade viral activity on a regular basis. Some have more recognizable viral syndromes. Others are simply prone to catching bugs easily and get sore throats often, including waking up in the morning with them.

Numerous studies in the last two years are making a viral-cancer connection. From a cell's point of view, a viral invasion is a form of stress. This activates NF-kappaB, as would any initial stress. Chronic viral infections learn to coexist inside of cells, literally hijacking cells and altering their genetic function.[734] Unfortunately, the viruses specifically stimulate the excess production of NF-kappaB.[735]

Considerable evidence for this is mounting:

1) Hepatitis B and C both excessively raise NF-kappaB, leading to increased risk for liver cancer. Several labs around the world re-

cently confirmed the Hepatitis C and cancer connection[736] involving elevated NF-kappaB.[737,738] In a like manner, several other labs confirmed the Hepatitis B and cancer connection.[739,740]

2) The Epstein Barr Virus (EBV) activates NF-kappaB in lymph cells, causing lymphoma.[741]

3) Human T-cell leukemia virus type I is the cause of adult T-cell leukemia/lymphoma. It is activated by excess NF-kappaB production.[742,743]

4) Human papillomavirus (HPV), a commonly sexually transmitted viral infection that can lead to cervical cancer, actively promotes excess NF-kappaB.[744]

5) The Kaposi's sarcoma herpes virus induces problems by excessively activating NF-kappaB.[745]

Mounting a more efficient immune response against viruses and not getting so run down that viral issues flare up are key factors in cancer-risk reduction. It is evident that if a person is overweight and has extra leptin, TNFa, and NF-kappaB already circulating, then a viral infection has an easier time because it is hijacking a defense system that is already handicapped.

SOLUTIONS

Making sure one's body is in a less inflammatory condition is the fundamental way to prevent problems with excess NF-kappaB. Following the *Five Rules*, getting regular exercise, managing stress, and maintaining optimum body weight are keys to reducing risk for disease. Adopting a lifestyle conducive to healthy rhythms and feeling in sync is essential.

As a person gets into higher levels of ongoing inflammation and wear and tear, there is a concurrent excess production of TNFa and NF-kappaB. If a person is overweight, the fat cells make this problem worse by generating increased amounts of these signals into the body, on top of other stress factors.

Excess TNFa and NF-kappaB problems reflect a general lack of antioxidants, as NF-kappaB sits underneath the antioxidant system.

Improved antioxidant status is likely to cool down the tendency toward excess NF-kappaB production. This is why a variety of antioxidants, such as vitamin E, show improvement for issues such as Alzheimer's.[746] Having enough antioxidants prevents toxins from inducing liver damage. They do this by helping to prevent excess NF-kappaB.[747] Even getting enough vitamin C can help reduce TNFa and NF-kappaB.[748]

While antioxidants alone may not fully solve an NF-kappaB problem, they are the first line of defense. The more "antioxidant reserves" individuals have, the greater their ability to tolerate issues that would otherwise lead to excessive production of NF-kappaB. A comprehensive array of basic antioxidant nutrients is helpful for everyone, specifically for the prevention of disease. Even the *Journal of the American Medical Association* agrees with this fundamental recommendation for disease prevention.[749]

In chapters 46 and chapter 47, on breast and prostate cancer, we list additional nutrients that have powerful NF-kappaB regulating effects. These apply not only to cancer issues; they apply to offsetting the wear and tear of life as well. The greater the degree of stressful wear and tear a person experiences, the greater the need for protection. This is not hard to figure out. Use enough support to stay in balance, in sync, and keep up with the demands of life.

SUMMARY

Excess leptin causes many problems relating to body weight and the ability to attain and maintain a proper body weight.

Additionally, excess leptin is a major risk factor for disease. This is because it raises and reinforces the excess production of TNFa and NF-kappaB. Carrying extra pounds of body fat that cranks out these inflammatory signals is a major risk factor for any disease. Whether individuals get cancer, heart disease, Alzheimer's, or some disease depends on genetic risk as well as on other stress factors that contribute to their health picture.

Antioxidants form the first line of defense against stress-related generation of excess NF-kappaB. Those who have been advocating antioxidants for years, based on their ability to deactivate free radicals, now have far more powerful scientific information to back up their use. Antioxidants are the primary bank account of natural compounds that act as a buffer for the tolerance of stress. When the buffer is lacking or is used up by too much stress, then excess activation of the panic-stricken NF-kappaB can wreak havoc with health.

The jigsaw puzzle of who gets what and why, as well as how to exactly solve the problems of disease, will foster the great scientific discoveries of this century. Meanwhile, it is apparent that reducing body fat to a healthy level and keeping the body in a state of natural balance are the keys to disease-free aging.

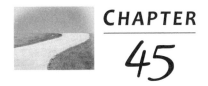

CHAPTER 45

A Major Breakthrough for Bones

PROPERLY FUNCTIONING LEPTIN is essential for the formation and health of bones. It is a primary hormone that must work properly for bone health.

Drug companies want to have a drug for everything. They see a big market in bone-loss issues, in which drugs are used for prevention. Current drugs to help prevent bone loss have adverse side effects and are not even directed at the real issue – making new bone. They only address a secondary factor in bone loss. A recent scientific article seeking to promote new areas for bone-loss drug design stated the following about current bone-loss drugs:

These drugs have been identified by serendipity rather than rational drug design and are not ideal because of limited bioavailability, mode of administration, or other unwanted effects. There is still a place for even more suitable and effective resorption inhibitors than those currently available. The more compelling need in this field is an acceptable drug that is anabolic for bone, that safely and acceptably increases bone mass, and improves the disturbances in bone microarchitecture that characterize established and advanced osteoporosis.[750]

As it turns out, leptin fits the description of this ideal drug. A primary factor in bone health is to maintain leptin in good working order and to avoid leptin resistance and having too little leptin.

STARVATION METABOLISM AND BONE LOSS

Underweight women are prone to osteopenia and osteoporosis.[751] It is documented that underweight women lose significant bone.[752] Bone loss can occur during dieting as leptin levels drop, a more significant issue for older women.[753,754] This is one reason why proper leptin management and following the *Five Rules* is so important.

Bone loss occurs when the anorexic-like starvation metabolism is present. It accelerates in the presence of excess inflammation of any type.

LEPTIN HELPS BONE WORK PROPERLY

Healthy bones are a more complex issue than simply the amount of bone mass. Leptin is involved with the healthy workings of bone metabolism. Leptin is involved with the formation of blood cells, both red cells and white cells. This activity takes place inside of bones.[755] Leptin acts as a powerful hormone inside of bone which stimulates the formation of new bone.[756]

In fact, not only does leptin act inside of bones to help make bone, recent information shows that when leptin binds to the hypothalamus gland in the brain, it facilitates the gland to initiate new bone formation.[757,758] Omega 3 fatty acids are essential for this leptin-regulated bone building to take place.[759]

HOW BONE BUILDING WORKS

There are two main types of cells in bone that act to repair and build bone; osteoblasts and osteoclasts. Osteoclasts work by taking down old bone or stressed bone. Essentially, this is demolition work. Osteoblasts work by building up new bone. They take raw materials, such as protein and calcium, and construct bone.

Proper bone health involves a synergistic balance between osteoclasts and osteoblasts. As older or stressed bone is removed, new bone is built in its place. This process goes on throughout life.

Problems occur when factors speed up the rate of bone loss or when there is difficulty making new bone.

The current bone-loss drugs are targeted at osteoclasts, hoping to slow down the rate at which bone is removed. This may slow down inappropriate bone loss, but it does not solve the problem of building new bone or the problem of why bone loss accelerates. Such medications are second-rate, temporary solutions.

As we have mentioned above, leptin is the key hormonal signal that works on bone as well as coordinates a signal from the brain to build bone. Leptin is the key anabolic hormone for bone building, helping osteoblasts to form new bone.

This is why starvation metabolism causes bone loss. Bone is not made fast enough because there is not enough leptin to help stimulate the formation of new bone.

INFLAMMATION AND BONES

A number of factors cause the loss of bone to accelerate in the first place. These factors speed up the rate at which osteoclasts take down bone. They fall under the general umbrella of stress and inflammation, issues we have discussed throughout this book.

A large body of scientific evidence shows that excess IL-6, TNFa, and NF-kappaB speed up the activity of osteoclasts, causing bone to be lost at an excessive rate.[760,761,762,763,764]

Vitamin D helps bones by protecting the bone-building cells, osteoblasts, from inappropriate cell death.[765] However, excess TNFa and NF-kappaB block the ability of vitamin D to protect osteoblasts, leading to excess osteoblast cell death.[766] These inflammatory signals interfere with bone building and at the same time accelerate bone loss.

SOLUTIONS FOR HEALTHY BONES

Tocotrienols, a special form of vitamin E, help improve bone mineral density.[767] Unlike regular vitamin E, tocotrienols work by lowering excess TNFa and NF-kappaB, the true source of the accelerated bone loss.

Another important nutrient is magnesium. A lack of magnesium causes depressed osteoblast bone building and accelerated osteoclast bone loss. It has been shown that with a lack of magnesium, growth plate of bone decreased thirty-three percent, indicating a lack of bone building. At the same time, TNFa activity inside of osteoclasts increased up to five hundred percent of normal. The lack of magnesium permits excessive inflammation in the bone, a problem that prevents calcium from building bone.[768]

The results of a four-year study with adults ranging in age from sixty-nine to ninety-seven confirmed the value of magnesium, potassium, fruits, and vegetables in the diet in terms of significantly helping preserve bone mass in these older individuals.

This study also laid to rest one of the oldest arguments among nutritionists; that is, is dietary protein good or bad for bone? Researchers thought that too much protein would be bad for bone because it would cause an acid pH, which would work against the alkalizing minerals, fruits, and vegetables. Much to their surprise, they found that higher protein consumption facilitated better bone density.[769]

This result is not at all surprising to us. For years, we have told our clients the value of protein to help build bone.

Strength-bearing exercise helps bones because it applies stress to bones, in essence promoting them to break down so they can be built up. It is based on the common principle, "if you do not use it, you lose it." This strategy works well only if a person has the energetic and nutritional capacity to repair bone and form new bone. This includes adequate dietary protein.

SUMMARY

Building healthy bone requires the proper activity of bone-building hormones, cells, and nutrients. These are the anabolic bone-building factors. They include proper function of the hormone leptin and various nutrients such as calcium, vitamin D, omega 3 fatty acids, and protein.

Maintaining bone requires an absence of inflammation, which interferes with bone building and accelerates bone loss. Nutrients proven to specifically help this issue are magnesium, tocotrienols, and alkalizing fruits and vegetables.

There are many nutrient suggestions throughout this book that help reduce excess inflammation. There are also numerous lifestyle and dietary tips to reduce stress and inflammation. A person needs to do enough to get out of the wear-and-tear trend. The inflammatory wear-and-tear trend is the actual cause of accelerated bone loss.

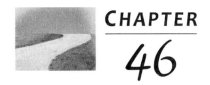

CHAPTER

46

Leptin, NF kappaB
and Prostate Cancer

RESEARCHERS, at this point, have found that insulin resistance is more predictive than are leptin levels of significantly increased risk for prostate cancer.[770] This is consistent with how insulin resistance coexists with problems of excess IGF1. It is excess IGF1 that helps fuel the production of prostate cancer. We explained this mechanism in chapter 34 on growth hormone.

However, a close analysis of prostate-cancer cells shows that they have active leptin receptors in them. Furthermore, it may require only moderate levels of excess leptin to stimulate prostate cancer.[771] The more advanced and aggressive the prostate cancer is, the higher the level of leptin fueling its growth.[772]

We know that leptin resistance and insulin resistance work together to generate excess amounts of TNFa and NF-kappaB. We have explained that cancer which is resistant to medical therapy shows excess production of NF-kappaB. This is certainly true of prostate cancer.[773,774,775,776,777]

Studies show that excess NF-kappaB activity is the mechanism that makes prostate cancer resistant to treatment. Furthermore, it is not a passive factor that happens to be occurring at the same time as prostate cancer. It is the prime cause.

NF-KAPPAB CAUSES TESTOSTERONE PROBLEMS
On a cellular basis, NF-kappaB means survival. On a male-body basis,

the hormone testosterone means survival. In prostate cancer, even in cancer that does not require testosterone for growth, testosterone is used to make the cancer resistant to death.[778] The mechanism that enables this hijacking of testosterone to work against a man is the improperly elevated level of NF-kappaB.

The level of severity and invasiveness of prostate cancer is related to how much excess NF-kappaB there is. The greater the amount of NF-kappaB, the more severe the cancer.[779] Additionally, if NF-kappaB is blocked, then the prostate cancer stops growing and spreading.[780]

It is recognized that excess NF-kappaB causes excess TNFa and IL-6, the two classic excess immune signals coming from fat cells that are in higher circulation due to leptin resistance. Once the NF-kappaB is knocked down, the TNFa and IL-6 go down. This makes a previously untreatable disease susceptible to treatment.[781]

The bottom line of any prostate cancer, and especially prostate cancer that cannot be stopped, is a hijacking of testosterone by NF-kappaB and excessive NF-kappaB, that is used by the cancer to aid its own survival. The two most important survival systems in the male body have been turned against the body.

This opens the door to new solutions never before possible, focusing on reducing NF-kappaB so that cancer can be killed. For example, researchers have demonstrated that a deficiency of zinc enables excess production of NF-kappaB and prostate cancer. When zinc is replenished, the excess NF-kappaB decreases. The cancer cells that were resistant to medical drugs are now susceptible to being killed by medical drugs.[782]

RISK FACTORS FOR PROSTATE CANCER

There are a variety of irritants that can induce excess NF-kappaB in the prostate. They include estrogenic chemicals in the food supply, pollution, fungal infections, excess alcohol consumption, among others. There may be a combination of irritants that set the stage for wear and tear and create a situation in which NF-kappaB increases excessively.

As we mentioned above, there is evidence linking leptin resistance to the severity of prostate cancer. While it is certainly possible to contract prostate cancer from factors other than leptin, leptin resistance creates a situation that seriously weakens the male body and sets the stage for prostate cancer. This leptin-resistance situation is a prime risk factor for a great majority of American men.

Leptin resistance causes excess fat to form around internal body organs, including the prostate gland. This excess fat generates pro-inflammatory immune signals, TNFa and IL-6. The excess fat also reduces normal circulation to the prostate, tilting the pH of the prostate to a more acidic condition in which infections can thrive and healthy enzymes do not work correctly.

These inflammatory immune signals also ramp up NF-kappaB, causing it to be overactive on a continuous basis, a chemistry issue essential for cancer to prosper. The excess leptin also depresses testosterone, causing a weakness in the male system. Throw in some environmental-toxin irritants, and we have a recipe for problems.

NATURAL OPTIONS

A key to preventing prostate cancer and maintaining optimum male function is to keep the body in overall natural balance. The most fundamental issues in this regard are eating properly and exercise. This is the foundation of a healthy program for anyone and the cornerstone of a treatment plan for those with a health problem.

We previously raised the issue of what the minimum daily need is for various nutrients. We proposed that needs are based on functional results. Thus, there may be a need for supplemental nutrients that enable the body to maintain optimum weight loss or even to initiate the possibility of weight loss.

While such nutrients are often beyond what is needed to prevent basic nutritional deficiencies – for example, vitamin C to prevent scurvy – specific nutrients may be essential to help a person overcome leptin resistance. This need varies from person to person.

What about the nutritional needs of someone who is at high risk for prostate cancer or who has prostate cancer?

In the preventive sense, there are two ways to look at this. One way is to use nutrition to help correct leptin resistance and insulin resistance, in turn, lowering the risk factor for the problem. The other way is to use nutrition to lower NF-kappaB.

Traditional cancer therapy does not work on resistant cancer cells because of excess NF-kappaB. Nutritional support is one of the most effective and side-effect-free ways to lower NF-kappaB.

Nature has already provided answers. The scientific evidence is clear that nutritional supplements can lower NF-kappaB and thereby make cancer cells more susceptible to being killed. We have already mentioned the importance of zinc. In this chapter, we have talked specifically about prostate cancer; however, this information applies to any type of cancer.

In a scientific review of over eighty case-controlled studies, it was demonstrated that the greater the amount of cruciferous vegetables in the diet, the lower the risk for cancer. The proposed mechanism of action is the I3C (Indole-3-carbinol) content of the cruciferous vegetables and its effect on detoxification and estrogen metabolism.[783]

Eating three half-cup servings of cruciferous vegetables per week cuts the risk of prostate cancer by forty-one percent.[784] Even eating a small amount helps, and it is clear that more is better. New research shows that I3C helps to induce cell death in cancer cells.[785] Part of the mechanism is a reduction in NF-kappaB. This led the researchers to conclude that "I3C may be an effective chemo preventive or therapeutic agent against prostate cancer."[786]

Another promising nutrient is curcumin, a natural spice. Curcumin can directly turn off NF-kappaB in hormone-sensitive and hormone-independent types of prostate cancer, leading to the death of prostate-cancer cells.[787] A recent study showed that curcumin made prostate cancer cells more susceptible to being killed. This enabled chemotherapy to work when before it could not. This led researchers to conclude that "the incorporation of curcumin into cytotoxic therapies may be a promising strategy for the treatment of androgen-independent prostate cancer."[788]

Other nutrient strategies are also backed by solid science. Silymarin, an herb we mentioned for liver support, has the ability to lower NF-kappaB and cause prostate-cancer cells to become susceptible to medical treatment. Researchers conclude, "These results indicate that silibinin, the active component of silymarin, can be used to enhance the effectiveness of TNFalpha-based chemotherapy in advanced prostate cancer."[789]

Another nutrient, NAC (N-acetyl-cysteine) is known to suppress NF-kappaB. Scientists recently reported that it can be an effective compound for helping chemotherapy to work more effectively during prostate-cancer treatment.[790]

When it comes to prostate cancer, or any cancer, for that matter, there is no longer any reason for nutritional and drug therapies to be at odds with each other. Nutritional supplements not only excel at reducing risk for individuals living with extra pounds of fat, they can also make a medical treatment work that would otherwise have little or no chance of succeeding.

SUMMARY

Leptin resistance and extra body fat are important risk factors that cause wear and tear to the male system, weakening it and setting the stage for prostate cancer risk.

Taking effective steps to clear leptin resistance and lose unneeded body weight are at the forefront of quality of life for any man.

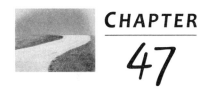

CHAPTER

47

Leptin, NF kappaB
and Breast Cancer

IT WAS REPORTED in 1999 that leptin activity is present in breast-cancer cells.[791] There was a report in 2000 showing that patients with breast cancer were found to have higher circulating leptin and TNFa.[792] Another 2000 study also confirmed higher circulating leptin correlating to higher breast cancer in premenopausal women.[793]

Studies in 2002 distinctly characterized leptin as a growth promoter of breast cancer. One study, using human breast-cancer MCF-7 cells, showed that leptin fueled the growth of this type of breast-cancer cell.[794] In another study, with cells from twenty breast-cancer biopsies, all twenty were found to have active leptin activity.

Additionally, this study showed that leptin significantly fueled the growth of another breast-cancer cell line, T47-D.[795] The most recent study shows that high leptin and high blood sugar, due to insulin resistance, fuel breast-cancer cell growth.[796] It is clear that leptin activity is associated with breast cancer, and that leptin activity fuels the growth of breast cancer.

This information does not prove that leptin causes breast cancer; it simply means that leptin is involved in the process. Since leptin is essential for reproduction and is associated with fat, leptin will always be present in breast tissue. A key question becomes, at what point does leptin shed its helpful role and start becoming a life-threatening problem?

NF-KAPPAB AND BREAST CANCER

Excess and ongoing NF-kappaB activation must be present for breast cancer to occur.[797] For example, breast cells can induce cell death in themselves if they start to become cancerous. If a mutant breast cell escapes self-imposed death, then it can go on to cause cancer.

What enables breast cancer to occur is excessive and ongoing production of NF-kappaB. This is what makes breast cancer resistant to normal body checks and balances. It is also what makes breast cancer resistant to drug treatment.[798]

It is unlikely that we will ever discover a single irritant that causes breast cancer. There are many estrogenic chemicals in the environment that can easily bind to breast cells and induce extra NF-kappaB activation. Too much emotional distress activates excess NF-kappaB. So does physical wear and tear. Insulin resistance leads to excess IGF1, in turn stimulating the growth of breast-cancer cells. Combine this with higher estrogens and higher leptin associated with higher body fat, and/or a certain time in a woman's life, and we have an overall situation that can tilt the body into chronic NF-kappaB activation. It is not one issue; it is a combination of factors that disrupted natural balance.

Some women have better genetic tolerance for these issues and never have a problem. Other women have poor genetic tolerance and are more susceptible to problems even from lower amounts of "stressors." Therefore, family history is a predictive factor in a woman's genetic ability to control NF-kappaB.

Regardless of genetic predisposition, keeping leptin in natural balance is a key way to reduce risk factors associated with breast cancer.

A COMMENT ON TAMOXIFEN

Tamoxifen is a favored drug used to suppress estrogen activity following breast cancer. The hope is that it will stop breast cancer from returning by reducing estrogenic activity in breast tissue. On the surface, this argument sounds reasonable. A closer look, based on new information, raises doubts regarding the safety of the drug.

It was found that Tamoxifen raises the production of leptin from fat cells, with a steady increase during the first six months of use. Twenty-one out of the thirty women in the study also experienced an increase in body fat as a result of the treatment.[799]

In a study comparing fifty-eight women who had breast cancer to fifty-eight women who did not, it was found that the cancer patients had higher leptin levels. Furthermore, within the cancer-patient group, those taking Tamoxifen had higher levels of leptin than those not taking Tamoxifen. This was true even after correcting for body fat. The researchers concluded, "high-serum leptin levels seen in breast-cancer patients are not related to the stage of the disease or to cancer itself but may be associated with the use of Tamoxifen."[800]

This information is alarming because a drug that elevates leptin levels promotes leptin resistance. In turn, this can increase inflammation and NF-kappaB anywhere in the body. This has the net effect of increasing general cancer risk.

We have already explained that leptin resistance promotes insulin resistance. Women with insulin resistance are much more likely to get a recurrence of breast cancer than women who do not have insulin resistance.[801]

Tamoxifen increases fatty congestion in the liver, a primary problem of leptin resistance. We have discussed the nature of fatty liver problems, including the magnification of liver damage from toxic exposure. The problem goes away when the drug is stopped.[802]

Tamoxifen causes abnormal estrogenic cell metabolism on the endometrial lining of the uterus.[803] The initial results of a major Tamoxifen study have been released. Notable side effects of the therapy include endometrial cancer, vaginal bleeding and discharge, cerebrovascular events, venous thromboembolic events, and hot flashes.[804]

This is a typical situation in which the medical profession feels that the benefits outweigh the risks. More pointedly, the drug has numerous adverse side effects, but it is going to be recommended until there is a more effective drug to sell, which is likely to be years away.[805]

Unlike the drug trial that halted the widespread use of estrogen replacement, it is unlikely that the use of Tamoxifen will be halted until there is a better drug. Tamoxifen has a degree of workability, and thus there is a degree of justification for its use. However, it only moderately addresses one potential cause of breast-cancer recurrence. It also has many side effects, some very serious. In terms of the numbers game played by medical statisticians, continued use can be rationalized. What this means to the health of an individual taking the drug is not so clear.

THE MOMENTUM FOR A NEW APPROACH

There is adequate science already available to put a variety of nutritional supplements to rigorous medical testing. Most of these nutrients have very few, if any, adverse side effects. The nutrients can be used in combination with Tamoxifen and other breast-cancer treatments. In some cases they may work better, which needs more clarification.

What follows is a significant array of compelling information that is sure to open new doors for breast-cancer risk reduction. It will also lend a hand in helping medical doctors more effectively treat breast cancer, as well as help prevent a recurrence of the problem.

An individual reading this book will understand that reducing excess inflammation is a good idea. However, think twice before reaching for a bottle of acetaminophen. Acetaminophen increases the growth of breast-cancer cells by forty percent, specifically due to increased production of NF-kappaB.[806]

Tocotrienols, a special form of vitamin E, have powerful anti-proliferative and cancer-cell killing capability, an ability that regular vitamin E (d alpha tocopherol) does not have.[807] Numerous cell studies show the ability of tocotrienols to reduce the spreading of breast-cancer cells or to knock them out.[808,809,810,811]

Unlike Tamoxifen, tocotrienols can block both estrogen-receptor positive and estrogen-receptor negative breast-cancer cells. When tocotrienols are combined with Tamoxifen, there is synergistic benefit.[812,813] Tocotrienols have a far superior advantage over regular vitamin E because they are much better at lowering TNFa and NF-kappaB.[814]

Green tea is a natural option to reduce both TNFa and NF-kappaB.[823] Green tea modulates, in a positive manner, genetic signals that otherwise lead to an excess production of NF-kappaB in breast-cancer cells.[824] Therefore, green tea has the ability to help the body kill cancerous breast cells, while leaving healthy breast cells undamaged.[825]

Trans-resveratrol, a powerful antioxidant found in some red wines and available as a nutritional supplement, binds to estrogen receptors in breast tissue and interferes with cancer.[826] Scientists have proven that resveratrol works by reducing NF-kappaB, thereby stopping the breast-cancer activity.[827] There is plenty of science to show that resveratrol is a highly protective nutrient and against breast cancer.[828,829,830,831]

The bioflavonoid quercetin, found in fresh vine-ripened fruit and available as a nutritional supplement, induces death in breast-cancer cells.[832] Quercetin has been shown to prevent environmental chemicals from promoting estrogen driven breast cancer.[833]

Interestingly, quercetin is shown to be more effective than Tamoxifen at binding to type II EBS receptors. The same study also shows it to be very effective at stopping the progression of a human breast-cancer cell line.[834] There is data to support the use of quercetin and Tamoxifen together, helping to synergistically make cancer more susceptible to medical treatment.[835]

Indole-3-carbinol (I3C) is the active component of cruciferous vegetables, mentioned in our discussion of prostate cancer. Several studies conducted in the early 1990s demonstrated that 400 milligrams of I3C per day in women can normalize the way estrogen is metabolized, so that it will not go down a pathway that could stimulate cancer.[836,837,838]

When researchers injected I3C directly into breast-cancer cells, I3C halted the cancer-cell division by blocking cancer-cell DNA duplication.[839] This led to another study, to explore whether the I3C was as effective as Tamoxifen. Researchers injected one group of human breast-cancer cells with I3C, another group with Tamoxifen, and a third with I3C and Tamoxifen. The cells injected with Tamoxifen alone experienced a sixty percent inhibition in DNA synthesis, the cells injected with I3C had a ninety percent inhibition, and the combination had a ninety-five percent reduction.[840]

If there were drugs that could knock out NF-kappaB, while leaving healthy cells alone, they would be the "gold standard" of cancer treatment and heralded on the front page of every paper and magazine as the greatest breakthrough ever made for the treatment of cancer. The fact that nature already provides a wide array of such substances should be of more than passing interest, even to the worst skeptic.

Adequate science now exists for any women to incorporate special nutritional support as part of a breast-cancer risk-reduction program or to assist in a positive outcome of medical treatment. This use of nutrition goes a good deal beyond basic nutritional needs. This is nutritional use based on the most recent genetic discoveries relating to how natural function turns against the individual.

This data shows that reducing NF-kappaB slows down cancer and makes cancer that is resistant to medical treatment much more responsive to medical treatment. This is accomplished by restoring a normal gene signal back into a state of balance. Because these nutrients do not have adverse side effects, there is good reason for consumers and medical professionals to gain a better working understanding of these nutrients in actual practice.

SUMMARY

Leptin is essential for female health, reproduction, and proper estrogen balance. Problems with leptin cause problems in the female system, including increased risk for breast cancer.

Leptin resistance leads to an inflammatory condition of excess TNFa and NF-kappaB, increasing cancer risk and the potential for cancer that is not responsive to medical treatment.

Mastering leptin is the answer to this problem.

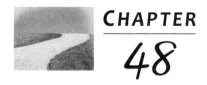

The Anti-Aging Skills of the Health Asset Manager™

IT TAKES A CONSIDERABLE AMOUNT of skill and personal knowledge about the human body to be a competent *Health Asset Manager*. It takes an additional level of personal strength and integrity to make daily choices to keep oneself on track and in a healthy pattern.

The *Five Rules* are the key points about how to eat in order to have a good energy level and avoid developing problems with leptin resistance.

Our emphasis is on establishing an entire lifestyle that facilitates a condition of natural balance. When people have a good underlying base of healthy habits, they have much more potential to tolerate stress, perform at a higher level of efficiency, and have an overall higher quality of health.

Leptin is a hormone signal relating to long-term survival. A program for mastering leptin must, by definition, be a program for the long haul. This means a way of approaching life in which true success is measured not only by the ability to overcome acute challenges but also by the true quality of health as years go by.

Individuals need a basic way to approach life that facilitates this result. The *Five Rules* are not a diet plan to follow for a few weeks in order to drop a few pounds only to return to previous poor habits. Those who implement the *Five Rules* as a way of life will have a tremendous advantage in maintaining their health.

Relaxing exercise, adequate sleep, and good stress-management skills are other key factors essential to the basic leptin-management plan.

In essence, mastering leptin is an issue of managing energy. If the body gets out of balance, the subconscious brain may enforce misguided survival instincts. This leads to weight gain and other health issues.

The far-reaching impact of leptin on all hormones is a significant health breakthrough. Leptin is the single most important hormone in the body. Although leptin was not discovered until 1994, what first seemed like a key hormone that regulated the response to starvation soon became the superstar of hormones. Leptin is in control; all other hormones answer to leptin. Leptin is the energy broker for the body, literally providing the financial energy to make metabolism work.

It takes considerable skill to manage leptin effectively. If done well, a person's health will benefit dramatically. Serious issues with leptin resistance, including obesity, sex-hormone issues, weight gain around the middle, fatty liver disease, addiction problems, memory and brain problems, cardiovascular issues, and cancer risk can all be improved with an effective leptin-management plan.

In addition to good diet and exercise, there are nutrient solutions that help resolve leptin resistance, increase the metabolism of fat, and reduce excess levels of leptin.

If leptin issues are left unresolved, there is eventually an increased risk for cancer. This is because the genetic signal NF-kappaB gets overworked and stays in a chronic state of activation. This is a serious consequence of the failure to master leptin. The risk for any disease of aging is significantly increased.

Failing to master leptin as the years go by increases internal friction, therefore increasing the rate of aging. Initially, this is an out-of-rhythm feeling that goes along with increased wear and tear. It can develop into an exhaustion of the metabolic system, such as fibromyalgia, or it can end up in a condition where the body's own natural and essential survival systems turn against the body. The excess production of TNFa, NF-kappaB, as well as cancer causation, and accelerated aging all share the same common features.[841]

Generally, this does not happen over a period of a few weeks or months. It happens as a result of a lifestyle based on leptin mismanagement over a number of years. This results in a loss of the natural balance of the systems of health. This causes aging to occur faster than it should. If natural balance is restored, in many cases the aging process can be slowed down. In some cases, damage can be repaired and reflect "reverse aging."

BECOMING A *HEALTH ASSET MANAGER*™

Who taught us to put our health solely in the hands of our doctors? Why were we never educated to take charge of our own health? If we received any health education at all as children and teens, was it so simplistic it failed to arm us with vital information?

The top priority of the pharmaceutical-based medical world is the sale of drugs. The top priority of public-health officials appears to be the dispensing and enforcement of immunizations. Could more knowledge and education keep us off the drug path and on a health path, in which drugs were not needed in the first place? The person with the biggest vested interest in your health is you. Quality of health is at stake, your single most important asset.

Knowledge is power. As a reader of this book, you are empowered with knowledge of immense personal value – knowledge that is also practical and can be implemented as a lifestyle. Using this knowledge can have a profound effect on overall health, both in terms of fixing existing issues and preventing serious health conditions. It will not only benefit individuals, but it will also result in reduced health-care costs for society. This is truly information that can be used as a life tool, and it enables us to educate our family as well. This is where the change begins.

The ability to skillfully return the body to a state of natural balance is the key to a healthy future. *Mastering* leptin is the single most important skill of the *Health Asset Manager*. Our information opens the doors to healthy solutions that have never before been realized.

Mastering Leptin
ONLINE RESOURCES

- Tips for success
- Nutritional supplements
- Free e-newsletter from Byron J. Richards
- Latest findings on leptin and weight loss
- Take the Leptin Quiz
- Watch free videos online
- Leptin Diet approved recipes

Visit:
www.WellnessResources.com/leptin
or call: 800-717-9355 for more information.

REFERENCES

[1] Surgeon General's Report on Nutrition and Health. US Department of Health and Human Services. www.mcsspotlight.org/media/reports/surgen_rep.html

[2] http://www.cdc.gov/nccdphp/factsheets/death_causes2000.htm

[3] Mokdad AH, Bowman BA, Ford ES, Vinico F, Marks JS, Koplan JP. The continuing epidemics of obesity and diabetes in the United States. *JAMA* 2001 Sep12;286(10):1195-200

[4] Bridges EJ, Woods SL. Cardiovascular chronobiology: do you know what time it is? *Prog Cardiovasc Nurs* 2001 Spring;16(2):65-79.

[5] Smith DH. Pharmacology of cardiovascular chronotherapeutic agents. *Am J Hypertens* 2001 Sep;14(9Pt 2):296S-301S.

[6] Levi F. Giacchetti S, Zidani R, Brezault-Bonnet C, Tigaud JM, Goldwasser F, Misset JL. Chronotherapy of colorectal cancer metastases. *Hepatogastroenterology* 2001 Mar-Apr;48(38):320-2.

[7] Vandel P, Boiteux J, Sechter D. Bilogicial rhythms and psychiatric syndromes. *Rev Prat* 1997 Nove 1;47(17):1878-83.

[8] Nagayama H. Influences of biological rhythms on the effects of psychotropic drugs. *Pyschosom Med* 1999 Set-Oct;61(5):618-29.

[9] Okawa M, Uchiyama M, Ozaki S, Shibui K, Ichikawa H. Circadian rhythm sleep disorders in adolescents: clinical trial of combined treatments based on chronobiology/ *Psychiatry Clin Neurosci* 1998 Oct;52(5):483-90.

[10] Kagami M, Tomioka H, Nakazawa T, Yoshida S. Chronotherapy of bronchial asthma: circadian rhythms in asthmatic symptoms. Report I: Survey on chronobiology acrophase of asthmatic symptoms. *Arerugi* 2001 Jun;50(6):528-34.

[11] Kraft M. Corticosteroids and leukotrienes: chronobiology and chronotherapy. *Chronobiol Int* 1999 Sep;16(5):683-93.

[12] Turkoski BB. Medication timing for the elderly: the impact of biorhythms on effectiveness. *Geriatr Nurs* 1998 May-June;19(3):146-51.

[13] Stefanov R, Dimitrov BD. Cytomegalovirus infection in infants: an example of a chronopharmacological approach. *Folia Med (Plovdiv)* 1999;41(1):20-4.

[14] Fyfe AI. Transplant atherosclerosis: the clinical syndrome, pathogenesis and possible model of spontaneous atherosclerosis. *Can J Cardiol* 1992 Jun;8(5):509-19

[15] Stockfleth E, Ulrich C, Meyer T, Christophers E. Epithelial malignancies in organ transplant patients: clinical presentation and new methods of treatment. *Recent Results Cancer Res* 2002;160:251-8

[16] Zackheim HS, Koo J, LeBoit PE, McCalmont TH, Bowman PH, Kashani-Sabet M, Jones C, Zehnder J. Psoriasiform mycosis fungoides with fatal outcome after treatment with cyclosporine. *J Am Acad Dermatol* 2002 Jul;47(1):155-7

[17] Pielop JA, Jones D, Duvic M. Transient CD30+ nodal transformation of cutaneous T-cell lymphoma associated with cyclosporine treatment. *Int J Dermatol* 2001 Aug;40(8):505-11

[18] Zhang Y, Proenca R, Maffei M, Barone M, Leopold L & Friedman JM. (1994) Positional cloning of the mouse obese gene and its human homologue. *Nature* 372, 425-432.

[19] Trayhurn P, Beattie JH. Physiological role of adipose tissue: white adipose tissue as an endocrine and secretory organ *Nutrition Society* (2001) 60, 329-339.

[20] Wilding JP. Leptin and the control of obesity. *Curr Opin Pharmacol* 2001 Dec;1(6):656-61.

[21] Scarpace PJ, Tumer N. Peripheral and hypothalamic leptin resistance with age-related obesity. *Physiol Behav* 2001 Nov-Dec;74(4-5):721-7.

[22] Schwartz MW. Brain pathways controlling food intake and body weight. *Exp Biol Med Vol.* 226(11):978-981, 2001.

[23] Trayhurn P, Beattie JH. Physiological role of adipose tissue: white adipose tissue as an endocrine and secretory organ *Nutrition Society* (2001) 60, 329-339.

[24] Cannon WB Bodily changes in pain, hunger, fear, and rage. New York and London:D.Appleton and Co. 1929.

[25] Trayhurn P, Duncan JS, & Rayner DV (1995a) Acute cold-induced suppression of ob(obese) expression and circulating heptin levels in lean mice by the beta 3-adrenoceptor agonists BRL 35135A and ZD2079. *Biochemical and Biophysical Research Communications* 228, 605-610.

[26] Satoh N, Ogawa Y, Katsuura G, Numata Y, Tsuji T, Hayase M, Ebihara K, Masuzaki H, Hosoda K, Yoshimasa Y & Nakao K. (1999) Sympathetic activation of leptin via the ventromedial hypothalamus – Leptin-induced increase in catecholamine secretion. *Diabetes* 48, 1787-1793.

[27] Sinha MK, Ohannesian JP, Heiman ML< Kriauciunas A, Stephens TW, Magosin S, Marco C & Caro JF. (1996) Nocturnal rise of leptin in lean, obese, and non-insulin-dependent diabetes mellitus subjects. *Journal of Clinical Investigation* 97, 1344-1347.

[28] Licinio J, Mantzoros C, Negrao AB, Cizza G, Wong ML, Bongiorno PB, Chrousos GP, Karp B, Allen C, Flier JS & Gold PW. (1997) Human leptin levels are pulsatile and inversely related to pituitary-adrenal function. *Nature Medicine* 3, 575-579.

[29] Herrmann TS, Bean ML, Black TM, Wang P, Coleman RA. High glycemic index carbohydrate diet alters the diurnal rhythm of leptin but not insulin concentrations. *Exp Biol Med* (Maywood) 2001 Dec;226(11):1037-44

[30] Kalsbeek A, Fliers E, Romijn JA, La Fleur SE, Wortel J, Bakker O, Endert E, Buijs RM. The suprachiasmatic nucleus generates the diurnal changes in plasma leptin levels. *Endocrinology* 2001 Jun;142(6):2677-85

[31] Himms-Hagen J. (1999) Physiological roles of the leptin endocrine system: Differences between ice and humans. *Critical Reviews in Clinical and Laboratory Sci-*

ence 36, 575-655.

[32] Licinio J, Caglayan S, Ozata M, Yildiz BO, De Miranda PB, O'Kirwan F, Whitby R, Liang L, Cohen P, Bhasin S, Krauss RM, Veldhuis JD, Wagner AJ, DePaoli AM, McCann SM, Wong ML. Phenotypic effects of leptin replacement on morbid obesity, diabetes mellitus, hypogonadism, and behavior in leptin-deficient adults. *Proc Natl Acad Sci U S A.* 2004 Mar 30;101(13):4531-4536. Epub 2004 Mar 09.

[33] Trayhurn P, Hoggard N, Mercer JG & Rayner DV. (1999) Leptin: fundamental aspects. *International Journal of Obesity* 23, 22-28.

[34] Kieffer TJ, Heller RS, Leech CA, Holz GG, Habener JF. Leptin suppression of insulin secretion by te activation of the ATP-sensitive K channels in pancreatic B-cells. *Diabetes* 46: 1087-1093, 1997.

[35] Van Gaal Lf, Wauters MA, Mertens IL, Considine RV, De Leeuw IH: Clinical endocrinology of human leptin. *Int J Obes Relat Metab Disord* 23 (Suppl 1): 29-36, 1999.

[36] Tatti P, Masselli L, Buonanno A, Di Mauro P, Strollo F. Leptin levels in diabetic and nondiabetic subjects. *Endocrine* 2001 Aug;15(3):305-8.

[37] Celi F, Bini V, Papi F, Contessa G, Santilli E, Falorni A. Leptin serum levels are involved in the relapse after weight excess reduction in obese children and adolescents. *Diabetes Nutr Metab.* 2003 Oct-Dec;16(5-6):306-11.

[38] Naimi TS, Brewer RD, Mokdad A, Denny C, Serdula MK, Marks JS. Binge Drinking Among US Adults. *JAMA* 2003 Jan 1;289(1):70-5

[39] Mokdad AH, Ford ES, Bowman BA, Dietz WH, Vinicor F, Bales VS, Marks JS. Prevalence of obesity, diabetes, and obesity-related health risk factors, 2001. *JAMA* 2003 Jan 1;289(1):76-9

[40] Kiefer F, Jahn H, Wolf K, Kampf P, Knaudt K, Wiedemann K. Free-choice alcohol consumption in mice after application of the appetite regulating peptide leptin. *Alcohol Clin Exp Res* 2001 May;25(5):787-9

[41] Kiefer F, Jahn H, Jaschinski M, Holzbach R, Wolf K, Naber D, Wiedemann K. Leptin: a modulator of alcohol craving? *Biol Psychiatry* 2001 May 1;49(9):782-7

[42] Nicolas JM, Fernandez-Sola J, Fatjo F, Casamitjana R, Bataller R, Sacanella E, Tobias E, Badia E, Estruch R. Increased circulating leptin levels in chronic alcoholism. Alcohol Clin Exp Res 2001 Jan;25(1):83-8

[43] Rojdmark S, Calissendorff J, Brismar K. Alcohol ingestion decreases both diurnal and nocturnal secretion of leptin in healthy individuals. *Clin Endocrinol* (Oxf) 2001 Nov;55(5):639-47

[44] Campillo B, Sherman E, Richardet JP, Bories PN. Serum leptin levels in alcoholic liver cirrhosis: relationship with gender, nutritional status, liver function and energy metabolism. *Eur J Clin Nutr* 2001 Nov;55(11):980-8

[45] Lin HZ, Yang SQ, Zeldin G, Diehl AM. Chronic ethanol consumption induces the production of tumor necrosis factor-alpha and related cytokines in liver and adipose tissue. *Alcohol Clin Exp Res* 1998 Aug;22(5 Suppl):231S-237S

[46] Kiefer F, Jahn H, Schick M, Wiedemann K ALCOHOL INTAKE, TUMOUR NECROSIS FACTOR-alpha, LEPTIN AND CRAVING: FACTORS OF A POSSIBLY VICIOUS CIRCLE? *Alcohol* 2002

Jul-Aug;37(4):401-4

[47] Hill DB, Barve S, Joshi-Barve S, McClain C. Increased monocyte nuclear factor-kappaB activation and tumor necrosis factor production in alcoholic hepatitis. *J Lab Clin Med* 2000 May;135(5):387-95

[48] Jokelainen K, Reinke LA, Nanji AA. NF kappaB activation is associated with free radical generation and endotoxemia and precedes pathological liver injury in experimental alcoholic liver disease. *Cytokine* 2001 Oct 7;16(1):36-9

[49] Nanji AA, Jokelainen K, Fotouhinia M, Rahemtulla A, Thomas P, Tipoe GL, Su GL, Dannenberg AJ. Increased severity of alcoholic liver injury in female rats: role of oxidative stress, endotoxin, and chemokines. *Am J Physiol Gastrointest Liver Physiol* 2001 Dec;281(6): G1348-56

[50] Saller R, Meier R, Brignoli R. The use of silymarin in the treatment of liver diseases. *Drugs* 2001;61(14):2035-63

[51] Nawrot U, Grzybek-Hryncewicz K, Czarny A. The ability of Candida spp. strains to induce production of tumor necrosis factor and interleukin-6 by whole blood cells. *Acta Microbiol Pol.* 2003;52(1):87-91.

[52] Pietruski JK, Pietruska MD, Jablonska E, Sacha P, Zaremba M, Stokowska W. Interleukin 6, tumor necrosis factor alpha and their soluble receptors in the blood serum of patients with denture stomatitis and fungal infection. *Arch Immunol Ther Exp (Warsz).* 2000;48(2):101-5.

[53] Bajaj JS, Singh A, Aggarwal SK, Chattopadhya D, Baveja UK. Synergistic immunosuppression by candida in HIV infection: a cytokine based analysis. *J Commun Dis.* 2000 Mar;32(1):1-9.

[54] Orozco AS, Zhou X, Filler SG. Mechanisms of the proinflammatory response of endothelial cells to Candida albicans infection. *Infect Immun.* 2000 Mar;68(3):1134-41.

[55] Choi JH, Ko HM, Kim JW, Lee HK, Han SS, Chun SB, Im SY. Platelet-activating factor-induced early activation of NF-kappa B plays a crucial role for organ clearance of Candida albicans. *J Immunol.* 2001 Apr 15;166(8):5139-44.

[56] Farah CS, Gotjamanos T, Seymour GJ, Ashman RB. Cytokines in the oral mucosa of mice infected with Candida albicans. *Oral Microbiol Immunol.* 2002 Dec;17(6):375-8.

[57] Rodriguez-Galan MC, Sotomayor C, Costamagna ME, Cabanillas AM, Renteria BS, Masini-Repiso AM, Correa S. Immunocompetence of macrophages in rats exposed to Candida albicans infection and stress. *Am J Physiol Cell Physiol.* 2003 Jan;284(1):C111-8. Epub 2002 Aug 28.

[58] Yordanov M, Deleva A, Ivanovska N. Host resistance against Candida alibcans infection in mice with adjuvant induced arthritis. *Mycopathologia.* 2002;153(2):77-82.

[59] Noverr MC, Phare SM, Toews GB, Coffey MJ, Huffnagle GB. Pathogenic yeasts Cryptococcus neoformans and Candida albicans produce immunomodulatory prostaglandins. *Infect Immun.* 2001 May;69(5):2957-63.

[60] Yemma JJ, Berk MP. Chemical and physiological effects of Candida albicans toxin on tissues. *Cytobios.* 1994;77(310):147-58.

[61] Deva R, Shankaranarayanan P, Ciccoli R, Nigam S. Candida albicans induces selectively transcriptional activation of cyclooxygenase-2 in HeLa cells: pivotal roles of Toll-like receptors, p38 mitogen-activated protein kinase, and NF-kappa B. J Immunol. 2003 Sep 15;171(6):3047-55.

[62] Ivanovska N, Hristova M. Treatment with oxoglaucine can enhance host resistance to Candida albicans infection of mice with adjuvant arthritis. Diagn Microbiol Infect Dis. 2000 Sep;38(1):17-20.

[63] Catania A, Cutuli M, Garofalo L, Carlin A, Airaghi L, Barcellini W, Lipton JM. The neuropeptide alpha-MSH in host defense. Ann N Y Acad Sci. 2000;917:227-31.

[64] Tillonen J, Homann N, Rautio M, Jousimies-Somer H, Salaspuro M. Role of yeasts in the salivary acetaldehyde production from ethanol among risk groups for ethanol-associated oral cavity cancer. Alcohol Clin Exp Res. 1999 Aug;23(8):1409-15.

[65] Narvhus JA, Gadaga TH. The role of interaction between yeasts and lactic acid bacteria in African fermented milks: a review. Int J Food Microbiol. 2003 Sep 1;86(1-2):51-60.

[66] Hammer T, Bode R. Enzymatic production of alpha-aminoadipate-delta-semialdehyde and related compounds by lysine epsilon-dehydrogenase from Candida albicans. Zentralbl Mikrobiol. 1992;147(1-2):65-70.

[67] Polson DA, Thompson MP. Macronutrient composition of the diet differentially affects leptin and adiponutrin mRNA expression in response to meal feeding. J Nutr Biochem. 2004 Apr;15(4):242-6.

[68] Capasso A. Involvement of nuclear factor-kB in the expression of opiate withdrawal. Prog Neuropsychopharmacol Biol Psychiatry 2001 Aug;25(6):1259-68

[69] Shalev U, Yap J, Shaham Y. Leptin attenuates acute food deprivation-induced relapse to heroin seeking. J Neurosci 2001 Feb 15;21(4):RC129

[70] Lee YW, Hennig B, Yao J, Toborek M. Methamphetamine induces AP-1 and NF kappaB binding and transactivation in human brain endothelial cells. J Neurosci Res 2001 Nov 15;66(4):583-91

[71] Larsen PJ, Vrang N, Tang-Christensen M, Jensen PB, Hay-Schmidt A, Romer J, Bjerre-Knudsen L, Kristensen P. Ups and downs for neuropeptides in body weight homeostasis: pharmacological potential of cocaine amphetamine regulated transcript and preproglucagon-derived peptides. Eur J Pharmacol 2002 Apr 12;440(2-3):159-72

[72] Kristensen P, Judge ME, Thim L, Ribel U, Christjansen KN, Wulff BS, Clausen JT, Jensen PB, Madsen OD, Vrang N, Larsen PJ, Hastrup S. Hypothalamic CART is a new anorectic peptide regulated by leptin. Nature 1998 May 7;393(6680):72-6

[73] Ludvigsen S, Thim L, Blom AM, Wulff BS. Solution structure of the satiety factor, CART, reveals new functionality of a well-known fold. Biochemistry 2001 Aug 7;40(31):9082-8

[74] Tsuruta Y, Yoshimatsu H, Hidaka S, Kondou S, Okamoto K, Sakata T. Hyperleptinemia in A(y)/a mice upregulates arcuate cocaine- and amphetamine-regulated transcript expression. Am J Physiol Endocrinol Metab 2002 Apr;282(4):E967-73

[75] Kask A, Schioth HB, Mutulis F, Wikberg JE, Rago L. Anorexigenic cocaine- and amphetamine-regulated transcript peptide intensifies fear reactions in rats. Brain Res 2000 Feb 28;857(1-2):283-5

[76] Kastin AJ, Akerstrom V. Entry of CART into brain is rapid but not inhibited by excess CART or leptin. Am J Physiol 1999 Nov;277(5 Pt 1):E901-4

[77] Brandon CL, Marinelli M, White FJ. Adolescent exposure to methylphenidate alters the activity of rat midbrain dopamine neurons. Comment in: Biol Psychiatry. 2003 Dec 15;54(12):1307-9. Biol Psychiatry. 2003 Dec 15;54(12):1310-1. Biol Psychiatry. 2003 Dec 15;54(12):1338-44.

[78] Volkow ND, Wang GJ, Ma Y, Fowler JS, Zhu W, Maynard L, Telang F, Vaska P, Ding YS, Wong C, Swanson JM. Expectation enhances the regional brain metabolic and the reinforcing effects of stimulants in cocaine abusers. J Neurosci. 2003 Dec 10;23(36):11461-8.

[79] Carlezon WA Jr, Mague SD, Andersen SL. Enduring behavioral effects of early exposure to methylphenidate in rats. Comment in: Biol Psychiatry. 2003 Dec 15;54(12):1307-9. Biol Psychiatry. 2003 Dec 15;54(12):1310-1. Biol Psychiatry. 2003 Dec 15;54(12):1330-7.

[80] Bolanos CA, Barrot M, Berton O, Wallace-Black D, Nestler EJ. Methylphenidate treatment during pre- and periadolescence alters behavioral responses to emotional stimuli at adulthood. Comment in: Biol Psychiatry. 2003 Dec 15;54(12):1307-9. Biol Psychiatry. 2003 Dec 15;54(12):1310-1. Biol Psychiatry. 2003 Dec 15;54(12):1317-29.

[81] Whitfield JF. Leptin: brains and bones. Expert Opin Investig Drugs 2001 Sep;10(9):1617-22

[82] Figenschau Y, Knutsen G, Shahazeydi S, Johansen O, Sveinbjornsson B. Human articular chondrocytes express functional leptin receptors. Biochem Biophys Res Commun 2001 Sep 14;287(1):190-7

[83] Hardwick JC, Van Den Brink GR, Offerhaus GJ, Van Deventer SJ, Peppelenbosch MP. Leptin is a growth factor for colonic epithelial cells. Gastroenterology 2001 Jul;121(1):79-90

[84] Chen HC, Smith SJ, Tow B, Elias PM, Farese RV Jr. Leptin modulates the effects of acyl CoA:diacylglycerol acyltransferase deficiency on murine fur and sebaceous glands. J Clin Invest 2002 Jan;109(2):175-81

[85] Christou H, Serdy S, Mantzoros CS. Leptin in relation to growth and developmental processes in the fetus. Semin Reprod Med 2002;20(2):123-30

[86] Shanley LJ, Irving AJ, Harvey J. Leptin enhances NMDA receptor function and modulates hippocampal synaptic plasticity. J Neurosci 2001 Dec 15;21(24): RC186

[87] Dicou E, Attoub S, Gressens P. Neuroprotective effects of leptin in vivo and in vitro. Neuroreport 2001 Dec 21;12(18):3947-51

[88] Sriram K, Benkovic SA, Miller DB, O'Callaghan JP. Obesity exacerbates chemically induced neurodegeneration. Neuroscience 2002;115(4):1335-46

[89] Masuo K, Mikami H, Ogihara T, Tuck ML. Familial obesity, sympathetic activation and blood pressure level. Blood Press 2001;10(4):199-204.

[90] Breier BH, Vickers MH, Ikenasio BA, Chan KY, Wong WP. Fetal programming of appetite and obesity. Mol Cell Endocrinol 2001 Dec 20;185(1-2):73-9.

[91] Law C. Adult obesity and growth in childhood. *BMJ* 2001 Dec 8;323(7325):1320-1.

[92] Qiu C, Williams MA, Vadachkoria S, Frederick IO, Luthy DA. Increased maternal plasma leptin in early pregnancy and risk of gestational diabetes mellitus. *Obstet Gynecol.* 2004 Mar;103(3):519-25.

[93] Atamer Y, Erden AC, Demir B, KoCyigit Y, Atamer A. The relationship between plasma levels of leptin and androgen in healthy and preeclamptic pregnant women. *Acta Obstet Gynecol Scand.* 2004 May;83(5):425-30.

[94] Lepercq J, Guerre-Millo M, Andre J, Cauzac M, Hauguel-de Mouzon S. Leptin: a potential marker of placental insufficiency. *Gynecol Obstet Invest.* 2003;55(3):151-5.

[95] Bartha JL, Romero-Carmona R, Escobar-Llompart M, Comino-Delgado R. The relationships between leptin and inflammatory cytokines in women with preeclampsia. *BJOG.* 2001 Dec;108(12):1272-6.

[96] Diaz E, Halhali A, Luna C, Diaz L, Avila E, Larrea F. Newborn birth weight correlates with placental zinc, umbilical insulin-like growth factor I, and leptin levels in preeclampsia. *Arch Med Res.* 2002 Jan-Feb;33(1):40-7.

[97] Vatten LJ, Skjaerven R. Is pre-eclampsia more than one disease? *BJOG.* 2004 Apr;111(4):298-302.

[98] Cedergren MI. Maternal morbid obesity and the risk of adverse pregnancy outcome. *Obstet Gynecol.* 2004 Feb;103(2):219-24.

[99] Sattar N, Ramsay J, Crawford L, Cheyne H, Greer IA. Classic and novel risk factor parameters in women with a history of preeclampsia. *Hypertension.* 2003 Jul;42(1):39-42. Epub 2003 May 12.

[100] Haukkamaa L, Salminen M, Laivuori H, Leinonen H, Hiilesmaa V, Kaaja R. Risk for subsequent coronary artery disease after preeclampsia. *Am J Cardiol.* 2004 Mar 15;93(6):805-8.

[101] Duley L. Pre-eclampsia and the hypertensive disorders of pregnancy. *Br Med Bull.* 2003;67:161-76.

[102] Raijmakers MT, Roes EM, Zusterzeel PL, Steegers EA, Peters WH. Thiol status and antioxidant capacity in women with a history of severe pre-eclampsia. *BJOG.* 2004 Mar;111(3):207-12.

[103] Chappell LC, Seed PT, Kelly FJ, Briley A, Hunt BJ, Charnock-Jones DS, Mallet A, Poston L. Vitamin C and E supplementation in women at risk of preeclampsia is associated with changes in indices of oxidative stress and placental function. *Am J Obstet Gynecol.* 2002 Sep;187(3):777-84.

[104] Lipid-Soluble Antioxidants and Pregnancy: Maternal Serum Levels of Coenzyme Q(10), alpha-Tocopherol and gamma-Tocopherol in Preeclampsia and Normal Pregnancy. *Gynecol Obstet Invest.* 2004;58(1):8-13. Epub 2004 Feb 25.

[105] Babay ZA, Warsy AS, El-Hazmi MA, Addar MH. Leptin level in pregnant mothers at term and cord blood and the effect of newborns gender. *Saudi Med J.* 2004 Feb;25(2):212-4.

[106] El-Haddad MA, Desai M, Gayle D, Ross MG. In utero development of fetal thirst and appetite: potential for programming. *J Soc Gynecol Investig.* 2004 Apr;11(3):123-30.

[107] Gopalakrishnan GS, Gardner DS, Rhind SM, Rae MT, Kyle CE, Brooks AN, Walker RM, Ramsay MM, Keisler DH, Stephenson T, Symonds ME.

PROGRAMMING OF ADULT CARDIOVASCULAR FUNCTION AFTER EARLY MATERNAL UNDERNUTRITION IN SHEEP. *Am J Physiol Regul Integr Comp Physiol.* 2004 Feb 19

[108] Bouret SG, Draper SJ, Simerly RB. Formation of projection pathways from the arcuate nucleus of the hypothalamus to hypothalamic regions implicated in the neural control of feeding behavior in mice. *J Neurosci.* 2004 Mar 17;24(11):2797-805.

[109] Bouret SG, Draper SJ, Simerly RB. Trophic action of leptin on hypothalamic neurons that regulate feeding. *Science.* 2004 Apr 2;304(5667):108-10.

[110] Pinto S, Roseberry AG, Liu H, Diano S, Shanabrough M, Cai X, Friedman JM, Horvath TL. Rapid rewiring of arcuate nucleus feeding circuits by leptin. *Science.* 2004 Apr 2;304(5667):110-5.

[111] Bonnet M, Delavaud C, Laud K, Gourdou I, Leroux C, Djiane J, Chilliard Y. Mammary leptin synthesis, milk leptin and their putative physiological roles. *Reprod Nutr Dev.* 2002 Sep-Oct;42(5):399-413.

[112] Casabiell X, Pineiro V, Tome MA, Peino R, Dieguez C, Casanueva FF. Presence of leptin in colostrum and/or breast milk from lactating mothers: a potential role in the regulation of neonatal food intake. *J Clin Endocrinol Metab.* 1997 Dec;82(12):4270-3.

[113] Salimei E, Varisco G, Rosi F. Major constituents, leptin, and non-protein nitrogen compounds in mares' colostrum and milk. *Reprod Nutr Dev.* 2002 Jan-Feb;42(1):65-72.

[114] Chen ZG, Zhang XH, He ZX, Cai Y. [Correlation between plasma leptin level and premature infant weight loss] [Article in Chinese] *Zhonghua Er Ke Za Zhi.* 2004 Feb;42(2):121-4.

[115] Dawson R, Pelleymounter MA, Millard WJ, Liu S, Eppler B. Attenuation of leptin-mediated effects by monosodium glutamate-induced arcuate nucleus damage. *Am J Physiol.* 1997 Jul;273(1 Pt 1):E202-6.

[116] Hermanussen M, Tresguerres JA. Does high glutamate intake cause obesity? *J Pediatr Endocrinol Metab.* 2003 Sep;16(7):965-8.

[117] Macho L, Fickova M, Jezova D, Zorad S. Late effects of postnatal administration of monosodium glutamate on insulin action in adult rats. *Physiol Res.* 2000;49 Suppl 1:S79-85.

[118] Hermanussen M, Tresguerres JA. Does high glutamate intake cause obesity? *J Pediatr Endocrinol Metab.* 2003 Sep;16(7):965-8.

[119] Perello M, Gaillard RC, Chisari A, Spinedi E. Adrenal enucleation in MSG-damaged hyperleptinemic male rats transiently restores adrenal sensitivity to leptin. *Neuroendocrinology.* 2003 Sep;78(3):176-84.

[120] Miskowiak B, Kesa B, Limanowski A, Partyka M, Filipiak B. Long-term effect of neonatal monosodium glutamate (MSG) treatment on reproductive system of the female rat. *Folia Morphol (Warsz).* 1999;58(2):105-13.

[121] Butchko HH, Stargel WW, Comer CP, Mayhew DA, Benninger C, Blackburn GL, de Sonneville LM, Geha RS, Hertelendy Z, Koestner A, Leon AS, Liepa GU, McMartin KE, Mendenhall CL, Munro IC, Novotny EJ, Renwick AG, Schiffman SS, Schomer DL, Shaywitz BA, Spiers PA, Tephly TR, Thomas JA, Trefz FK. Aspartame: review of safety. *Regul Toxicol Pharmacol.* 2002 Apr;35(2 Pt 2):S1-93. Medical and Scientific Af-

fairs, The NutraSweet Company, Mt Prospect, Illinois 60056, USA.

[122] American Dietetic Association. Position of the American Dietetic Association: use of nutritive and nonnutritive sweeteners. *J Am Diet Assoc.* 2004 Feb;104(2):255-75.

[123] Smith JD, Terpening CM, Schmidt SO, Gums JG. Relief of fibromyalgia symptoms following discontinuation of dietary excitotoxins. *Ann Pharmacother.* 2001 Jun;35(6):702-6.

[124] Millichap JG, Yee MM. The diet factor in pediatric and adolescent migraine. *Pediatr Neurol.* 2003 Jan;28(1):9-15.

[125] Oyama Y, Sakai H, Arata T, Okano Y, Akaike N, Sakai K, Noda K. Cytotoxic effects of methanol, formaldehyde, and formate on dissociated rat thymocytes: a possibility of aspartame toxicity. *Cell Biol Toxicol.* 2002;18(1):43-50.

[126] Nakao H, Umebayashi C, Nakata M, Nishizaki Y, Noda K, Okano Y, Oyama Y. Formaldehyde-induced shrinkage of rat thymocytes. *J Pharmacol Sci.* 2003 Jan;91(1):83-6.

[127] Bjorbaek C, Kahn BB. Leptin signaling in the central nervous system and the periphery. *Recent Prog Horm Res.* 2004;59:305-31.

[128] Bjorbaek C, Kahn BB. Leptin Signaling in the Central Nervous System and the Periphery. *Recent Prog Horm Res.* 2004;59(1):305-331.

[129] Schrauwen P, Hesselink M. Uncoupling protein 3 and physical activity: the role of uncoupling protein 3 in energy metabolism revisited. *Proc Nutr Soc.* 2003 Aug;62(3):635-43.

[130] Cannon B, Nedergaard J. Brown adipose tissue: function and physiological significance. *Physiol Rev.* 2004 Jan;84(1):277-359.

[131] Klaus S. Adipose tissue as a regulator of energy balance. *Curr Drug Targets.* 2004 Apr;5(3):241-50.

[132] Cameron-Smith D, Burke LM, Angus DJ, Tunstall RJ, Cox GR, Bonen A, Hawley JA, Hargreaves M A short-term, high-fat diet up-regulates lipid metabolism and gene expression in human skeletal muscle. *Am J Clin Nutr.* 2003 Feb;77(2):313-8.

[133] Noland RC, Hickner RC, Jimenez-Linan M, Vidal-Puig A, Zheng D, Dohm GL, Cortright RN. Acute endurance exercise increases skeletal muscle uncoupling protein-3 gene expression in untrained but not trained humans. *Metabolism.* 2003 Feb;52(2):152-8.

[134] Iossa S, Lionetti L, Mollica MP, Crescenzo R, Botta M, Barletta A, Liverini G. Effect of high-fat feeding on metabolic efficiency and mitochondrial oxidative capacity in adult rats. *Br J Nutr.* 2003 Nov;90(5):953-60.

[135] Minokoshi Y, Kim YB, Peroni OD, Fryer LG, Muller C, Carling D, Kahn BB. Leptin stimulates fatty-acid oxidation by activating AMP-activated protein kinase. Comment in: Nature. 2002 Jan 17;415(6869):268-9. *Nature.* 2002 Jan 17;415(6869):339-43.

[136] Gong DW, He Y, Karas M, Reitman M. Uncoupling protein-3 is a mediator of thermogenesis regulated by thyroid hormone, beta3-adrenergic agonists, and leptin. *J Biol Chem.* 1997 Sep 26;272(39):24129-32.

[137] Vettor R, Mingrone G, Manco M, Granzotto M, Milan G, Scarda A, Lombardi A, Greco AV, Federspil G. Reduced expression of uncoupling proteins-2 and -3 in adipose tissue in post-obese patients submitted to biliopancreatic diversion. *Eur J Endocrinol.* 2003 May;148(5):543-50.

[138] Langin D. The role of uncoupling protein 2 in the development of type 2 diabetes. *Drugs Today (Barc).* 2003 Apr;39(4):287-95.

[139] Steinberg GR, Smith AC, Wormald S, Malenfant P, Collier C, Dyck DJ. Endurance training partially reverses dietary-induced leptin resistance in rodent skeletal muscle. *Am J Physiol Endocrinol Metab.* 2004 Jan;286(1):E57-63.

[140] Kahara T, Takamura T, Hayakawa T, Nagai Y, Yamaguchi H, Katsuki T, Katsuki K, Katsuki M, Kobayashi K. Prediction of exercise-mediated changes in metabolic markers by gene polymorphism. *Diabetes Res Clin Pract.* 2002 Aug;57(2):105-10.

[141] Tonkonogi M, Krook A, Walsh B, Sahlin K. Endurance training increases stimulation of uncoupling of skeletal muscle mitochondria in humans by non-esterified fatty acids: an uncoupling-protein-mediated effect? *Biochem J.* 2000 Nov 1;351 Pt 3:805-10.

[142] Schrauwen P, Hesselink MK, Vaartjes I, Kornips E, Saris WH, Giacobino JP, Russell A. Effect of acute exercise on uncoupling protein 3 is a fat metabolism-mediated effect. *Am J Physiol Endocrinol Metab.* 2002 Jan;282(1):E11-7.

[143] Zhou M, Lin BZ, Coughlin S, Vallega G, Pilch PF. UCP-3 expression in skeletal muscle: effects of exercise, hypoxia, and AMP-activated protein kinase. *Am J Physiol Endocrinol Metab.* 2000 Sep;279(3):E622-9.

[144] Vidal-Puig AJ, Grujic D, Zhang CY, Hagen T, Boss O, Ido Y, Szczepanik A, Wade J, Mootha V, Cortright R, Muoio DM, Lowell BB. Energy metabolism in uncoupling protein 3 gene knockout mice. *J Biol Chem.* 2000 May 26;275(21):16258-66.

[145] MRC Dunn Human Nutrition Unit, Hills Road, CB2 2XY, Cambridge, UK. Talbot DA, Lambert AJ, Brand MD. Production of endogenous matrix superoxide from mitochondrial complex I leads to activation of uncoupling protein 3. *FEBS Lett.* 2004 Jan 2;556(1-3):111-5.

[146] Wallace DC. Animal models for mitochondrial disease. *Methods Mol Biol.* 2002;197:3-54.

[147] Li B, Nolte LA, Ju JS, Han DH, Coleman T, Holloszy JO, Semenkovich CF. Skeletal muscle respiratory uncoupling prevents diet-induced obesity and insulin resistance in mice. Comment in: Nat Med. 2000 Oct;6(10):1092-3. Nat Med. 2000 Oct;6(10):1115-20.

[148] Echtay KS, Winkler E, Frischmuth K, Klingenberg M. Uncoupling proteins 2 and 3 are highly active H(+) transporters and highly nucleotide sensitive when activated by coenzyme Q (ubiquinone). *Proc Natl Acad Sci U S A.* 2001 Feb 13;98(4):1416-21.

[149] Superoxide activates mitochondrial uncoupling protein 2 from the matrix side. Studies using targeted antioxidants. *J Biol Chem.* 2002 Dec 6;277(49):47129-35. Epub 2002 Oct 07.

[150] Suzuki K, Ito Y, Ochiai J, Kusuhara Y, Hashimoto S, Tokudome S, Kojima M, Wakai K, Toyoshima H, Tamakoshi K, Watanabe Y, Hayakawa N, Maruta M, Watanabe M, Kato K, Ohta Y, Tamakoshi A; JACC Study Group. Relationship between obesity and serum markers of oxidative stress and inflammation in Japanese. *Asian Pac J Cancer Prev.* 2003

Jul-Sep;4(3):259-66

[151] Iritani N, Sugimoto T, Fukuda H, Tomoe K. Changes in UCP family expressions in rat tissues due to diet and aging. *J Nutr Sci Vitaminol* (Tokyo). 2002 Oct;48(5):410-6.

[152] Ren J. Leptin and hyperleptinemia - from friend to foe for cardiovascular function. *J Endocrinol*. 2004 Apr;181(1):1-10.

[153] Zamboni M, Zoico E, Fantin F, Panourgia MP, Di Francesco V, Tosoni P, Solerte B, Vettor R, Bosello O. Relation between leptin and the metabolic syndrome in elderly women. *J Gerontol A Biol Sci Med Sci*. 2004 Apr;59(4):M396-400.

[154] Valsamakis G, McTernan Pg P, Chetty R, Al Daghri N, Field A, Hanif W, Barnett Ah A, Kumar S. Modest weight loss and reduction in waist circumference after medical treatment are associated with favorable changes in serum adipocytokines. *Metabolism*. 2004 Apr;53(4):430-4.

[155] Ferrier KE, Nestel P, Taylor A, Drew BG, Kingwell BA. Diet but not aerobic exercise training reduces skeletal muscle TNF-alpha in overweight humans. *Diabetologia*. 2004 Mar 26

[156] Pasanisi F, Contaldo F, de Simone G, Mancini M. Benefits of sustained moderate weight loss in obesity. *Nutr Metab Cardiovasc Dis*. 2001 Dec;11(6):401-6.

[157] Martins D, Tareen N, Pan D, Norris K. The relationship between body mass index, blood pressure and pulse rate among normotensive and hypertensive participants in the third National Health and Nutrition Examination Survey (NHANES*). Cell Mol Biol (Noisy-le-grand)*. 2003 Dec;49(8):1305-9.

[158] Tsuda K, Nishio I. Leptin and membrane fluidity of erythrocytes in essential hypertension; an electron paramagnetic resonance investigation. *Am J Hypertens*. 2004 Apr;17(4):375-9.

[159] Beltowski J, Wojcicka G, Marciniak A, Jamroz A. Oxidative stress, nitric oxide production, and renal sodium handling in leptin-induced hypertension. *Life Sci*. 2004 Apr 30;74(24):2987-3000.

[160] Rahmouni K, Haynes WG. Leptin and the cardiovascular system. *Recent Prog Horm Res*. 2004;59:225-44.

[161] Baranowska B, Wolinska-Witort E, Wasilewska-Dziubinska E, Roguski K, Martynska L, Chmielowska M. The role of neuropeptides in the disturbed control of appetite and hormone secretion in eating disorders. *Neuroendocrinol Lett*. 2003 Dec;24(6):431-4.

[162] Vanpatten S, Karkanias GB, Rossetti L, Cohen DE. Intracerebroventricular leptin regulates hepatic cholesterol metabolism. *Biochem J*. 2004 Apr 15;379(Pt 2):229-33.

[163] Jung CH, Sung KC, Shin HS, Rhee EJ, Lee WY, Kim BS, Kang JH, Kim H, Kim SW, Lee MH, Park JR, Kim SW. Thyroid dysfunction and their relation to cardiovascular risk factors such as lipid profile, hsCRP, and waist hip ratio in Korea. *Korean J Intern Med*. 2003 Sep;18(3):146-53.

[164] Surks MI, Ortiz E, Daniels GH, Sawin CT, Col NF, Cobin RH, Franklyn JA, Hershman JM, Burman KD, Denke MA, Gorman C, Cooper RS, Weissman NJ. Subclinical thyroid disease: scientific review and guidelines for diagnosis and management. Comment in: *JAMA*. 2004 Apr 7;291(13):1562; author reply 1562-3. JAMA. 2004 Jan 14;291(2):228-38.

[165] Guo F, Bakal K, Minokoshi Y, Hollenberg AN. Leptin Signaling Targets the Thyrotropin-Releasing Hormone Gene Promoter In Vivo. *Endocrinology*. 2004 Feb 5

[166] Huo L, Munzberg H, Nillni EA, Bjorbaek C. Role of STAT3 in Regulation of Hypothalamic trh Gene-Expression by Leptin. *Endocrinology*. 2004 Feb 5

[167] Gong DW, He Y, Karas M, Reitman M. Uncoupling protein-3 is a mediator of thermogenesis regulated by thyroid hormone, beta3-adrenergic agonists, and leptin. *J Biol Chem*. 1997 Sep 26;272(39):24129-32.

[168] Thompson PD, Clarkson P, Karas RH. Statin-associated myopathy. Comment in: JAMA. 2003 Aug 20;290(7):888; author reply 888-9. JAMA. 2003 Aug 20;290(7):888; author reply 888-9. *JAMA*. 2003 Apr 2;289(13):1681-90.

[169] Gotto AM Jr. Risks and benefits of continued aggressive statin therapy. *Clin Cardiol*. 2003 Apr;26(4 Suppl 3):III3-12.

[170] De Pinieux G, Chariot P, Ammi-Said M, Louarn F, Lejonc JL, Astier A, Jacotot B, Gherardi R. Lipid-lowering drugs and mitochondrial function: effects of HMG-CoA reductase inhibitors on serum ubiquinone and blood lactate/pyruvate ratio. *Br J Clin Pharmacol*. 1996 Sep;42(3):333-7.

[171] Passi S, Stancato A, Aleo E, Dmitrieva A, Littarru GP. Statins lower plasma and lymphocyte ubiquinol/ubiquinone without affecting other antioxidants and PUFA. *Biofactors*. 2003;18(1-4):113-24.

[172] Langsjoen PH, Langsjoen AM. The clinical use of HMG CoA-reductase inhibitors and the associated depletion of coenzyme Q10. A review of animal and human publications. *Biofactors*. 2003;18(1-4):101-11.

[173] Silver MA, Langsjoen PH, Szabo S, Patil H, Zelinger A. Statin cardiomyopathy? A potential role for Co-Enzyme Q10 therapy for statin-induced changes in diastolic LV performance: description of a clinical protocol. *Biofactors*. 2003;18(1-4):125-7.

[174] Pettit FH, Harper RF, Vilaythong J, Chu T, Shive W. Reversal of statin toxicity to human lymphocytes in tissue culture. *Drug Metabol Drug Interact*. 2003;19(3):151-60.

[175] Celi F, Bini V, Papi F, Contessa G, Santilli E, Falorni A. Leptin serum levels are involved in the relapse after weight excess reduction in obese children and adolescents. *Diabetes Nutr Metab*. 2003 Oct-Dec;16(5-6):306-11.

[176] Radic R, Nikolic V, Karner I, Kosovic P, Kurbel S, Selthofer R, Curkovic M. Circadian rhythm of blood leptin level in obese and non-obese people. *Coll Antropol*. 2003 Dec;27(2):555-61.

[177] Dunbar JC, Lu H. Chronic intracerebroventricular insulin attenuates the leptin-mediated but not alpha melanocyte stimulating hormone increase in sympathetic and cardiovascular responses. *Brain Res Bull* 2000 May 15;52(2):123-6

[178] Masuo K. Obesity-related hypertension: role of the sympathetic nervous system, insulin, and leptin. *Curr Hypertens Rep* 2002 Apr;4(2):112-8

[179] Esler M, Rumantir M, Wiesner G, Kaye D, Hastings J, Lambert G. Sympathetic nervous system and insulin resistance: from obesity to diabetes. *Am J Hypertens* 2001 Nov;14(11 Pt 2):304S-309S

[180] Bratanova-Tochkova TK, Cheng H, Daniel S,

Gunawardana S, Liu YJ, Mulvaney-Musa J, Schermer-horn T, Straub SG, Yajima H, Sharp GW. Triggering and augmentation mechanisms, granule pools, and biphasic insulin secretion. Diabetes 2002 Feb;51 Suppl 1:S83-90

[181] Radziuk J, Pye S. Hepatic glucose uptake, gluco-neogenesis and the regulation of glycogen synthesis. *Diabetes Metab Res Rev* 2001 Jul-Aug;17(4):250-72

[182] Powers, MA Handbook of Diabetes Medical Nutrition Therapy *Aspen Publishers* 1996:8-9

[183] Buczkowska EO, Jarosz-Chobot P. Insulin effect on metabolism in skeletal muscles and the role of muscles in regulation of glucose homeostasis *Przegl Lek* 2001;58(7-8):782-7

[184] Powers, MA Handbook of Diabetes Medical Nutrition Therapy *Aspen Publishers* 1996:8

[185] Zammit VA, Waterman IJ, Topping D, McKay G. Insulin stimulation of hepatic triacylglycerol secrection and the etiology of insulin resistance. J Nutr 2001 Aug;131(8);2074-7

[186] Diraison F, Dusserre E, Vidal H, Sothier M, Bey-lot M. Increased hepatic lipogenesis but decreased expression of lipogenic gene in adipose tissue in human obesity. *Am J Physiol Endocrinol Metab* 2002 Jan;282(1):E46-51

[187] Zhao AZ, Shinohara MM, Huang D, Shimizu M, Eldar-Finkelman H, Krebs EG, Beavo JA, Bornfeldt KE. Leptin induces insulin-like signaling that antago-nizes cAMP elevation by glucagon in hepatocytes. *J Biol Chem* 2000 Apr 14;275(15):11348-54

[188] Seppala-Lindroos A, Vehkavaara S, Hakkinen AM, Goto T, Westerbacka J, Sovijarvi A, Halavaara J, Yki-Jarvinen H. Fat accumulation in the liver is as-sociated with defects in insulin suppression of glucose production and serum free Fatty acids independent of obesity in normal men. *J Clin Endocrinol Metab* 2002 Jul;87(7):3023-8

[189] Nemecz M, Preininger K, Englisch R, Furnsinn C, Schneider B, Waldhausl W, Roden M. Acute effect of leptin on hepatic glycogenolysis and gluconeogenesis in perfused rat liver.*Hepatology* 1999 Jan;29(1):166-72

[190] Harris RB. Acute and chronic effects of leptin on glucose utilization in lean mice. *Biochem Biophys Res Commun* 1998 Apr 17;245(2):502-9

[191] Hanefeld M, Kohler C. The metabolic syndrome and its epidemiologic dimensions in historical perspective *Z Arztl Fortbild Qualitatssich* 2002 Mar;96(3):183-8

[192] Gomez-Ambrosi J, Salvador J, Paramo JA, Orbe J, de Irala J, Diez-Caballero A, Gil MJ, Cienfuegos JA, Fruhbeck G. Involvement of leptin in the association between percentage of body fat and cardiovascular risk factors. Clin Biochem 2002 Jun;35(4):315-20

[193] Unger RH. Lipotoxic diseases. *Annu Rev Med* 2002;53:319-36

[194] Hosker JP, Burnett MA, Mathews DR, Turner RC. Suppression of insulin secretion by falling plasma glucose levels is impaired in type 2 diabetes. *Diabetic Med* 1988;5:856

[195] Gerich JE. Is reduced first-phase insulin release the earliest detectable abnormality in individuals destined to develop type 2 diabetes? *Diabetes* 2002 Feb;51 Suppl 1:S117-21

[196] Trayhurn P, Hoggard N, Mercer JG & Rayner DV. (1999) Leptin: fundamental aspects. *International Journal of Obesity* 23, 22-28.

[197] Kieffer TJ, Heller RS, Leech CA, Holz GG, Habener JF. Leptin suppression of insulin secretion by te acti-vation of the ATP-sensitive K channels in pancreatic B-cells. *Diabetes* 46: 1087-1093, 1997.

[198] Lam NT, Cheung AT, Riedel MJ, Light PE, Cheese-man CI, Kieffer TJ. Leptin reduces glucose transport and cellular ATP levels in INS-1 beta-cells. *J Mol Endocrinol*. 2004 Apr;32(2):415-24.

[199] Van Gaal Lf, Wauters MA, Mertens IL, Considine RV, DE Leeuw IH: Clinical endocrinology of human leptin. *Int J Obes Relat Metab Disord* 23 (Suppl 1): 29-36, 1999.

[200] Seufert J. Leptin effects on pancreatic beta-cell gene expression and function. *Diabetes*. 2004 Feb;53 Suppl 1:S152-8.

[201] Masuo K, Mikami H, Ogihara T, Tuck ML. Familial obesity, sympathetic activation and blood pressure level. *Blood Press* 2001;10(4):199-204.

[202] Law C. Adult obesity and growth in childhood. *BMJ* 2001 Dec 8;323(7325):1320-1.

[203] Breier BH, Vickers MH, Ikenasio BA, Chan KY, Wong WP. Fetal programming of appetite and obesity. *Mol Cell Endocrinol* 2001 Dec 20;185(1-2):73-9.

[204] Wang J, Obici S, Morgan K, Barzilai N, Feng Z, Ros-setti L. Overfeeding rapidly induced leptin and insulin resistance. *Diabetes* 2001 Dec;50(12):2786-91.

[205] Huang BW, Chiang MT, Yao HT, Chiang W. The effect of high-fat and high-fructose diets on glucose tolerance and plasma lipid and leptin levels in rats. *Diabetes Obes Metab*. 2004 Mar;6(2):120-6.

[206] Busserolles J, Gueux E, Rock E, Demigne C, Mazur A, Rayssiguier Y. Oligofructose protects against the hypertriglyceridemic and pro-oxidative effects of a high fructose diet in rats. *J Nutr*. 2003 Jun;133(6):1903-8.

[207] Bray GA, Nielsen SJ, Popkin BM. Consumption of high-fructose corn syrup in beverages may play a role in the epidemic of obesity. *Am J Clin Nutr*. 2004 Apr;79(4):537-43.

[208] Polson DA, Thompson MP. Macronutrient com-position of the diet differentially affects leptin and adiponutrin mRNA expression in response to meal feeding. *J Nutr Biochem*. 2004 Apr;15(4):242-6.

[209] Rolls,BJ, Morri,ER and Roe LS Portion size of food affects energy intake in normal-weight and overweight men and women *Am J Clin Nutr* 2002;76:1207–13.

[210] Guyton A. Specific dynamic action of protein. *Textbook of Medical Physiology* WB Saunders Company 1991:793-4.

[211] Polson DA, Thompson MP. Macronutrient com-position of the diet differentially affects leptin and adiponutrin mRNA expression in response to meal feeding. *J Nutr Biochem*. 2004 Apr;15(4):242-6.

[212] Receputo G, Rapisarda R, Motta L. Centenarians: health status and life conditions *Ann Ital Med Int* 1995 Jan-Mar;10(1):41-5

[213] Bray GA. Reciprocal relation of food intake and sympathetic activity: experimental observations and clinical implications. *Int J Obes Relat Metab Disord* 2000 Jun;24 Suppl 2:S8-17

[214] Astrup A. Thermogenic drugs as a strategy for treat-ment of obesity. *Endocrine* 2000 Oct;13(2):207-12

[215] Boozer CN, Daly PA, Homel P, Solomon JL, Blanchard D, Nasser JA, Strauss R, Meredith T.

Herbal ephedra/caffeine for weight loss: a 6-month randomized safety and efficacy trial. *Int J Obes Relat Metab Disord* 2002 May;26(5):593-604

[216] Cammisotto PG, Bukowiecki LJ. Mechanisms of leptin secretion from white adipocytes. *Am J Physiol Cell Physiol.* 2002 Jul;283(1):C244-50.

[217] Zheng G, Sayama K, Okubo T, Juneja LR, Oguni I. Anti-obesity effects of three major components of green tea, catechins, caffeine and theanine, in mice. *In Vivo.* 2004 Jan-Feb;18(1):55-62.

[218] Sachan DS, Hongu N. Increases in VO(2)max and metabolic markers of fat oxidation by caffeine, carnitine, and choline supplementation in rats. *0955-2863* 2000 Oct;11(10):521-526

[219] Ryu S, Choi SK, Joung SS, Suh H, Cha YS, Lee S, Lim K. Caffeine as a lipolytic food component increases endurance performance in rats and athletes. *J Nutr Sci Vitaminol* (Tokyo) 2001 Apr;47(2):139-46

[220] McCarty MF. Modulation of adipocyte lipoprotein lipase expression as a strategy for preventing or treating visceral obesity. *Med Hypotheses* 2001 Aug;57(2):192-200

[221] Sakamoto W, Nishihira J, Fujie K, Mizuno S, Ozaki M, Yukawa S. Coffee and fitness-coffee suppresses lipopolysaccharide-induced liver injury in rats. *J Nutr Sci Vitaminol* (Tokyo) 2000 Dec;46(6):316-20

[222] Lindaman BA, Hinkhouse MM, Conklin JL, Cullen JJ. The effect of phosphodiesterase inhibition on gallbladder motility in vitro. *J Surg Res* 2002 Jun 15;105(2):102-8

[223] Boekema PJ, Samsom M, van Berge Henegouwen GP, Smout AJ. Coffee and gastrointestinal function: facts and fiction. A review. *Scand J Gastroenterol Suppl* 1999;230:35-9

[224] Cammisotto PG, Bukowiecki LJ. Mechanisms of leptin secretion from white adipocytes. *Am J Physiol Cell Physiol* 2002 Jul;283(1):C244-50

[225] Ramsey JJ, Colman RJ, Swick AG, Kemnitz JW. Energy expenditure, body composition, and glucose metabolism in lean and obese rhesus monkeys treated with ephedrine and caffeine. *Am J Clin Nutr* 1998 Jul;68(1):42-51

[226] van Dam RM, Feskens EJ. Coffee consumption and risk of type 2 diabetes mellitus. *Lancet* 2002 Nov 9;360(9344):1477-8

[227] Lieberman HR, Tharion WJ, Shukitt-Hale B, Speckman KL, Tulley R. Effects of caffeine, sleep loss, and stress on cognitive performance and mood during U.S. Navy SEAL training. *Psychopharmacology* (Berl) 2002 Nov;164(3):250-61

[228] Yeomans MR, Ripley T, Davies LH, Rusted JM, Rogers PJ. Effects of caffeine on performance and mood depend on the level of caffeine abstinence. *Psychopharmacology* (Berl) 2002 Nov;164(3):241-9

[229] McClellan Stine M, O'Connor RJ, Yatko BR, Grunberg NE, Cousino Klein L. Evidence for a relationship between daily caffeine consumption and accuracy of time estimation. *Hum Psychopharmacol* 2002 Oct;17(7):361-7

[230] Kruger S, Braunig P. Abuse of body weight reducing agents in bulimia nervosa *Nervenarzt* 1995 Jan;66(1):66-9

[231] Sours JA. Case reports of anorexia nervosa and caffeinism. *Am J Psychiatry* 1983 Feb;140(2):235-6

[232] Shaul PW, Farrell MK, Maloney MJ. Caffeine toxicity as a cause of acute psychosis in anorexia nervosa. *J Pediatr* 1984 Sep;105(3):493-5 Shaul PW, Farrell MK, Maloney MJ. Caffeine toxicity as a cause of acute psychosis in anorexia nervosa. *J Pediatr* 1984 Sep;105(3):493-5

[233] Forman J, Aizer A, Young CR. Myocardial infarction resulting from caffeine overdose in an anorectic woman. *Ann Emerg Med* 1997 Jan;29(1):178-80

[234] Keijzers GB, De Galan BE, Tack CJ, Smits P. Caffeine can decrease insulin sensitivity in humans. *Diabetes Care* 2002 Feb;25(2):364-9

[235] Hartley TR, Lovallo WR, Whitsett TL. Cardiovascular effects of caffeine in men and women. *Am J Cardiol.* 2004 Apr 15;93(8):1022-6.

[236] Lane JD, Pieper CF, Phillips-Bute BG, Bryant JE, Kuhn CM. Caffeine affects cardiovascular and neuroendocrine activation at work and home. *Psychosom Med* 2002 Jul-Aug;64(4):595-603

[237] Baranowska B, Wolinska-Witort E, Wasilewska-Dziubinska E, Roguski K, Martynska L, Chmielowska M. The role of neuropeptides in the disturbed control of appetite and hormone secretion in eating disorders. *Neuroendocrinol Lett.* 2003 Dec;24(6):431-4.

[238] Halford JC, Blundell JE. Separate systems for serotonin and leptin in appetite control. *Ann Med* 2000 Apr;32(3):222-32

[239] Christensen L, Pettijohn L. Mood and carbohydrate cravings. *Appetite* 2001 Apr;36(2):137-45

[240] Christenese L, Somers S. Comparison of nutrient intake among depressed and nondepressed individuals. *Int J Eat Disord* 1996 July;20(1):105-9

[241] Sayegh R, Schiff I, Wurtman J, Spiers P, McDermott J, Wurtman R. The effect of carbohydrate rich beverage on mood, appetite, and cognitive function in women with premenstrual syndrome. *Obstet Gynecol* 1995 Oct;86(4 Pt 1):520-8

[242] Yoshimatsu H, Chiba S, Tajima D, Akehi Y, Sakata T. Histidine suppresses food intake through its conversion into neuronal histamine. *Exp Biol Med* (Maywood) 2002 Jan;227(1):63-8

[243] Mollet A, Lutz TA, Meier S, Riediger T, Rushing PA, Scharrer E. Histamine H1 receptors mediate the anorectic action of the pancreatic hormone amylin. *Am J Physiol Regul Integr Comp Physiol* 2001 Nov;281(5): R1442-8

[244] Morimoto T, Yamamoto Y, Yamatodani A. Brain histamine and feeding behavior. *Behav Brain Res* 2001 Oct 15;124(2):145-50

[245] Watanabe T, Yanai K. Studies on functional roles of the histaminergic neuron system by using pharmacological agents, knockout mice and positron emission tomography. *Tohoku J Exp Med* 2001 Dec;195(4):197-217

[246] Kang JH, Kim KS, Choi SY, Kwon HY, Won MH, Kang TC. Carnosine and related dipeptides protect human ceruloplasm against peroxyl radical mediated modification. *Mol Cells* 2002 Jun 30:13(3):498-502

[247] Tabakman R, Lazarovici P, Kohen R. Neuroprotective effects of carnosine and homocarnosine on pheochromocytoma PC12 cells exposed to ischemia. *J Neurosci Res* 2002 May 15;68(4):463-9

[248] Boldyrev AA, Yuneva MO, Sorokina EV, Kramarenko GG, Fedorova TN, Konovalova GG, Lankin VZ.

Antioxidant systems in tissues of senescence accelerated mice. *Biochemestry (Mosc)* 2001 Oct;66(10):1157-63

[249] Dukic-Stefanovic S, Schinzel R, Riederer P, Munch G. AGES in brain aging: AGE-inhibitors as neuroprotective and anti-dementia drugs? *Biogerontology* 2001;2(1):19-334

[250] Horning MS, Blakemore LJ, Trombley PQ. Endogenous mechanisms of neuroprotection; role of zinc, copper, and carnosine. *Brain Res* 2000 Jan 3;852 (1) :56-61

[251] Niijima A, Okui T, Matsumura Y, Yamano T, Tsuruoka N, Kiso Y, Nagai K. Effects of L carnosine on renal sympathetic nerve activity in DOCA-salt hypertensive rats. *Auton Neurosci* 2002 May 31;97(2):99-102

[252] Wilding JP. Neuropeptides and appetite control. *Diabet Med* 2002 Aug;19(8):619-27

[253] Fekete C, Sarkar S, Rand WM, Harney JW, Emerson CH, Bianco AC, Lechan RM. Agouti-related protein (AGRP) has a central inhibitory action on the hypothalamic-pituitary-thyroid (HPT) axis; comparisons between the effect of AGRP and neuropeptide Y on energy homeostasis and the HPT axis. *Endocrinology* 2002 Oct;143(10):3846-53

[254] Claycombe KJ, Xue BZ, Mynatt RL, Zemel MB, Moustaid-Moussa N. Regulation of leptin by agouti. *Physiol Genomics* 2000 Apr 27;2(3):101-5.

[255] Zemel MB. Agouti/melanocortin interaction with leptin pathways in obesity. *Nutr Rev* 1998 Sep;56(9):271-4.

[256] Zemel MB, Shi H, Greer B, Dirienzo D, Zemel PC. Regualtion of adiposity by dietary calcium. *FASEB J* 2000 Jun;14(9):1132-8.

[257] Makimura H, Mizuno TM, Mastaitis JW, Agami R, Mobbs CV. Reducing hypothalamic AGRP by RNA interference increases metabolic rate and decreases body weight without influencing food intake. *BMC Neurosci* 2002 Nov 7;3(1):18

[258] Zemel MB. Caluium modulation of hypertension and obesity mechanisms and implications. *J Am Coll Nutr* 2001 Oct;20(5 Suppl):428S-435;discussion 440S-442S.

[259] Shi H, Dirienzo D, Zemel MB. Effects of dietary calcium on adipocyte lipid metabolism and body weight regulation in energy-restricted aP2-agouti transgenic mice. *FASEB J* 2001 Feb;15(2):291-3.

[260] Menendez C, Lage M, Peino R, Baldelli R, Concheiro P, Dieguez C, Casanueva FF. Retinoic acid and vitamin D(3) powerfully inhibit in vitro leptin secretion by human adipose tissue. *J Endocrinol* 2001 Aug;170(2):425-31.

[261] Holst JJ, Orskov C. Incretin hormones—an update. Scand J Clin Lab Invest Suppl 2001;(234):75-85

[262] Miyawaki K, Yamada Y, Ban N, Ihara Y, Tsukiyama K, Zhou H, Fujimoto S, Oku A, Tsuda K, Toyokuni S, Hiai H, Mizunoya W, Fushiki T, Holst JJ, Makino M, Tashita A, Kobara Y, Tsubamoto Y, Jinnouchi T, Jomori T, Seino Y. Inhibition of gastric inhibitory polypeptide signaling prevents obesity. Nat Med 2002 Jul;8(7):738-42

[263] Ninomiya Y, Shigemura N, Yasumatsu K, Ohta R, Sugimoto K, Nakashima K, Lindemann B. Leptin and sweet taste. *Vitam Horm* 2002;64:221-48

[264] Cone RD, Cowley MA, Butler AA, Fan W, Marks DL, Low MJ. The arcuate nucleus as a conduit for diverse signals relevant to energy homeostasis. *Int J Obes Relat Metab Disord* 2001 Dec;25 Suppl 5:S63-7

[265] Tschop M, Flora DB, Mayer JP, Heiman ML. Hypophysectomy prevents ghrelin-induced adiposity and increases gastric ghrelin secretion in rats. *Obes Res* 2002 Oct;10(10):991-9

[266] Beck B, Musse N, Stricker-Krongrad A. Ghrelin, macronutrient intake and dietary preferences in long-evans rats. *Biochem Biophys Res Commun* 2002 Apr 12;292(4):1031-5

[267] Caixas A, Bashore C, Nash W, Pi-Sunyer F, Laferrere B. Insulin, unlike food intake, does not suppress ghrelin in human subjects. *J Clin Endocrinol Metab* 2002 Apr;87(4):1902

[268] Volante M, Allia E, Gugliotta P, Funaro A, Broglio F, Deghenghi R, Muccioli G, Ghigo E, Papotti M. Expression of ghrelin and of the GH secretagogue receptor by pancreatic islet cells and related endocrine tumors. *J Clin Endocrinol Metab* 2002 Mar;87(3):1300-8

[269] Trudel L, Tomasetto C, Rio MC, Bouin M, Plourde V, Eberling P, Poitras P. Ghrelin/motilin-related peptide is a potent prokinetic to reverse gastric postoperative ileus in rat. *Am J Physiol Gastrointest Liver Physiol* 2002 Jun;282(6):G948-52

[270] Papotti M, Cassoni P, Volante M, Deghenghi R, Muccioli G, Ghigo E. Ghrelin-producing endocrine tumors of the stomach and intestine. *J Clin Endocrinol Metab* 2001 Oct;86(10):5052-9

[271] Volante M, Allia E, Gugliotta P, Funaro A, Broglio F, Deghenghi R, Muccioli G, Ghigo E, Papotti M. Expression of ghrelin and of the GH secretagogue receptor by pancreatic islet cells and related endocrine tumors. *J Clin Endocrinol Metab* 2002 Mar;87(3):1300-8

[272] Kanamoto N, Akamizu T, Hosoda H, Hataya Y, Ariyasu H, Takaya K, Hosoda K, Saijo M, Moriyama K, Shimatsu A, Kojima M, Kangawa K, Nakao K. Substantial production of ghrelin by a human medullary thyroid carcinoma cell line. *J Clin Endocrinol Metab* 2001 Oct;86(10):4984-90

[273] Cummings DE, Purnell JQ, Frayo RS, Schmidova K, Wisse BE, Weigle DS. A preprandial rise in plasma ghrelin levels suggests a role in meal initiation in humans. *Diabetes* 2001 Aug;50(8):1714-9

[274] Traebert M, Riediger T, Whitebread S, Scharrer E, Schmid HA. Ghrelin acts on leptin-responsive neurones in the rat arcuate nucleus. *J Neuroendocrinol* 2002 Jul;14(7):580-6

[275] Tschop M, Weyer C, Tataranni PA, Devanarayan V, Ravussin E, Heiman ML. Circulating ghrelin levels are decreased in human obesity. *Diabetes* 2001 Apr;50(4):707-9

[276] English PJ, Ghatei MA, Malik IA, Bloom SR, Wilding JP. Food fails to suppress ghrelin levels in obese humans. *J Clin Endocrinol Metab* 2002 Jun;87(6):2984

[277] Bagnasco M, Kalra PS, Kalra SP. Ghrelin and leptin pulse discharge in fed and fasted rats. *Endocrinology* 2002 Feb;143(2):726-9

[278] Mustonen AM, Nieminen P, Hyvarinen H. Preliminary evidence that pharmacologic melatonin treatment decreases rat ghrelin levels. *Endocrine* 2001 Oct;16(1):43-6

[279] Patten SB. Major depressive episodes and diet pills. *Expert Opin Pharmacother* 2002 Oct;3(10):1405-9

[280] Patten SB. "Diet pills" and major depression

in the Canadian population. *Can J Psychiatry* 2001 Jun;46(5):438-40

[281] Orlistat: a second look. At best, a minor adjunct to dietary measures. *Prescrire Int* 2002 Feb;11(57):10-2

[282] Binkley K, Knowles SR. Sibutramine and panic attacks. Am J Psychiatry 2002 Oct;159(10):1793-4

[283] Nisoli E, Carruba MO. An assessment of the safety and efficacy of sibutramine, an anti-obesity drug with a novel mechanism of action. *Obes Rev* 2000 Oct;1(2):127-39

[284] Birkenfeld AL, Schroeder C, Boschmann M, Tank J, Franke G, Luft FC, Biaggioni I, Sharma AM, Jordan J. Paradoxical effect of sibutramine on autonomic cardiovascular regulation. *Circulation* 2002 Nov 5;106(19):2459-65

[285] Wen W, Shu XO, Potter JD, Severson RK, Buckley JD, Reaman GH, Robison LL. Parental medication use and risk of childhood acute lymphoblastic leukemia. *Cancer* 2002 Oct 15;95(8):1786-94

[286] Samenuk D, Link MS, Homoud MK, Contreras R, Theohardes TC, Wang PJ, Estes NA Adverse cardiovascular events temporally associated with ma huang, an herbal source of ephedrine. *Mayo Clin Proc* 2002 Jan;77(1):12-6

[287] Fobi M, Lee H, Igwe D, Felahy B, James E, Stanczyk M, Fobi N. Prophylactic cholecystectomy with gastric bypass operation: incidence of gallbladder disease. *Obes Surg* 2002 Jun;12(3):350-3

[288] Melinek J, Livingston E, Cortina G, Fishbein MC. Autopsy findings following gastric bypass surgery for morbid obesity. *Arch Pathol Lab Med* 2002 Sep;126(9):1091-5

[289] Blachar A, Federle MP, Pealer KM, Ikramuddin S, Schauer PR. Gastrointestinal complications of laparoscopic Roux-en-Y gastric bypass surgery: clinical and imaging findings. *Radiology* 2002 Jun;223(3):625-32

[290] Goldner WS, O'Dorisio TM, Dillon JS, Mason EE. Severe metabolic bone disease as a long-term complication of obesity surgery. *Obes Surg* 2002 Oct;12(5):685-92

[291] Cummings DE, Weigle DS, Frayo RS, Breen PA, Ma MK, Dellinger EP, Purnell JQ. Plasma ghrelin levels after diet-induced weight loss or gastric bypass surgery. *N Engl J Med* 2002 May 23;346(21):1623-30

[292] Pombo M, Pombo CM, Garcia A, Caminos E, Gualillo O, Alvarez CV, Casanueva FF, Dieguez C. Hormonal control of growth hormone secretion. *Horm Res* 2001;55 Suppl 1:11-6

[293] Cui GL, Syversen U, Zhao CM, Chen D, Waldum HL. Long-term omeprazole treatment suppresses body weight gain and bone mineralization in young male rats. *Scand J Gastroenterol* 2001 Oct;36(10):1011-5

[294] McNamara DJ. Eggs and heart disease risk: perpetuating the misperception. Comment on: Am J Clin Nutr. 2001 May;73(5):885-91. *Am J Clin Nutr.* 2002 Feb;75(2):333-5.

[295] Kritchevsky SB, Kritchevsky D. Egg consumption and coronary heart disease: an epidemiologic overview. *J Am Coll Nutr.* 2000 Oct;19(5 Suppl):549S-555S.

[296] McNamara DJ. The impact of egg limitations on coronary heart disease risk: do the numbers add up? Comment in: *J Am Coll Nutr.* 2001 Feb;20(1):93-4. J Am Coll Nutr. 2000 Oct;19(5 Suppl):540S-548S.

[297] Zeisel SH, Mar MH, Howe JC, Holden JM. Concentrations of choline-containing compounds and betaine in common foods. Erratum in: J Nutr. 2003 Sep;133(9):2918. *J Nutr.* 2003 May;133(5):1302-7.

[298] Warensjo E, Jansson JH, Berglund L, Boman K, Ahren B, Weinehall L, Lindahl B, Hallmans G, Vessby B. Estimated intake of milk fat is negatively associated with cardiovascular risk factors and does not increase the risk of a first acute myocardial infarction. A prospective case-control study. *Br J Nutr.* 2004 Apr;91(4):635-42.

[299] Fontana L, Meyer TE, Klein S, Holloszy JO. Long-term calorie restriction is highly effective in reducing the risk for atherosclerosis in humans. *Proceedings of the National Academy of Sciences*, April 27, 2004.

[300] Bayes B, Pastor MC, Bonal J, Junca J, Hernandez JM, Riutort N, Foraster A, Romero R. Homocysteine, C-reactive protein, lipid peroxidation and mortality in haemodialysis patients. *Nephrol Dial Transplant* 2003 Jan;18(1):106-12

[301] Hasegawa T, Negishi T, Deguchi M. WBC Count, Atherosclerosis and Coronary Risk Factors. *J Atheroscler Thromb* 2002;9(5):219-23

[302] Kowalewski M, Urban M, Mroczko B, Szmitkowski M. Pro-inflammatory cytokines (IL-6, TNF-alpha) and cardiac troponin I (cTnI) in serum of young people with ventricular arrhythmias. *Pol Arch Med Wewn* 2002 Jul;108(1):647-51

[303] Riboldi P, Gerosa M, Luzzana C, Catelli L. Cardiac involvement in systemic autoimmune diseases. *Clin Rev Allergy Immunol* 2002 Dec;23(3):247-61

[304] Koenig W. Insulin resistance, heart disease and inflammation. Identifying the 'at-risk' patient: the earlier the better? The role of inflammatory markers. *Int J Clin Pract Suppl* 2002 Oct;(132):23-30

[305] Park A. Beyond cholesterol. Inflammation is emerging as a major risk factor—and not just in heart disease. *Time* 2002 Nov 25;160(22):74-5

[306] Sewter CP, Digby JE, Blows F, Prins JB & O'Rahilly S (1999) Regulation of tumour necrosis factor-alpha release from human adipose tissue in vitro. *Journal of Endocrinology* 163, 33-38.

[307] Hotamisligil GS, Arner P, Caro JF, Atkinson RL & Speigelman BaM (1995) Increased adipose tissue expression of tumor necrosis factor-x in human obesity and insulin resistance. *Journal of Clinical Investigation* 95, 2409-2415.

[308] Hotamisligil GS, (1999) The role of TNFx and TNF receptors in obesity and insulin resistance. *Journal of Internal Medicine* 245, 612-625.

[309] Coppack SW. Pro-inflammatory cytokines and adipose tissue. *Nutrition Society*(2001), 60, 349-356.

[310] Stephens JM & Pakala PH (1991) Transcriptional regression of the GLUT4 and C/EBP genes in 3T3-L1 adipocytes by tumor necrosis factor-alpha.

[311] Mohamed-Ali V, Pinkney JH & Coppack SW (1998) Adipose tissueas an endocrine and paracrine organ. *International Journal of Obesity and Related Metabolic Disorders* 22, 1145-1158.

[312] Plata-Salaman CR (1999) Central nervous system mechanisms contributing to the cachexia-anorexia syndrome. *Nutrition* 16, 1009-1012.

[313] Konstantinides S, Schafer K, Koschnick S, Loskutoff DJ. Leptin-dependent platelet aggregation and arterial thrombois suggests a mechanism for

atherothrombotic disease in obesity. *J Clin Invest* 2001 Nov;108(10):1533-40.

[314] Monk TH, Reynolds CF 3rd, Kupfer DJ, Hoch CC, Carrier J, Houck PR. Differences over the life span in daily life-style regularity. *Chronobiol Int* 1997 May;14(3):295-306

[315] Wang Q, Chen M, Hu R, Tang J, Li F, Luo B. The effects of glucocorticoids and insulin on serum leptin level and its diurnal rhythmicity *Zhonghua Nei Ke Za Zhi* 2002 Feb;41(2):104-8

[316] Szucs N, Varga I, Jakab C, Patocs A, Glaz E, Toth M, Kiss R, Racz K. Leptin inhibits cortisol and corticosterone secretion in pathologic human adrenocortical cells. *Pituitary* 2001 Jan-Apr;4(1-2):71-7

[317] Wang Q, Chen M, Hu R, Tang J, Li F, Luo B. The effects of glucocorticoids and insulin on serum leptin level and its diurnal rhythmicity *Zhonghua Nei Ke Za Zhi* 2002 Feb;41(2):104-8

[318] Gualillo O, Eiras S, Lago F, Dieguez C, Casanueva FF. Elevated serum leptin concentrations induced by experimental acute inflammation. *Life Sci* 2000 Oct 6;67(20):2433-41

[319] Fantuzzi G, Faggioni R. Leptin in the regulation of immunity, inflammation, and hematopoiesis. *J Leukoc Biol* 2000 Oct;68(4):437-46

[320] Maruna P, Gurlich R, Frasko R. Leptin—a new acute phase reactant *Vnitr Lek* 2001 Jul;47(7):478-83

[321] Finck BN, Johnson RW. Tumor necrosis factor-alpha regulates secretion of the adipocyte-derived cytokine, leptin. *Microsc Res Tech* 2000 Aug 1;50(3):209-15

[322] Gerhardt CC, Romero IA, Cancello R, Camoin L, Strosberg AD. Chemokines control fat accumulation and leptin secretion by cultured human adipocytes. *Mol Cell Endocrinol* 2001 Apr 25;175(1-2):81-92

[323] Voegeling S, Fantuzzi G. Regulation of free and bound leptin and soluble leptin receptors during inflammation in mice. *Cytokine* 2001 Apr 21;14(2):97-103

[324] Das UN. Is obesity an inflammatory condition? *Nutrition* 2001 Nov-Dec;17(11-12):953-66

[325] Chiellini C, Bertacca A, Novelli SE, Gorgun CZ, Ciccarone A, Giordano A, Xu H, Soukas A, Costa M, Gandini D, Dimitri R, Bottone P, Cecchetti V Increased leptin concentrations correlate with increased concentrations of inflammatory markers in morbidly obese individuals. *Int J Obes Relat Metab Disord* 2001 Dec;25(12):1759-66

[326] P, Pardini E, Perego L, Navalesi R, Folli F, Benzi L, Cinti S, Friedman JM, Hotamisligil GS, Maffei M. Obesity modulates the expression of haptoglobin in the white adipose tissue via TNFalpha. *J Cell Physiol* 2002 Feb;190(2):251-8

[327] Joussen AM, Poulaki V, Mitsiades N, Kirchhof B, Koizumi K, Dohmen S, Adamis AP. Nonsteroidal anti-inflammatory drugs prevent early diabetic retinopathy via TNF-alpha suppression. *FASEB J* 2002 Mar;16(3):438-40

[328] Nishiyama M, Makino S, Suemaru S, Nanamiya W, Asaba K, Kaneda T, Mimoto T, Nishioka T, Takao T, Hashimoto K. Glucocorticoid effects on the diurnal rhythm of circulating leptin levels. *Horm Res* 2000;54(2):69-73

[329] Leal-Cerro A, Soto A, Martinez MA, Dieguez C, Casanueva FF. Influence of cortisol status on leptin secretion. *Pituitary* 2001 Jan-Apr;4(1-2):111-6

[330] Fruhbeck G, Gomez-Ambrosi J. Depot-specific differences in the lipolytic effect of leptin on isolated white adipocytes. *Med Sci Monit* 2002 Feb;8(2):BR47-55

[331] Bjorntorp P. Do stress reactions cause abdominal obesity and comorbidities? *Obes Rev* 2001 May;2(2):73-86

[332] Bjorntorp P, Rossner S, Udden J. "Consolatory eating" is not a myth. Stress-induced increased cortisol levels result in leptin-resistant obesity *Lakartidningen* 2001 Nov 28;98(48):5458-61

[333] Gabriely I, Ma XH, Yang XM, Atzmon G, Rajala MW, Berg AH, Scherer P, Rossetti L, Barzilai N. Removal of visceral fat prevents insulin resistance and glucose intolerance of aging: an adipokine-mediated process? *Diabetes* 2002 Oct;51(10):2951-8

[334] Atkinson LL, Fischer MA, Lopaschuk GD. Leptin activates cardiac fatty acid oxidation independent of changes in the AMP-activated protein kinase - acetyl-CoA carboxylase - malonyl-CoA Axis. *J Biol Chem* 2002 Jun 10

[335] Lopes IM, Forga L, Martinez JA. Effects of leptin resistance on acute fuel metabolism after a high carbohydrate load in lean and overweight young men. *J Am Coll Nutr* 2001 Dec;20(6):643-8

[336] Ukropec J, Sebokova E, Klimes I. Nutrient sensing, leptin and insulin action. *Arch Physiol Biochem* 2001 Feb;109(1):38-51

[337] Fletcher RH, Fairchild KM Vitamins for chronic disease prevention in adults:clinical applications. *JAMA* June 19, 2002;287:3217-3219

[338] Nisoli E, Carruba MO, Tonello C, Macor C, Federspil G & Vettor R (2000b) Induction of fatty acid translocase/CD36, peroxisome proliferators-activated receptor, leptin, uncoupling proteins 2 and 3, and tumor necrosis factor-x gene expression in human sub-cutaneous fat by lipid infusion. *Diabetes* 49, 319-324.

[339] Simopoulos AP. Omega-3 Fatty acids in inflammation and autoimmune diseases. *J Am Coll Nutr* 2002 Dec;21(6):495-505

[340] James MJ, Gibson RA, Cleland LG. Dietary polyunsaturated fatty acids and inflammatory mediator production. *Am J Clin Nutr* 2000 Jan;71(1 Suppl):343S-8S

[341] Storlien LH, Higgins JA, Thomas TC, et al. Diet composition and insulin action in animal models. *Br J Nutr* 2000;83:S85-S90.

[342] Storlien LH, Kraegen EW, Chrisholm DJ, et al. Fish oil prevents insulin resistance induced by high-fat feeding in rats. *Science* 1987;237:885-888.

[343] Storlien LH, Jenkins AB, Chrisholm DJ, et al. Influence of dietary fat composition on development of insulin resistance in rats. Relationship to muscle triglyceride and omega-3 fatty acids in muscle phospholipids. *Diabetes* 1991;40:280-289.

[344] Wellhoener P, Fruehwald-Schultes B, Kern W, Dantz D, Kerner W, Bom J, Fehm HL, Peters A. Glucose metabolism rather than insulin is a main determinant of leptin secretion in humans. *J Clin Endocrinol Metab* 85:1267-1271, 2000.

[345] Thies F, Nebe-von-Caron G, Powell JR, Yaqoob P, Newsholme EA, Calder PC. Dietary supplementation with gamma-linolenic acid or fish oil decreases T lymphocyte proliferation in healthy older humans. *J Nutr* 2001 Jul;131(7):1928-27.

[346] Gaddi A, Descovich GC, Noseda G, et al. Controlled evaluation of pantethine, a natural hypolipidemic compound, in patients with different forms of hyperlipoproteinemia. *Atherosclerosis* 1984;50:73-83.

[347] Murai A, Miyahara T, Tanaka T, Sako Y, Nishimura N, Kameyama M. The effects of pantethine on lipid and lipoprotein abnormalities in survivors of cerebral infarction. *Artery* 1985;12(4):234-43

[348] Hiramtsu K, Nozaki H, Arimori S. Influence of pantethine on platelet volume, microviscosity, lipid composition and functions in diabetes mellitus with hyperlipdimia. *Tokai J Exp Clin Med* 1981 Jan;6(1):49-57.

[349] Gensini GF, Prisco D, Rogasi PG, Matucci M, Neri Serneri GG. Changes in fatty acid composition of the single platelet phospholipids induced by pantethine treatment. *Int J Clin Pharmacol Res* 1985;5(5):309-18

[350] Arsenio L, Bodria P, Magnati G, Strata A, Trovato R. Effectiveness of long-term treatment with pantethine in patients with dyslipidemia. *Clin Ther* 1986;8(5):537-45

[351] Donati C, Bertieri RS, Barbi G. [Pantethine, diabetes mellitus and atherosclerosis. Clinical study of 1045 patients] *Clin Ter* 1989 Mar 31;128(6):411-22.

[352] Prisco D, Rogasi PG, Matucci M, Paniccia R, Abbate R, Gensini GF, Neri Serneri GG. Effect of oral treatment with pantethine on platelet and plasma phospholipids in IIa hyperlipoproteinemia. *Angiology* 1987 Mar;38(3):241-7

[353] Noma A, Kita M, Okamiya T. Effect of pantethine on post-heparin plasma lipolytic activities and adipose tissue lipoprotein lipase in rats. *Horm Metab Res* 1984 May;16(5):233-6.

[354] Osono Y, Hirose N, Nakajima K, Hata Y. The effects of pantethine on fatty liver and fat distribution. *J Atheroscler Thromb* 2000;7(1):55-8

[355] Katsuki A, Sumida Y, Gabazza EC, Murashima S, Tanaka T, Furuta M, Araki-Sasaki R, Hori Y, Nakatani K, Yano Y, Adachi Y. Plasma levels of agouti-related protein are increased in obese men. *J Clin Endocrinol Metab* 2001 May;86(5):1921-4

[356] Weimann E. Gender-related differences in elite gymnasts: the female athlete triad. *J Appl Physiol* 2002 May;92(5):2146-52

[357] Nandi J, Meguid MM, Inui A, Xu Y, Makarenko IG, Tada T, Chen C. Central mechanisms involved with catabolism. *Curr Opin Clin Nutr Metab Care* 2002 Jul;5(4):407-18

[358] Saris WH. The concept of energy homeostasis for optimum health during training. *Can J Appl Physiol* 2001;26 Suppl:S167-75

[359] Nandi J, Meguid MM, Inui A, Xu Y, Makarenko IG, Tada T, Chen C. Central mechanisms involved with catabolism. *Curr Opin Clin Nutr Metab Care* 2002 Jul;5(4):407-18

[360] Monteleone P, Martiadis V, Colurcio B, Maj M. Leptin secretion is related to chronicity and severity of the illness in bulimia nervosa. *Psychosom Med* 2002 Nov-Dec;64(6):874-9

[361] Kraus T, Haack M, Schuld A, Hinze-Selch D, Pollmacher T. Low leptin levels but normal body mass indices in patients with depression or schizophrenia. *Neuroendocrinology* 2001 Apr;73(4):243-7

[362] Charnay Y, Cusin I, Vallet PG, Muzzin P, Rohner-Jeanrenaud F, Bouras C. Intracerebroventricular infusion of leptin decreases serotonin transporter binding sites in the frontal cortex of the rat. *Neurosci Lett* 2000 Apr 7;283(2):89-92

[363] Barker ME, Blumsohn A. Is weight loss in obese premenopausal women associated with a decline in bone mass? *J Bone Miner Res* 2002 Apr;17(4):746-9

[364] Morley JE. Anorexia, body composition, and ageing. *Curr Opin Clin Nutr Metab Care* 2001 Jan;4(1):9-13

[365] Diehl AM. Nonalcoholic steatosis and steatohepatitis IV. Nonalcoholic fatty liver disease abnormalities in macrophage function and cytokines. *Am J Physiol Gastrointest Liver Physiol* 2002 Jan;282(1):G1-5

[366] Andrico S, Gambera A, Specchia C, Pellegrini C, Falsetti L, Sartori E. Leptin in functional hypothalamic amenorrhoea. *Hum Reprod* 2002 Aug;17(8):2043-8

[367] Unkila-Kallio L, Andersson S, Koistinen HA, Karonen SL, Ylikorkala O, Tiitinen A. Leptin during assisted reproductive cycles: the effect of ovarian stimulation and of very early pregnancy. *Hum Reprod* 2001 Apr;16(4):657-62

[368] Barton BE. IL-6-like cytokines and cancer cachexia: consequences of chronic inflammation. *Immunol Res* 2001;23(1):41-58

[369] Nowicki M, Bryc W, Kokot F. Hormonal regulation of appetite and body mass in patients with advanced prostate cancer treated with combined androgen blockade. *J Endocrinol Invest* 2001 Jan;24(1):31-6

[370] Schols AM, Creutzberg EC, Buurman WA, Campfield LA, Saris WH, Wouters EF. Plasma leptin is related to pro-inflammatory status and dietary intake in patients with chronic obstructive pulmonary disease. *Am J Respir Crit Care Med* 1999 Oct;160(4):1220-6

[371] Marti A, Marcos A, Martinez JA. Obesity and immune function relationships. *Obes Rev* 2001 May;2(2):131-40

[372] Fantuzzi G, Faggioni R. Leptin in the regulation of immunity, inflammation, and hematopoiesis. *J Leukoc Biol* 2000 Oct;68(4):437-46

[373] Faggioni R, Feingold KR, Grunfeld C. Leptin regulation of the immune response and the immunodeficiency of malnutrition. *FASEB J* 2001 Dec;15(14):2565-71

[374] Mancuso P, Gottschalk A, Phare SM, Peters-Golden M, Lukacs NW, Huffnagle GB. Leptin-deficient mice exhibit impaired host defense in Gram-negative pneumonia. *J Immunol* 2002 Apr 15;168(8):4018-24

[375] Busso N, So A, Chobaz-Peclat V, Morard C, Martinez-Soria E, Talabot-Ayer D, Gabay C. Leptin signaling deficiency impairs humoral and cellular immune responses and attenuates experimental arthritis. *J Immunol* 2002 Jan 15;168(2):875-82

[376] Savino W. The thymus gland is a target in malnutrition. *Eur J Clin Nutr* 2002 Aug;56 Suppl 3:S46-9

[377] Matarese G, La Cava A, Sanna V, Lord GM, Lechler RI, Fontana S, Zappacosta S. Balancing susceptibility to infection and autoimmunity: a role for leptin? *Trends Immunol* 2002 Apr 1;23(4):182-7

[378] Matarese G, Sanna V, Di Giacomo A, Lord GM, Howard JK, Bloom SR, Lechler RI, Fontana S, Zappacosta S. Leptin potentiates experimental autoimmune encephalomyelitis in SJL female mice and confers susceptibility to males. *Eur J Immunol* 2001 May;31(5):1324-32

[379] Heer M, Mika C, Grzella I, Drummer C, Herpertz-Dahlmann B. Changes in bone turnover in patients with anorexia nervosa during eleven weeks of inpatient dietary treatment. JW.1: Clin Chem 2002 May;48(5):754-60

[380] Barber MD, Fearon KC, Tisdale MJ, McMillan DC, Ross JA. Effect of a fish oil-enriched nutritional supplement on metabolic mediators in patients with pancreatic cancer cachexia. *Nutr Cancer* 2001;40(2):118-24

[381] Tannhauser PP. Anorexia nervosa: a multifactorial disease of nutritional origin? Int J Adolesc Med Health 2002 Jul-Sep;14(3):185-91

[382] Patrick L. Eating disorders: a review of the literature with emphasis on medical complications and clinical nutrition. *Altern Med Rev* 2002 Jun;7(3):184-202

[383] Su JC, Birmingham CL. Zinc supplementation in the treatment of anorexia nervosa. *Eat Weight Disord* 2002 Mar;7(1):20-2

[384] Koivisto VA, Yki-Jarvinen H, DeFronzo RA. Physical training and insulin sensitivity. *Diabetes Metab Rev* 1986;1:445-481

[385] Henriksen EJ. Invited Review: Effects of acute exercise and exercise training on insulin resistance. *J Appl Physiol* 2002 Aug;93(2):788-96

[386] Bogardus C, Ravussin E, Robbins DC, et al. Effects of physical training and diet therapy on carbohydrate metabolism in patients with glucose intolerance and non-insulin dependent diabetes. *Diabetes* 1984;33:311-318

[387] Wasserman DH, Lacy DB, Goldstein RE, Williams PE, Cherington AD. Exercise-induced fall in insulin and the increase in fat metabolism during prolonged exercise. Diabetes 1989;38:484-490

[388] Baba T, Kanda T, Yoshida A, Tsukui S, Nara M, Inukai T, Umeda T, Tamura J, Kobayashi I. Reciprocal changes in leptin and tumor necrosis factor-alpha with exercise in insulin resistant rats. *Res Commun Mol Pathol Pharmacol* 2000 Jul-Aug;108(1-2):133-43

[389] Kahara T, Takamura T, Hayakawa T, Nagai Y, Yamaguchi H, Katsuki T, Katsuki K, Katsuki M, Kobayashi K. Prediction of exercise-mediated changes in metabolic markers by gene polymorphism. *Diabetes Res Clin Pract* 2002 Aug;57(2):105-10

[390] Rozzano, MI. Arrhythmia risk stratification in patients with heart failure according to drug treatment and its effects *Ital Heart J* 2001 Dec;2(12 Suppl):1278-83

[391] Adigun AQ, Asiyanbola B, Ajayi AA. Cardiac autonomic function in Blacks with congestive heart failure: vagomimetic action, alteration in sympathovagal balance, and the effect of ACE inhibition on central and peripheral vagal tone. *Cell Mol Biol* (Noisy-le-gland) 2001 Sep;47(6):1063-7.

[392] Billman GE. Aerobic exercise conditioning: a non-pharmacological antiarrhythmic intervention. *J Appl Physiol* 2002 Feb;92(2):446-54.

[393] Ito H, Ohshima A, Tsuzuki M, Ohto N, Yanagawa M, Maruyama T, Kaji Y, Kanaya S, Nishioka K. Effects of increased physical activity and mild calorie restriction on heart rate variability in obese women. *Jpn Heart J* 2001 Jul;42(4):459-69.

[394] Matsushita T, Tanaka Y, Horinouchi O, Sonoda M, Arima T. Heart rate decline after exercise in patients with hypertrophic cardiomyopathy. *J Electrocardiol* 2001 Apr;34(2(:141-6.

[395] Rosenwinkel ET, Bloomfield DM, Arwady MA, Goldsmith RL. Exercise and autonomic function in health and cardiovascular disease. *Cardiol Clin* 2001 Aug;19(3):369-87.

[396] Goldsmith RL, Bloomfield DM, Rosenwinkel ET. Exercise and autonomic function. *Coron Artery Dis* 2000 Mar;11(2):129-35.

[397] Sartorio A, Narici MV, Fumagalli E, Faglia G, Lafortuna CL. Aerobic and anaerobic performance before and after a short-term body mass reduction program in obese subjects. *Diabetes Nutr Metab* 2001 Feb;14(1):51-7.

[398] Iwane M, Arita M, Tomimoto S, Satani O, Matsumoto M, Miyashita K, Nishio I. Walking 10,000 steps/day or more reduces blood pressure and sympathetic nerve activity in mild essential hypertension. *Hypertens Res* 2000 Nov;23(6):573-80.

[399] Amano M, Kanda T, Ue H, Moritani T. Exercise training and autonomic nervous system activity in obese individuals. *Med Sci Sports Exerc* 2001 Aug;33(8):1287-91.

[400] Collins HL, Rodenbaugh DW, Dicarlo SE. Dialy exercise attenuated the sympathetic component of the spontaneous arterial baroreflex control of heart rate in hypertensive rats. *Clin Exp Hypertens* 2000 Aug;22(6):607-22.

[401] Gutin B, Barbeau P, Litaker MS, Ferguson M, Owens S. Heart rate variability in obese children: relations to total body and visceral adiposity, and changes with physical training and detraining. *Obes Res* 2000 Jan;8(1):12-9.

[402] Nindl BC, Kraemer WJ, Arciero PJ, Samatallee N, Leone CD, Mayo MF, Hafeman DL. Leptin concentrations experience a delayed reduction after resistance exercise in men. *Med Sci Sports Exerc* 2002 Apr;34(4):608-13

[403] Kanaley JA, Fenicchia LM, Miller CS, Ploutz-Synder LL, Weinstock RS, Carhart R, Azevedo JL Jr. Resting leptin responses to acute and chronic resistance training in type 2 diabetic men and women. *Int J Obes Relat Metab Disord* 2001 Oct;25(10):1474-80

[404] Gippini A, Mato A, Pazos R, Suarez B, Vila B, Gayoso P, Lage M, Casanueva FF. Effect of long-term strength training on glucose metabolism. Implications for individual impact of high lean mass and high fat mass on relationship between BMI and insulin sensitivity. *J Endocrinol Invest* 2002 Jun;25(6):520-5

[405] Hayase H, Nomura S, Abe T, Izawa T. Relation between fat distributions and several plasma adipocytokines after exercise training in pre-menopausal and postmenopausal women. *J Physiol Anthropol Appl Human Sci* 2002 Mar;21(2):105-13

[406] Van Someren EJ. More than a marker: interaction between the circadian regulation of temperature and sleep, age-related changes, and treatment possibilities. *Chronobiol Int* 2000 May;17(3):313-54

[407] Krauchi K, Wirz-Justice A. Circadian clues to sleep onset mechanisms. *Neuropsychopharmacology* 2001 Nov;25(5 Suppl):S92-6

[408] Carrier J, Paquet J, Morettini J, Touchette E. Phase advance of sleep and temperature circadian rhythms in the middle years of life in humans. *Neurosci Lett* 2002 Mar 1;320(1-2):1-4

[409] Baydas G, Gursu F, Canpolat S, Konar V, Yasar A, Canatan H, Kelestimur H. Effects of pinealectomy on the circadian release pattern of leptin in male rat. *Neuroendocrinol Lett* 2001 Dec;22(6):449-52

[410] Canpolat S, Sandal S, Yilmaz B, Yasar A, Kutlu S, Baydas G, Kelestimur H. Effects of pinealectomy and exogenous melatonin on serum leptin levels in male rat. *Eur J Pharmacol* 2001 Sep 28;428(1):145-8

[411] Wolden-Hanson T, Mitton DR, McCants RL, Yellon SM, Wilkinson CW, Matsumoto AM, Rasmussen DD. Daily melatonin administration to middle-aged male rats suppresses body weight, intraabdominal adiposity, and plasma leptin and insulin independent of food intake and total body fat. *Endocrinology* 2000 Feb;141(2):487-97

[412] Nishida S, Segawa T, Murai I, Nakagawa S. Long-term melatonin administration reduces hyperinsulinemia and improves the altered fatty-acid compositions in type 2 diabetic rats via the restoration of Delta-5 desaturase activity. *J Pineal Res* 2002 Jan;32(1):26-33

[413] Kraus T, Haack M, Schuld A, Hinze-Selch D, Pollmacher T. Low leptin levels but normal body mass indices in patients with depression or schizophrenia. *Neuroendocrinology* 2001 Apr;73(4):243-7

[414] Charnay Y, Cusin I, Vallet PG, Muzzin P, Rohner-Jeanrenaud F, Bouras C. Intracerebroventricular infusion of leptin decreases serotonin transporter binding sites in the frontal cortex of the rat. *Neurosci Lett* 2000 Apr 7;283(2):89-92

[415] Nedvidkova J, Papezova H, Haluzik M, Schreiber V. Interaction between serum leptin levels and hypothalamo-hypophyseal-thyroid axis in patients with anorexia nervosa. *Endocr Res* 2000 May;26(2):219-30

[416] Sasaki M, Jordan P, Joh T, Itoh M, Jenkins M, Pavlick K, Minagar A, Alexander SJ. Melatonin reduces TNF-a induced expression of MAdCAM-1 via inhibition of NF kappaB. *BMC Gastroenterol* 2002 Apr 24;2(1):9

[417] Nava M, Quiroz Y, Vaziri ND, Rodriguez-Iturbe B. MELATONIN REDUCES RENAL INTERSTITIAL INFLAMMATION AND IMPROVES HYPERTENSION IN SPONTANEOUSLY HYPERTENSIVE RATS. *Am J Physiol Renal Physiol* 2002 Nov 19;

[418] Clasey JL, Weltman A, Patrie J, Weltman JY, Pezzoli S, Bouchard C, Thorner MO,Hartman ML. Abdominal visceral fat and fasting insulin are important predictors of 24-hour GH release independent of age, gender, and other physiological factors. *J Clin Endocrinol Metab* 2001 Aug;86(8):3845-52

[419] McCallum RW, Petrie JR, Dominiczak AF, Connell JM. Growth hormone deficiency and vascular risk. *Clin Endocrinol* (Oxf) 2002 Jul;57(1):11-24

[420] Moretti C, Mencacci C, Frajese GV, Cerilli M, Frajese G. Growth hormone-releasing hormone and pituitary adenylate cyclase-activating polypeptide in the reproductive system. *Trends Endocrinol Metab* 2002 Dec;13(10):428-35

[421] Monzavi R, Cohen P. IGFs and IGFBPs: role in health and disease. *Best Pract Res Clin Endocrinol Metab* 2002 Sep;16(3):433-47

[422] Furstenberger G, Senn HJ. Insulin-like growth factors and cancer. *Lancet Oncol* 2002 May;3(5):298-302

[423] van Garderen E, Schalken JA. Morphogenic and tumorigenic potentials of the mammary growth hormone/growth hormone receptor system. *Mol Cell Endocrinol* 2002 Nov 29;197(1-2):153-65

[424] Sandhu MS, Dunger DB, Giovannucci EL. Insulin, insulin-like growth factor-I (IGF-I), IGF binding proteins, their biologic interactions, and colorectal cancer. *J Natl Cancer Inst* 2002 Jul 3;94(13):972-80

[425] Chatzistamou I, Schally AV, Pafiti A, Kiaris H, Koutselini H. Expression of growth hormone-releasing hormone in human primary endometrial carcinomas. *Eur J Endocrinol* 2002 Sep;147(3):381-6

[426] Moretti C, Mencacci C, Frajese GV, Cerilli M, Frajese G. Growth hormone-releasing hormone and pituitary adenylate cyclase-activating polypeptide in the reproductive system. *Trends Endocrinol Metab* 2002 Dec;13(10):428-35

[427] Laban C, Bustin SA, Jenkins PJ. The GH-IGF-I axis and breast cancer. *Trends Endocrinol Metab* 2002 Dec;14(1):28-34

[428] Zeitler P, Siriwardana G. Antagonism of endogenous growth hormone-releasing hormone (GHRH) leads to reduced proliferation and apoptosis in MDA231 breast cancer cells. *Endocrine* 2002 Jun;18(1):85-90

[429] Halmos G, Schally AV, Czompoly T, Krupa M, Varga JL, Rekasi Z. Expression of growth hormone-releasing hormone and its receptor splice variants in human prostate cancer. *J Clin Endocrinol Metab* 2002 Oct;87(10):4707-14

[430] Chopin LK, Veveris-Lowe TL, Philipps AF, Herington AC. Co-expression of GH and GHR isoforms in prostate cancer cell lines. *Growth Horm IGF* Res 2002 Apr;12(2):126-36

[431] Swerdlow AJ, Higgins CD, Adlard P, Preece MA. Risk of cancer in patients treated with human pituitary growth hormone in the UK, 1959-85: a cohort study. *Lancet* 2002 Jul 27;360(9329):273-7 Comment in: Lancet. 2002 Jul 27;360(9329):268-9.

[432] Engelson ES, Glesby MJ, Mendez D, Albu JB, Wang J, Heymsfield SB, Kotler DP. Effect of recombinant human growth hormone in the treatment of visceral fat accumulation in HIV infection. *J Acquir Immune Defic Syndr* 2002 Aug 1;30(4):379-91

[433] Monzavi R, Cohen P. IGFs and IGFBPs: role in health and disease. *Best Pract Res Clin Endocrinol Metab* 2002 Sep;16(3):433-47

[434] Rose DR, Clemmons DR. Growth hormone receptor antagonist improves insulin resistance in acromegaly. *Growth Horm IGF Res* 2002 Dec;12(6):418-24

[435] Gravholt CH, Naeraa RW, Brixen K, Kastrup KW, Mosekilde L, Jorgensen JO, Christiansen JS. Short-term growth hormone treatment in girls with turner syndrome decreases fat mass and improves insulin sensitivity: a randomized, double-blind, placebo-controlled, cross-over study. *Pediatrics* 2002 Nov;110(5):889-96

[436] Van Pareren YK, De Muinck Keizer-Schrama SM, Stijnen T, Sas TC, Drop SL. Effect of Discontinuation of Long-Term Growth Hormone Treatment on Carbohydrate Metabolism and Risk Factors for Cardiovascular Disease in Girls with Turner Syndrome. *J Clin Endocrinol Metab* 2002 Dec 1;87(12):5442-5448

[437] Blackman MR, Sorkin JD, Munzer T, Bellantoni MF, Busby-Whitehead J, Stevens TE, Jayme J, O'Connor KG, Christmas C, Tobin JD, Stewart KJ, Cottrell E, St Clair C, Pabst KM, Harman SM. Growth

hormone and sex steroid administration in healthy aged women and men: a randomized controlled trial. *JAMA* 2002 Nov 13;288(18):2282-92

[438] Roelfsema F, Biermasz NR, Veldman RG, Veldhuis JD, Frolich M, Stokvis-Brantsma WH, Wit JM. Growth hormone (GH) secretion in patients with an inactivating defect of the GH-releasing hormone (GHRH) receptor is pulsatile: evidence for a role for non-GHRH inputs into the generation of GH pulses. *J Clin Endocrinol Metab* 2001 Jun;86(6):2459-64

[439] Maheshwari HG, Pezzoli SS, Rahim A, Shalet SM, Thorner MO, Baumann G. Pulsatile growth hormone secretion persists in genetic growth hormone-releasing hormone resistance. *Am J Physiol Endocrinol Metab* 2002 Apr;282(4):E943-51

[440] Pombo M, Pombo CM, Garcia A, Caminos E, Gualillo O, Alvarez CV, Casanueva FF, Dieguez C. Hormonal control of growth hormone secretion. *Horm Res* 2001;55 Suppl 1:11-6

[441] Isozaki O, Tsushima T, Miyakawa M, Demura H, Seki H. Interaction between leptin and growth hormone (GH)/IGF-I axis. *Endocr J* 1999 Mar;46 Suppl:S17-24

[442] Isozaki O, Tsushima T, Miyakawa M, Nozoe Y, Demura H, Seki H. Growth hormone directly inhibits leptin gene expression in visceral fat tissue in fatty Zucker rats. *J Endocrinol* 1999 Jun;161(3):511-6

[443] Lee KN, Jeong IC, Lee SJ, Oh SH, Cho MY. Regulation of leptin gene expression by insulin and growth hormone in mouse adipocytes. *Exp Mol Med* 2001 Dec 31;33(4):234-9

[444] Dunger D, Ahmed L, Ong K. Growth and body composition in type 1 diabetes mellitus. *Horm Res* 2002;58 Suppl 1:66-71

[445] Heptulla R, Smitten A, Teague B, Tamborlane WV, Ma YZ, Caprio S. Temporal patterns of circulating leptin levels in lean and obese adolescents: relationships to insulin, growth hormone, and free fatty acids rhythmicity. *J Clin Endocrinol Metab* 2001 Jan;86(1):90-6

[446] Soderberg S, Ahren B, Eliasson M, Dinesen B, Brismar K, Olsson T. Circulating IGF binding protein-1 is inversely associated with leptin in non-obese men and obese postmenopausal women. *Eur J Endocrinol* 2001 Mar;144(3):283-90

[447] Furuhata Y, Kagaya R, Hirabayashi K, Ikeda A, Chang KT, Nishihara M, Takahashi M. Development of obesity in transgenic rats with low circulating growth hormone levels: involvement of leptin resistance. *Eur J Endocrinol* 2000 Oct;143(4):535-41

[448] Armellini F, Zamboni M, Bosello O. Hormones and body composition in humans: clinical studies. *Int J Obes Relat Metab Disord* 2000 Jun;24 Suppl 2:S18-21

[449] Garcia-Rudaz MC, Ropelato MG, Escobar ME, Veldhuis JD, Barontini M. Amplified and orderly growth hormone secretion characterizes lean adolescents with polycystic ovary syndrome. *Eur J Endocrinol* 2002 Aug;147(2):207-16

[450] Zaczek D, Hammond J, Suen L, Wandji S, Service D, Bartke A, Chandrashekar V, Coschigano K, Kopchick J. Impact of growth hormone resistance on female reproductive function: new insights from growth hormone receptor knockout mice. *Biol Reprod* 2002 Oct;67(4):1115-24

[451] Muller AF, Lamberts SW, Janssen JA, Hofland LJ, Koetsveld PV, Bidlingmaier M, Strasburger CJ, Ghigo E, Van der Lely AJ. Ghrelin drives GH secretion during fasting in man. *Eur J Endocrinol* 2002 Feb;146(2):203-7

[452] Cappiello V, Ronchi C, Morpurgo PS, Epaminonda P, Arosio M, Beck-Peccoz P, Spada A. Circulating ghrelin levels in basal conditions and during glucose tolerance test in acromegalic patients. *Eur J Endocrinol* 2002 Aug;147(2):189-94

[453] Muller EE, Rigamonti AE, Colonna Vde G, Locatelli V, Berti F, Cella SG. GH-related and extra-endocrine actions of GH secretagogues in aging. *Neurobiol Aging* 2002 Sep-Oct;23(5):907

[454] Tschop M, Weyer C, Tataranni PA, Devanarayan V, Ravussin E, Heiman ML. Circulating ghrelin levels are decreased in human obesity. *Diabetes* 2001 Apr;50(4):707-9

[455] English PJ, Ghatei MA, Malik IA, Bloom SR, Wilding JP. Food fails to suppress ghrelin levels in obese humans. *J Clin Endocrinol Metab* 2002 Jun;87(6):2984

[456] Bagnasco M, Kalra PS, Kalra SP. Ghrelin and leptin pulse discharge in fed and fasted rats. *Endocrinology* 2002 Feb;143(2):726-9

[457] Wang P, Li N, Li JS, Li WQ. The role of endotoxin, TNF-alpha, and IL-6 in inducing the state of growth hormone insensitivity. *World J Gastroenterol* 2002 Jun;8(3):531-6

[458] Yumet G, Shumate ML, Bryant P, Lin CM, Lang CH, Cooney RN. Tumor necrosis factor mediates hepatic growth hormone resistance during sepsis. *Am J Physiol Endocrinol Metab* 2002 Sep;283(3):E472-81

[459] Lieskovska J, Guo D, Derman E. IL-6-overexpression brings about growth impairment potentially through a GH receptor defect. *Growth Horm IGF Res* 2002 Dec;12(6):388-98

[460] Landis CA, Lentz MJ, Rothermel J, Riffle SC, Chapman D, Buchwald D, Shaver JL. Decreased nocturnal levels of prolactin and growth hormone in women with fibromyalgia. *J Clin Endocrinol Metab* 2001 Apr;86(4):1672-8

[461] Crown AL, Cottle K, Lightman SL, Falk S, Mohamed-Ali V, Armstrong L, Millar AB, Holly JM. What is the role of the insulin-like growth factor system in the pathophysiology of cancer cachexia, and how is it regulated? *Clin Endocrinol* (Oxf) 2002 Jun;56(6):723-33

[462] Belury MA. DIETARY CONJUGATED LINOLEIC ACID IN HEALTH: Physiological Effects and Mechanisms of Action. *Annu Rev Nutr* 2002;22:505-31

[463] Sugano M, Akahoshi A, Koba K, Tanaka K, Okumura T, Matsuyama H, Goto Y, Miyazaki T, Murao K, Yamasaki M, Nonaka M, Yamada K. Dietary manipulations of body fat-reducing potential of conjugated linoleic acid in rats. *Biosci Biotechnol Biochem* 2001 Nov;65(11):2535-41

[464] DeLany JP, Blohm F, Truett AA, Scimeca JA, West DB. Conjugated linoleic acid rapidly reduces body fat content in mice without affecting energy intake. *Am J Physiol* 1999 Apr;276(4 Pt 2):R1172-9

[465] Ryder JW, Portocarrero CP, Song XM, Cui L, Yu M, Combatsiaris T, Galuska D, Bauman DE, Barbano DM, Charron MJ, Zierath JR, Houseknecht KL. Isomer-specific antidiabetic properties of conjugated

linoleic acid. Improved glucose tolerance, skeletal muscle insulin action, and UCP-2 gene expression. *Diabetes* 2001 May;50(5):1149-57

[466] McCarty MF. Hepatothermic therapy of obesity: rationale and an inventory of resources. *Med Hypotheses* 2001 Sep;57(3):324-36

[467] Kang K, Pariza MW. trans-10,cis-12-Conjugated linoleic acid reduces leptin secretion from 3T3-L1 adipocytes. *Biochem Biophys Res Commun* 2001 Sep 21;287(2):377-82

[468] Rahman SM, Wang Y, Yotsumoto H, Cha J, Han S, Inoue S, Yanagita T. Effects of conjugated linoleic acid on serum leptin concentration, body-fat accumulation, and beta-oxidation of fatty acid in OLETF rats. *Nutrition* 2001 May;17(5):385-90

[469] Akahoshi A, Goto Y, Murao K, Miyazaki T, Yamasaki M, Nonaka M, Yamada K, Sugano M. Conjugated linoleic acid reduces body fats and cytokine levels of mice. *Biosci Biotechnol Biochem* 2002 Apr;66(4):916-20

[470] Akahoshi A, Goto Y, Murao K, Miyazaki T, Yamasaki M, Nonaka M, Yamada K, Sugano M. Conjugated linoleic acid reduces body fats and cytokine levels of mice. *Biosci Biotechnol Biochem* 2002 Apr;66(4):916-20

[471] Van Cauter EV, Polonsky KS, Blackman JD, Roland D, Sturis J, Byrne MM, Scheen AJ. Abnormal temporal patterns of glucose tolerance in obesity: relationship to sleep-related growth hormone secretion and circadian cortisol rhythmicity. *J Clin Endocrinol Metab* 1994 Dec;79(6):1797-805

[472] Van Cauter EV, Polonsky KS, Blackman JD, Roland D, Sturis J, Byrne MM, Scheen AJ. Abnormal temporal patterns of glucose tolerance in obesity: relationship to sleep-related growth hormone secretion and circadian cortisol rhythmicity. *J Clin Endocrinol Metab* 1994 Dec;79(6):1797-805

[473] Parr TB. A new technique to elevate night time growth hormone release and potential growth hormone feedback control loop. *Med Hypotheses* 2001 May;56(5):610-3.

[474] Bidzinska B, Petraglia F, Angioni S, Genazzani AD, Criscuolo M, Ficarra G, Gallinelli A, Trentini GP, Genazzani AR. Effect of different chronic intermittent stressors and acetyl-l-carnitine on hypothalamic beta-endorphin and GnRH and on plasma testosterone levels in male rats. *Neuroendocrinology* 1993 Jun;57(6):985-90.

[475] Iossa S, Mollica MP, Lionetti L, Crescenzo R, Botta M, Barletta A, Liverini G. Acetyl-L-carnitine supplementation differently influences nutrient partitioning, serum leptin concentration and skeletal muscle mitochondrial respiration in young and old rats. *J Nutr* 2002 Apr;132(4):636-42

[476] Spagnoli A, et al. Long-term acetyl-L-carnitine treatment in Alzheimer's disease. *Neurology* 41:1726-1732; 1991.

[477] Calvani M, et al. Action of acetyl-L-carnitine in neurodegeneration and Alzheimer's disease. *Ann NY Acad Sci* 663:483-486; 1992.

[478] Carta A, et al. Acetyl-L-carnitine and Alzheimer's disease: pharmacological considerations beyond the cholinergic sphere. *Ann NY Acad Sci* 695:324-326; 1993.

[479] Parnetti L, et al. Milticentre atudy of l-alpha-glyceryl-phosphorylcholine vs ST200 among patients with probable senile dementia of Alzheimer's type. *Drugs Aging* 3:159-164; 1993.

[480] Guarnascheiil C, Fugazza G, Pistarini C. Pathological brain ageing: evaluation of the efficacy of a pharmacological aid. *Drugs Exp Clin Res* 14:715-718; 1998.

[481] Rai G, et al. Doulbe-blind, placebo-controlled study of acetyl-L-carnitine in patients with Alzheimer's dementia. *Curr Med Res Opin* 11:638-647; 1990.

[482] Bella R, Biondi R, Raffaele R, Pennisi G. Effect of acetyl-L-carnitine on generic patients suffering from dysthymic disorders. *Int J Clin Pharmacol Res* 10:355-360; 1990.

[483] Gecele M, Francesetti G, Meluzzi A. Acetyl-L-carnitine in aged subjects with major depression: clinical efficacy and effects on the circadian rhythm of cortisol. *Dementia* 2:333-337; 1991.

[484] Tempesta E, et al. L-acetylcarnitine in depressed elderly subjects. A cross-over study vs placebo. *Drugs Exp Clin Res* 13:417-423; 1987.

[485] Carta A, et al. Acetyl-L-carnitine and Alzheimer's disease: pharmacological considerations beyond the cholinergic sphere. *Ann NY Acad Sci* 695:324-326; 1993.

[486] Aureli T, Puccetti C, Di Cocco ME, Arduini A, Ricciolini R, Scalibastri M, Manetti C, Conti F. entry of [(1,2-13C2)acetyl]-L-carnitine in liver tricarboxylic acid cycle and lipogenesis: a study by 13C NMR spectroscopy in conscious, freely moving rats. *Eur J Biochem* 1999 Jul;263(1):287-93.

[487] Aureli T, Di Cocco ME, Capuani G, Ricciolini R, Manetti C, Miccheli A, Conti F. Effect of long-term feeding with acetyl-L-carnitine on the age-related changes in rat brain lipid composition: a study by 31P NMR spectroscopy. *Neurochem Res* 2000 Mar;25(3):395-9

[488] Aureli T, Di Cocco ME, Puccetti C, Ricciolini R, Scalibastri M, Miccheli A, Manetti C, Conti F. Acetyl-L-carnitine modulates glucose metabolism and stimulates glycogen synthesis in rat brain. *Brain Res* 1998 Jun 15;796(1-2):75-81.

[489] Soneru IL, Khan T, Orfalian Z, Abraira C. Acetyl-L-Carnitine effects on nerve conduction and glycemic regulation in experimental diabetes. *Endocr Res* 1997 Feb-May;23(1-2):27-36.

[490] Kano M, Kawakami T, Hori H, Hashimoto Y, Tao Y, Ishikawa Y, Takenaka T. Effects of ALCAR on the fast axoplasmic transport in cultured sensory neurons of streptozotocin-induced diabetic rats. *Neurosci Res* 1999 Mar;33(3):207-13.

[491] Wideman L, Weltman JY, Hartman ML, Veldhuis JD, Weltman A. Growth hormone release during acute and chronic aerobic and resistance exercise: recent findings. *Sports Med* 2002;32(15):987-1004

[492] Deschenes MR, Kraemer WJ. Performance and physiologic adaptations to resistance training. *Am J Phys Med Rehabil* 2002 Nov;81(11 Suppl):S3-16

[493] Werlang Coelho O, Rebello Velloso C, Resende de Lima Oliveira Brasil R, Vaisman M, Gil Soares de Araujo C. Muscle power increases after resistance training in growth-hormone-deficient adults. *Med Sci Sports Exerc* 2002 Oct;34(10):1577-81

[494] Hakkinen K, Kraemer WJ, Pakarinen A, Triplett-McBride T, McBride JM, Hakkinen A, Alen M, McGuigan MR, Bronks R, Newton RU. Effects of

heavy resistance/power training on maximal strength, muscle morphology, and hormonal response patterns in 60-75-year-old men and women. *Can J Appl Physiol* 2002 Jun;27(3):213-31

[495] Heaton JP, Morales A. Andropause—a multisystem disease. *Can J Urol* 2001 Apr;8(2):1213-22

[496] Zmuda J, Cauley, J, Kriska, A, Glynn, N, Gutai, J, Kuller, L. Longitudinal relation between endogenous testosterone and cardiovascular disease risk factors in middle-aged men. *Am J Epidemiol.* 1997: 146:609-617.

[497] Edwards, E, Hamilton, J, Duntley, S. Testosterone propionate as a therapeutic agent in patients with organic disease of the peripheral vessels. *N Engl J Med.* 1939; 220 :865.

[498] Jaffee, M. Effect of testosterone cypionate on post-exercise St segment depression. *Br Heart J.* 1977; 39:1217-1222.

[499] Wu SZ, Weng XZ. Therapeutic effects of an androgenic preparation on myocardial ischemia and cardiac function in 62 elderly male coronary heart disease patients. *Chin Med J* (Engl). 1993; 106:415-418.

[500] Phillips, GB, Pinkernell, BH, Jing TY. The association of hypotestosteronemia with coronary artery disease in men. *Arterioscler Thromb.* 1994; 14:701-706.

[501] Barrett-Connor, EL. Testosterone and risk factors for cardiovascular disease in men. *Diabete Metab.* 1995: 21:156-161.

[502] Tenover, JL. Testosterone and the aging male. *J Androl.* 1997: 18:103-106.

[503] Rolf C, von Eckardstein S, Koken U, Nieschlag E. Testosterone substitution of hypogonadal men prevents the age-dependent increases in body mass index, body fat and leptin seen in healthy ageing men: results of a cross-sectional study. *Eur J Endocrinol* 2002 Apr;146(4):505-11

[504] Soderberg S, Olsson T, Eliasson M, Johnson O, Brismar K, Carlstrom K, Ahren B. A strong association between biologically active testosterone and leptin in non-obese men and women is lost with increasing (central) adiposity. *Int J Obes Relat Metab Disord* 2001 Jan;25(1):98-105

[505] Ogura T, Tobe K, Mimura Y, Otsuka F, Yamauchi T, Imai A, Tsukamoto C, Iwasaki Y, Matsuura K. Testosterone modulates serum leptin concentrations in a male patient with hypothalamic hypogonadism. *J Endocrinol Invest* 2000 Apr;23(4):246-50

[506] Tena-Sempere M, Barreiro ML. Leptin in male reproduction: the testis paradigm. *Mol Cell Endocrinol* 2002 Feb 25;188(1-2):9-13

[507] Casabiell X, Pineiro V, Vega F, De La Cruz LF, Dieguez C, Casanueva FF. Leptin, reproduction and sex steroids. *Pituitary* 2001 Jan-Apr;4(1-2):93-9

[508] Sih R, Morley JE, Kaiser FE, Perry HM 3rd, Patrick P, Ross C. Testosterone replacement in older hypogonadal men: a 12-month randomized controlled trial. *J Clin Endocrinol Metab* 1997 Jun;82(6):1661-7

[509] Glander HJ, Lammert A, Paasch U, Glasow A, Kratzsch J. Leptin exists in tubuli seminiferi and in seminal plasma. *Andrologia* 2002 Sep;34(4):227-33

[510] Abate N, Haffner SM, Garg A, Peshock RM, Grundy SM. Sex steroid hormones, upper body obesity, and insulin resistance. *J Clin Endocrinol Metab* 2002 Oct;87(10):4522-7

[511] Jansson PA, Eliasson B, Lindmark S, Eriksson JW. Endocrine abnormalities in healthy first-degree relatives of type 2 diabetes patients—potential role of steroid hormones and leptin in the development of insulin resistance. *Eur J Clin Invest* 2002 Mar;32(3):172-8

[512] Chan JL, Bluher S, Yiannakouris N, Suchard MA, Kratzsch J, Mantzoros CS. Regulation of circulating soluble leptin receptor levels by gender, adiposity, sex steroids, and leptin: observational and interventional studies in humans. *Diabetes* 2002 Jul;51(7):2105-12

[513] Prasad A. Zinc in growth and development and spectrum of human zinc deficiency. *J Am Coll Nutr* 7 377-384, 1988.

[514] Netter A, et al. Effects of zinc administration on plasma testosterone, dihydrotestosterone and sperm count. *Arch Androl* 7 69-73, 1981.

[515] Xu Z, Kawai M, Bandiera SM, Chang TK. Influence of dietary zinc deficiency during development on hepatic CYP2C11, CYP2C12, CYP3A2, CYP3A9, and CYP3A18 expression in postpubertal male rats. *Biochem Pharmacol* 2001 Nov 1;62(9):1283-91

[516] Gauthaman K, Adaikan PG, Prasad RN. Aphrodisiac properties of Tribulus Terrestris extract (Protodioscin) in normal and castrated rats. *Life Sci* 2002 Aug 9;71(12):1385-96

[517] Dimitrov, M, Gerogiev, P, Vitanov, S. Use of tribestan on rams with sexual disorders. *Vet Med Nauki.* 1987; 24(5): 102-110.

[518] Zarkova, S. Steroid saponins of Tribulus terrestris L. have a stimulant effect on the sexual function. *Rev Port Ciencias Vet* 1984; 79 (470): 117-126.

[519] Protich, M, Twvetkov, D, nalbanski, B, et al. Clinical trial of a preparation Tribestan in infertile men. *Akush Ginekol.* 1983; 22(4): 326-329. (in Bulgarian)

[520] Coleman, DL, Schwizer, RW, Leiter, EH. DHEA's Effects on Weight. *Diabetes.* Jan 1984; 33(1): 26-32.

[521] Regulation of the immune response by dehydroepiandrosterone and its metabolites. *Journal of Endocrinology (United Kingdom).* 1996;150/Suppl. S209-S220.

[522] Yen, SS, Morales, AJ, Khorram, O. Replacement of DHEA in aging men and women – Potential remedial effects. *Ann NY Acad Sci (U.S.)* . 1995; 774: 128-142.

[523] Brown GA, Vukovich MD, Martini ER, Kohut ML, Franke WD, Jackson DA, King DS. Effects of androstenedione-herbal supplementation on serum sex hormone concentrations in 30- to 59-year-old men. *Int J Vitam Nutr Res* 2001 Sep;71(5):293-301

[524] Kochakian, CD. Metabolites of testosterone, significance in the vital economy. *Steroids.* 1990; 55: 92-97.

[525] Mahesh, VB, Greenblatt, RB. The in-vivo conversion of dehydroepiandrosterone and androstenedione to testosterone in the human. Acta Endocrinol. 1962; 41: 400-406.

[526] Scordalakes EM, Imwalle DB, Rissman EF. Oestrogen's masculine side: mediation of mating in male mice. *Reproduction* 2002 Sep;124(3):331-8

[527] Cohen PG. Aromatase, adiposity, aging and disease. The hypogonadal-metabolic-atherogenic-disease and aging connection. *Med Hypotheses* 2001 Jun;56(6):702-8

[528] Machinal-Quelin F, Dieudonne MN, Pecquery R, Leneveu MC, Giudicelli Y. Direct in vitro effects of androgens and estrogens on ob gene expression and leptin secretion in human adipose tissue. *Endocrine*

2002 Jul;18(2):179-84

529 Dhawan K, Sharma A. Prevention of chronic alcohol and nicotine-induced azospermia, sterility and decreased libido, by a novel tri-substituted benzoflavone moiety from Passiflora incarnata Linneaus in healthy male rats. Life Sci 2002 Nov 15;71(26):3059-69

530 Bakker J, Honda S, Harada N, Balthazart J. Sexual partner preference requires a functional aromatase (cyp19) gene in male mice. Horm Behav 2002 Sep;42(2):158-71

531 Li X, Warri A, Makela S, Ahonen T, Streng T, Santti R, Poutanen M. Mammary gland development in transgenic male mice expressing human P450 aromatase. Endocrinology 2002 Oct;143(10):4074-83

532 Vermeulen A, Kaufman JM, Goemaere S, van Pottelberg I. Estradiol in elderly men. Aging Male 2002 Jun;5(2):98-102

533 Satoh K, Sakamoto Y, Ogata A, Nagai F, Mikuriya H, Numazawa M, Yamada K, Aoki N. Inhibition of aromatase activity by green tea extract catechins and their endocrinological effects of oral administration in rats. Food Chem Toxicol 2002 Jul;40(7):925-33

534 Atrazine is the most commonly used herbicide in the U.S. and probably the world.

535 Kato S, Mano T, Kobayashi T, Yamazaki N, Himeno Y, Yamamoto K, Itoh M, Harada N, Nagasaka A. A calcium-deficient diet caused decreased bone mineral density and secondary elevation of estrogen in aged male rats-effect of menatetrenone and elcatonin. Metabolism 2002 Oct;51(10):1230-4

536 Martin WJ, McGowan E, Cashen DE, Gantert LT, Drisko JE, Hom GJ, Nargund R, Sebhat I, Howard AD, Van der Ploeg LH, MacIntyre DE. Activation of melanocortin MC(4) receptors increases erectile activity in rats ex copula. Eur J Pharmacol 2002 Nov 1;454(1):71-9

537 Sainsbury A, Schwarzer C, Couzens M, Jenkins A, Oakes SR, Ormandy CJ, Herzog H. Y4 receptor knockout rescues fertility in ob/ob mice. Genes Dev 2002 May 1;16(9):1077-88

538 Martin LJ, Mahaney MC, Almasy L, MacCluer JW, Blangero J, Jaquish CE, Comuzzie AG. Leptin's sexual dimorphism results from genotype by sex interactions mediated by testosterone. Obes Res 2002 Jan;10(1):14-21

539 Casabiell X, Pineiro V, Vega F, De La Cruz LF, Dieguez C, Casanueva FF. Leptin, reproduction and sex steroids. Pituitary 2001 Jan-Apr;4(1-2):93-9

540 Cizza G, Dorn LD, Lotsikas A, Sereika S, Rotenstein D, Chrousos GP. Circulating plasma leptin and IGF-1 levels in girls with premature adrenarche: potential implications of a preliminary study. Horm Metab Res 2001 Mar;33(3):138-43

541 Tanaka M, Nakaya S, Kumai T, Watanabe M, Tateishi T, Shimizu H, Kobayashi S. Effects of estrogen on serum leptin levels and leptin mRNA expression in adipose tissue in rats. Horm Res 2001;56(3-4):98-104

542 Fedorcsak P, Storeng R, Dale PO, Tanbo T, Torjesen P, Urbancsek J, Abyholm T. Leptin and leptin binding activity in the preovulatory follicle of polycystic ovary syndrome patients. Scand J Clin Lab Invest 2000 Dec;60(8):649-55

543 Spritzer PM, Poy M, Wiltgen D, Mylius LS, Capp E. Leptin concentrations in hirsute women with polycystic ovary syndrome or idiopathic hirsutism: influence on LH and relationship with hormonal, metabolic, and anthropometric measurements. Hum Reprod 2001 Jul;16(7):1340-6

544 Gambineri A, Pelusi C, Vicennati V, Pagotto U, Pasquali R. Obesity and the polycystic ovary syndrome. Int J Obes Relat Metab Disord 2002 Jul;26(7):883-96

545 Veldhuis JD, Pincus SM, Garcia-Rudaz MC, Ropelato MG, Escobar ME, Barontini M. Disruption of the synchronous secretion of leptin, LH, and ovarian androgens in nonobese adolescents with the polycystic ovarian syndrome. J Clin Endocrinol Metab 2001 Aug;86(8):3772-8

546 Schofl C, Horn R, Schill T, Schlosser HW, Muller MJ, Brabant G. Circulating ghrelin levels in patients with polycystic ovary syndrome. J Clin Endocrinol Metab 2002 Oct;87(10):4607-10

547 Villa P, Soranna L, Mancini A, De Marinis L, Valle D, Mancuso S, Lanzone A. Effect of feeding on growth hormone response to growth hormone-releasing hormone in polycystic ovarian syndrome: relation with body weight and hyperinsulinism. Hum Reprod 2001 Mar;16(3):430-4

548 Van Dam EW, Roelfsema F, Helmerhorst FH, Frolich M, Meinders AE, Veldhuis JD,Pijl H. Low amplitude and disorderly spontaneous growth hormone release in obese women with or without polycystic ovary syndrome. J Clin Endocrinol Metab 2002 Sep;87(9):4225-30

549 Garcia-Rudaz MC, Ropelato MG, Escobar ME, Veldhuis JD, Barontini M. Amplified and orderly growth hormone secretion characterizes lean adolescents with polycystic ovary syndrome. Eur J Endocrinol 2002 Aug;147(2):207-16

550 Wu X, Sallinen K, Zhou S, Su Y, Pollanen P, Erkkola R. Androgen excess contributes to altered growth hormone/insulin-like growth factor-1 axis in nonobese women with polycystic ovary syndrome. Fertil Steril 2000 Apr;73(4):730-4

551 Anim-Nyame N, Domoney C, Panay N, Jones J, Alaghband-Zadeh J, Studd JW. Plasma leptin concentrations are increased in women with premenstrual syndrome. Hum Reprod 2000 Nov;15(11):2329-32

552 Messinis IE, Papageorgiou I, Milingos S, Asprodini E, Kollios G, Seferiadis K. Oestradiol plus progesterone treatment increases serum leptin concentrations in normal women. Hum Reprod 2001 Sep;16(9):1827-32

553 Maruyama S, Minami S, Kaseki H, Ishihara K, Araki S, Suzue R. A comparison of serum leptin concentrations in obese and normal weight Japanese women with regular menstrual cycle. J Nutr Sci Vitaminol (Tokyo) 2001 Feb;47(1):87-9

554 Poston L. Leptin and preeclampsia. Semin Reprod Med 2002;20(2):131-8

555 Kirwan JP, Hauguel-De Mouzon S, Lepercq J, Challier JC, Huston-Presley L, Friedman JE, Kalhan SC, Catalano PM. TNF-alpha is a predictor of insulin resistance in human pregnancy. Diabetes 2002 Jul;51(7):2207-13

556 Tsai EM, Yang CH, Chen SC, Liu YH, Chen HS, Hsu SC, Lee JN. Leptin affects pregnancy outcome of in vitro fertilization and steroidogenesis of human granulosa cells. J Assist Reprod Genet 2002 Apr;19(4):169-76

[557] Gogacz M, Polak G, Jakowicki J, Kotarski J. Peritoneal fluid leptin concentration in infertile patients. *J Reprod Immunol* 2001 Aug;51(2):159-65

[558] Unkila-Kallio L, Andersson S, Koistinen HA, Karonen SL, Ylikorkala O, Tiitinen A. Leptin during assisted reproductive cycles: the effect of ovarian stimulation and of very early pregnancy. *Hum Reprod* 2001 Apr;16(4):657-62

[559] Kitawaki J, Koshiba H, Ishihara H, Kusuki I, Tsukamoto K, Honjo H. Expression of leptin receptor in human endometrium and fluctuation during the menstrual cycle. *J Clin Endocrinol Metab* 2000 May;85(5):1946-50

[560] Matarese G, Alviggi C, Sanna V, Howard JK, Lord GM, Carravetta C, Fontana S, Lechler RI, Bloom SR, De Placido G. Increased leptin levels in serum and peritoneal fluid of patients with pelvic endometriosis. *J Clin Endocrinol Metab* 2000 Jul;85(7):2483-7

[561] Wu MH, Chuang PC, Chen HM, Lin CC, Tsai SJ. Increased leptin expression in endometriosis cells is associated with endometrial stromal cell proliferation and leptin gene up-regulation. *Mol Hum Reprod* 2002 May;8(5):456-64

[562] Lebovic DI, Chao VA, Martini JF, Taylor RN. IL-1beta induction of RANTES (regulated upon activation, normal T cell expressed and secreted) chemokine gene expression in endometriotic stromal cells depends on a nuclear factor-kappaB site in the proximal promoter. *J Clin Endocrinol Metab* 2001 Oct;86(10):4759-64

[563] Bidzinska B, Petraglia F, Angioni S, Genazzani AD, Criscuolo M, Ficarra G, Gallinelli A, Trentini GP, Genazzani AR. Effect of different chronic intermittent stressors and acetyl-l-carnitine on hypothalamic beta-endorphin and GnRH and on plasma testosterone levels in male rats. *Neuroendocrinology* 1993 Jun;57(6):985-90.

[564] Genazzani AD, Petraglia F, Algeri I, Gastaldi M, Calvani M, Botticelli G, Genazzani AR. Acetyl-l-carnitine as possible drug in the treatment of hypothalamic amenorrhea. *Acta Obstet Gynecol Scand* 1991;70(6):487-92.

[565] Iossa S, Mollica MP, Lionetti L, Crescenzo R, Botta M, Barletta A, Liverini G. Acetyl-L-carnitine supplementation differently influences nutrient partitioning, serum leptin concentration and skeletal muscle mitochondrial respiration in young and old rats. *J Nutr 2002* Apr;132(4):636-42

[566] Pearlstein T. Selective serotonin reuptake inhibitors for premenstrual dysphoric disorder: the emerging gold standard? *Drugs* 2002;62(13):1869-85

[567] Van Ameringen M, Mancini C, Pipe B, Campbell M, Oakman J. Topiramate treatment for SSRI-induced weight gain in anxiety disorders. *J Clin Psychiatry* 2002 Nov;63(11):981-4

[568] Masand PS, Gupta S. Selective serotonin-reuptake inhibitors: an update. *Harv Rev Psychiatry* 1999 Jul-Aug;7(2):69-84

[569] Silvestri R, Pace-Schott EF, Gersh T, Stickgold R, Salzman C, Hobson JA. Effects of fluvoxamine and paroxetine on sleep structure in normal subjects: a home-based Nightcap evaluation during drug administration and withdrawal. *J Clin Psychiatry* 2001 Aug;62(8):642-52

[570] Dagan Y. Circadian Rhythm Sleep Disorders (CRSD) in psychiatry—a review. *Isr J Psychiatry Relat Sci* 2002;39(1):19-27

[571] Writing Group for the Women's Health Initiative Investigators. Risks and benefits of estrogen plus progestin in healthy postmenopausal women: principal results From the Women's Health Initiative randomized controlled trial. *JAMA* 2002 Jul 17;288(3):321-33

[572] A. H. Follingstad M.D. Estriol, the forgotten estrogen. *JAMA*, Jan. 2 1978 Vol 239 No.1

[573] Lemon H, Wotiz H, Parsons L, Mozden P. Reduced Estriol secretion in patients with breast cancer prior to endocrine therapy. *JAMA* 1966; 196;112-120.

[574] Reyes-Romero MA. The physiological role of estriol during human fetal development is to act as antioxidant at lipophilic milieus of the central nervous system. *Med Hypotheses* 2001 Jan;56(1):107-9

[575] O'Hara MW, Schlechte JA, Lewis DA, Wright EJ. Prospective study of postpartum blues. Biologic and psychosocial factors. *Arch Gen Psychiatry* 1991 Sep;48(9):801-6

[576] Zeisler H, Jirecek S, Hohlagschwandtner M, Knofler M, Tempfer C, Livingston JC. Concentrations of estrogens in patients with preeclampsia. *Wien Klin Wochenschr* 2002 Jun 28;114(12):458-61

[577] Voskuhl RR, Palaszynski K. Sex hormones in experimental autoimmune encephalomyelitis: implications for multiple sclerosis. *Neuroscientist* 2001 Jun;7(3):258-70

[578] Sicotte NL, Liva SM, Klutch R, Pfeiffer P, Bouvier S, Odesa S, Wu TC, Voskuhl RR. Treatment of multiple sclerosis with the pregnancy hormone estriol. *Ann Neurol* 2002 Oct;52(4):421-8

[579] Buntner B, Rosciszewska D. Urinary excretion of estrogen fractions, alpha and beta pregnanediol and pregnanetriol in women with epileptic seizures during the premenstrual period. *urol Neurochir Pol* 1975 May-Jun;9(3):311-7

[580] Zemlyak I, Brooke SM, Sapolsky RM. Protection against gp120-induced neurotoxicity by an array of estrogenic steroids. *Brain Res* 2002 Dec 27;958(2):272-6

[581] Kajta M, Budziszewska B, Marszal M, Lason W. Effects of 17-beta estradiol and estriol on NMDA-induced toxicity and apoptosis in primary cultures of rat cortical neurons. *J Physiol Pharmacol* 2001 Sep;52(3):437-46

[582] Plaino L, Stomati M, Casarosa E, Artini PG, Santuz M, D'Ambrogio G, Cobellis L, Luisi M, Genazzani AR, Petraglia F. Ovarian follicular fluid contains immunoreactive estriol: lack of correlation with estradiol concentrations. *Gynecol Endocrinol* 2000 Aug;14(4):231-5

[583] Ghosh S, Kabir SN, Pakrashi A, Chatterjee S, Chakravarty B. Subclinical hypothyroidism: a determinant of polycystic ovary syndrome. *Horm Res* 1993;39(1-2):61-6 Comment in: Horm Res. 1994;41(1):43-4.

[584] Lee JR. *What Your Doctor May Not Tell You About Menopause*. New York. Warner Books, 1996

[585] Moen MH, Buajordet M, Leirstrand T. Progesterone cream—efficient in premenstrual syndrome and climacteric problems? *Tidsskr Nor Laegeforen* 2002 Jun 10;122(15):1477-8

[586] Triezenberg DJ, Ang J. Are progesterone or progestogens effective in managing premenstrual syndrome

(PMS) symptoms? *J Fam Pract* 2002 Feb;51(2):109
[587] Wyatt K, Dimmock P, Jones P, Obhrai M, O'Brien S. Efficacy of progesterone and progestogens in management of premenstrual syndrome: systematic review. *BMJ* 2001 Oct 6;323(7316):776-80
[588] O'Sullivan AJ, Martin A, Brown MA. Efficient fat storage in pre-menopausal women and in early pregnancy: a role for estrogen. *J Clin Endocrinol Metab* 2001 Oct;86(10):4951-6
[589] Li WL, Guo XY, Zhang JY, Peng P, Zhang YL. Serum leptin levels of menopausal women before and after hormone replacement therapy. Di Yi Jun Yi Da Xue Xue Bao 2002 Jul;22(7):635-6
[590] Ainslie DA, Morris MJ, Wittert G, Turnbull H, Proietto J, Thorburn AW. Estrogen deficiency causes central leptin insensitivity and increased hypothalamic neuropeptide Y. *Int J Obes Relat Metab Disord* 2001 Nov;25(11):1680-8
[591] Wyon YA, Spetz AC, Theodorsson GE, Hammar ML. Concentrations of calcitonin gene-related peptide and neuropeptide Y in plasma increase during flushes in postmenopausal women. *Menopause* 2000 Jan-Feb;7(1):25-30
[592] Kanaley JA, Sames C, Swisher L, Swick AG, Ploutz-Snyder LL, Steppan CM, Sagendorf KS, Feiglin D, Jaynes EB, Meyer RA, Weinstock RS. Abdominal fat distribution in pre- and postmenopausal women: The impact of physical activity, age, and menopausal status. *Metabolism* 2001 Aug;50(8):976-82
[593] Isidori AM, Strollo F, More M, Caprio M, Aversa A, Moretti C, Frajese G, Riondino G, Fabbri A. Leptin and aging: correlation with endocrine changes in male and female healthy adult populations of different body weights. *J Clin Endocrinol Metab* 2000 May;85(5):1954-62
[594] Martini G, Valenti R, Giovani S, Campagna S, Franci B, Nuti R. Leptin and body composition in healthy postmenopausal women. *Panminerva Med* 2001 Sep;43(3):149-54
[595] Cioffi M, Esposito K, Vietri MT, Gazzerro P, D'Auria A, Ardovino I, Puca GA,Molinari AM. Cytokine pattern in postmenopause. *Maturitas* 2002 Mar 25;41(3):187-92
[596] Schurman L, Sedlinsky C, Mangano A, Sen L, Leiderman S, Fernandez G, Theas S, Damilano S, Gurfinkel M, Seilicovich A. Estrogenic status influences nitric oxide-regulated TNF-alpha release from human peripheral blood monocytes. *Exp Clin Endocrinol Diabetes* 2001;109(6):340-4
[597] Sites CK, Toth MJ, Cushman M, L'Hommedieu GD, Tchernof A, Tracy RP, Poehlman ET. Menopause-related differences in inflammation markers and their relationship to body fat distribution and insulin-stimulated glucose disposal. *Fertil Steril* 2002 Jan;77(1):128-35
[598] Kano H, Hayashi T, Sumi D, Matusi-Hirai H, Tsunekawa T, Endo H, Iguchi A. Estriol retards and stabilizes atherosclerosis through an NO-mediated system. Life Sci 2002 May 24;71(1):31-42
[599] Ohata S, Ishibashi Y, Hirano Y, Sakane T, Takahashi N, Sugamori T, Inoue S, Katoh H, Ochiai K, Sano K, Murakami Y, Shimada T. Relationship between endothelial function and female hormone level in very old females: evaluation from ischemic reactive

hyperemic response in forearm vessels *J Cardiol* 2000 Jun;35(6):417-24
[600] Itoi H, Minakami H, Iwasaki R, Sato I. Comparison of the long-term effects of oral estriol with the effects of conjugated estrogen on serum lipid profile in early menopausal women. *Maturitas* 2000 Oct 31;36(3):217-22
[601] Hayashi T, Ito I, Kano H, Endo H, Iguchi A. Estriol (E3) replacement improves endothelial function and bone mineral density in very elderly women. *J Gerontol A Biol Sci Med Sci* 2000 Apr;55(4):B183-90; discussion B191-3
[602] Manonai J, Theppisai U. Effect of oral estriol on urogenital symptoms, vaginal cytology, and plasma hormone level in postmenopausal women. *J Med Assoc Thai* 2001 Apr;84(4):539-44
[603] Mandigers RJ, Nell T. Treatment of bitches with acquired urinary incontinence with oestriol. *Vet Rec* 2001 Dec 22-29;149(25):764-7
[604] Raz R. Postmenopausal women with recurrent UTI. *Int J Antimicrob Agents* 2001 Apr;17(4):269-71
[605] Yoshimura T, Okamura H. Short term oral estriol treatment restores normal pre-menopausal vaginal flora to elderly women. *Maturitas* 2001 Sep 28;39(3):253-7
[606] Kuczynska K, Wolczynski S, Janucik-Gacuta M, Zbroch T. Influence of hormonal replacement therapy on bacterial vaginosis in the group of peri- and postmenopausal women *Ginekol Pol* 2001 Oct;72(10):816-24
[607] Heimer G. Estriol in the postmenopausal. *Acta Obstet Gynecol Scand*. 1987; Suppl 139;1-23.
[608] Losif C. Effects of protracted administration of Estriol on the lower genito urinary tract in postmenopausal women. *Arch Gynecol Obstet* 1992; 251; 115-120.
[609] Ushiroyama T, Sakai M, Higashiyama T, Ikeda A, Ueki M. Estrogen replacement therapy in postmenopausal women: a study of the efficacy of estriol and changes in plasma gonadotropin levels. Gynecol Endocrinol 2001 Feb;15(1):74-80
[610] Granberg S, Eurenius K, Lindgren R, Wilhelmsson L. The effects of oral estriol on the endometrium in postmenopausal women. *Maturitas* 2002 Jun 25;42(2):149-56
[611] Lundstrom E, Wilczek B, von Palffy Z, Soderqvist G, von Schoultz B. Mammographic breast density during hormone replacement therapy: effects of continuous combination, unopposed transdermal and low-potency estrogen regimens. *Climacteric* 2001 Mar;4(1):42-85.
[612] Takahashi K, Okada M, Ozaki T, Kurioka H, Manabe A, Kanasaki H, Miyazaki K. Safety and efficacy of oestriol for symptoms of natural or surgically induced menopause. *Hum Reprod* 2000 May;15(5):1028-366.
[613] Son DS, Roby KF, Rozman KK, Terranova PF. Estradiol enhances and estriol inhibits the expression of CYP1A1 induced by 2,3,7,8-tetrachlorodibenzo-p-dioxin in a mouse ovarian cancer cell line. Toxicology 2002 Jul 15;176(3):229-43
[614] Lemon H. Oestriol and prevention of breast cancer. Lancet 1973; 546-547.
[615] Lemon H, Kumar P, Peterson C, Rodriguez-Sierra J, Abbo K. Inhibition of radiogenic mammary carcinoma in rats by Estriol or tamoxifen. cancer 1989;63:1685-

1692.

[616] Heimer G. Estriol in the postmenopausal. *Acta Obstet Gynecol Scand.* 1987; Suppl 139;1-23.

[617] Zang YC, Halder JB, Hong J, Rivera VM, Zhang JZ. Regulatory effects of estriol on T cell migration and cytokine profile: inhibition of transcription factor NF-kappa

[618] B. J Neuroimmunol 2002 Mar;124(1-2):106-14 8. Pasqualini JR, Gelly C, Nguyen BL, Vella C. Importance of estrogen sulfates in breast cancer. J Steroid Biochem 1989;34(1-6):155-63.

[619] Lauritzen C. Results of a 5-year prospective study of Estriol succinate treatment in patients with climacteric complaints. *Horm Metabol Res.* 1987; 19; 579-584.

[620] Matsubara M, Yoshizawa T, Morioka T, Katayose S. Serum leptin and lipids in patients with thyroid dysfunction. *J Atheroscler Thromb* 2000;7(1):50-4

[621] Wang JL, Chinookoswong N, Yin S, Shi ZQ. Caloreigenic actions of leptin are additive to, but not dependent on, those of thyroid hormones. *Am J Physiol Endocrinol Metab* 2000 Dec;279(6):E1278-85

[622] Chen MD, Song YM, Tsou CT, Lin WH, Sheu WH. Leptin concentration and the Zn/Cu ratio in plasma in women with thyroid disorder. *Biol Trace Elem Res* 2000 Summer;75(1-3):99-105

[623] Miyakawa M, Tsushima T, Murakami H, Isozaki O, Takano K. Serum leptin levels and bioelectrical impedance assessment of body composition in patients with Graves' disease and hypothyroidism. *Endocr J* 1999 Oct;46(5):665-73

[624] Guo F, Bakal K, Minokoshi Y, Hollenberg AN. Leptin Signaling Targets the Thyrotropin-Releasing Hormone Gene Promoter In Vivo. Endocrinology. 2004 Feb 5

[625] Huo L, Munzberg H, Nillni EA, Bjorbaek C. Role of STAT3 in Regulation of Hypothalamic trh Gene-Expression by Leptin. Endocrinology. 2004 Feb 5

[626] Tagliaferri M, Berselli ME, Calo G, Minocci A, Savia G, Petroni ML, Viberti GC, Liuzzi A. Subclinical hypothyroidism in obese patients: relation to resting energy expenditure, serum leptin, body composition, and lipid profile. *Obes Res* 2001 Mar;9(3):196-201

[627] Kautzky-Willer A, Ludwig C, Nowotny P, Roden A, Huemer C, Widhalm K, Vierhapper H, Waldhausl W, Roden M. Elevation of plasma leptin concentrations in obese hyperinsulinaemic hypothyroidism before and after treatment. Eur J Clin Invest 1999 May;29(5):395-403

[628] Iossa S, Lionetti L, Mollica MP, Crescenzo R, Barletta A, Liverini Fat balance and serum leptin concentrations in normal, hypothyroid, and hyperthyroid rats.G.*Int J Obes Relat Metab Disord* 2001 Mar;25(3):417-25

[629] Rubello D, Sonino N, Casara D, et al. Acute and chronic effects of high glucocorticoid levels on hypothalamic-pituitary-thyroid axis in man. *J Endocrinol Invest* 1992:15:437-441

[630] Bobek S, Sechman A, Niezgoda J, Jacek T. Reverse 3,3',5'-triiodothyronine suppresses increase in free fatty acids in chickens elicited by dexamethasone or adrenaline. *J Vet Med A Physiol Pathol Clin Med* 2002 Apr;49(3):121-4

[631] Silberman DM, Wald M, Genaro AM. Effects of chronic mild stress on lymphocyte proliferative response. Participation of serum thyroid hormones and corticosterone. *Int Immunopharmacol* 2002 Mar;2(4):487-97

[632] Servatius RJ, Natelson BH, Moldow R, Pogach L, Brennan FX, Ottenweller JE. Persistent neuroendocrine changes in multiple hormonal axes after a single or repeated stressor exposures. *Stress* 2000 Nov;3(4):263-74

[633] Stathatos N, Levetan C, Burman KD, Wartofsky L. The controversy of the treatment of critically ill patients with thyroid hormone. *Best Pract Res Clin Endocrinol Metab* 2001 Dec;15(4):465-78

[634] Alink GM, Brouwer A, Heussen GA. Effects of outdoor and indoor airborne particulate matter on thyroid hormone and vitamin A metabolism. *Toxicol Lett* 1994 Jun;72(1-3):73-81

[635] Zaitseva NV, Zemlianova MA, Kir'ianov DA. Identification of specific features of the development of iodine deficiency in children exposed to low-intensity ecological factors (in case of the Perm Region) *Vestn Ross Akad Med Nauk* 2001;(6):39-45

[636] Dodina LG. The clinical functional status of the thyroid and the cortisol level in those living in a region of ecological stress *Med Tr Prom Ekol* 1999;(10):8-10

[637] Langer P, Tajtakova M, Fodor G, Kocan A, Bohov P, Michalek J, Kreze A. Increased thyroid volume and prevalence of thyroid disorders in an area heavily polluted by polychlorinated biphenyls. *Eur J Endocrinol* 1998 Oct;139(4):402-9

[638] Osius N, Karmaus W. Thyroid hormone level in children in the area of a toxic waste incinerator in South Essen *Gesundheitswesen* 1998 Feb;60(2):107-12

[639] Porter WP, Jaeger JW, Carlson IH. Endocrine, immune, and behavioral effects of aldicarb (carbamate), atrazine (triazine) and nitrate (fertilizer) mixtures at groundwater concentrations. *Toxicol Ind Health* 1999 Jan-Mar;15(1-2):133-50

[640] Leatherland JF. Changes in thyroid hormone economy following consumption of environmentally contaminated Great Lakes fish. Toxicol Ind Health 1998 Jan-Apr;14(1-2):41-57

[641] Vladeva S, Gatseva P, Gopina G. Comparative analysis of results from studies of goitre in children from Bulgarian villages with nitrate pollution of drinking water in 1995 and 1998. *Cent Eur J Public Health* 2000 Aug;8(3):179-81

[642] Khmel'nitskii OK, Tret'iakova MS, Kiselev AV, Basinskii VA, Batashova VS, Vasil'ev IuB, Gorbachev AL, Derizhanova IS, Kovalenko VL, Kulaev IA, Konstantinov GS, Murochkin VV, Tararak, TIa, Ashanin BS, Troshin VP, Khodasevich LS, Maliavskii IIu. Morpho-ecological characteristics of thyroid diseases in various regions of Russia and Belorussia from surgical data *Arkh Patol* 2000 Jul-Aug;62(4):19-27

[643] Gasparoni A, Autelli M, Ravagni-Probizer MF, Bartoli A, Regazzi-Bonora M, Chirico G, Rondini G. Effect of passive smoking on thyroid function in infants. *Eur J Endocrinol* 1998 Apr;138(4):379-82

[644] Wade MG, Parent S, Finnson KW, Foster W, Younglai E, McMahon A, Cyr DG, Hughes C. Thyroid toxicity due to subchronic exposure to a complex mixture of 16 organochlorines, lead, and cadmium. *Toxicol Sci* 2002 Jun;67(2):207-18

[645] Schantz SL, Widholm JJ. Cognitive effects of endo-

crine-disrupting chemicals in animals. *Environ Health Perspect* 2001 Dec;109(12):1197-206

[646] Saxena NK, Ikeda K, Rockey DC, Friedman SL, Anania FA. Leptin in hepatic fibrosis: evidence for increased collagen production in stellate cells and lean littermates of ob/ob mice. *Hepatology* 2002 Apr;35(4):762-71

[647] Ikejima K, Honda H, Yoshikawa M, Hirose M, Kitamura T, Takei Y, Sato N. Leptin augments inflammatory and profibrogenic responses in the murine liver induced by hepatotoxic chemicals. *Hepatology* 2001 Aug;34(2):288-97

[648] Nicassio PM, Moxham EG, Schuman CE, Gevirtz RN. The contribution of pain, reported sleep quality, and depressive symptoms to fatigue in fibromyalgia. *Pain* 2002 Dec;100(3):271-9

[649] Lawson K. Tricyclic antidepressants and fibromyalgia: what is the mechanism of action? *Expert Opin Investig Drugs* 2002 Oct;11(10):1437-45

[650] Moldofsky H. Management of sleep disorders in fibromyalgia. *Rheum Dis Clin North Am* 2002 May;28(2):353-65

[651] Paulson M, Norberg A, Danielson E. Men living with fibromyalgia-type pain: experiences as patients in the Swedish health care system. *J Adv Nurs* 2002 Oct;40(1):87-95

[652] Schlienger JL, Perrin AE, Grunenberger F, Goichot B. Hormonal perturbations in fibromyalgia. *Ann Endocrinol* (Paris) 2001 Dec;62(6):542-8

[653] Tsigos C, Chrousos GP. Hypothalamic-pituitary-adrenal axis, neuroendocrine factors and stress. *J Psychosom Res* 2002 Oct;53(4):865-71

[654] Okifuji A, Turk DC. Stress and psychophysiological dysregulation in patients with fibromyalgia syndrome. *Appl Psychophysiol Biofeedback* 2002 Jun;27(2):129-41

[655] Geenen R, Jacobs JW, Bijlsma JW. Evaluation and management of endocrine dysfunction in fibromyalgia. *Rheum Dis Clin North Am* 2002 May;28(2):389-404

[656] Geenen R, Jacobs JW, Bijlsma JW. Evaluation and management of endocrine dysfunction in fibromyalgia. *Rheum Dis Clin North Am* 2002 May;28(2):389-404

[657] Bennett RM. Adult growth hormone deficiency in patients with fibromyalgia. *Curr Rheumatol Rep* 2002 Aug;4(4):306-12

[658] Paiva ES, Deodhar A, Jones KD, Bennett R. Impaired growth hormone secretion in fibromyalgia patients: evidence for augmented hypothalamic somatostatin tone. *Arthritis Rheum* 2002 May;46(5):1344-50

[659] Riedel W, Schlapp U, Leck S, Netter P, Neeck G Blunted ACTH and cortisol responses to systemic injection of corticotropin-releasing hormone (CRH) in fibromyalgia: role of somatostatin and CRH-binding protein. Ann N Y Acad Sci 2002 Jun;966:483-90

[660] Hein G, Franke S Are advanced glycation end-product-modified proteins of pathogenetic importance in fibromyalgia? *Rheumatology* (Oxford) 2002 Oct;41(10):1163-7

[661] Tsigos C, Chrousos GP. Hypothalamic-pituitary-adrenal axis, neuroendocrine factors and stress. *J Psychosom Res* 2002 Oct;53(4):865-71

[662] Rohr UD, Herold J. Melatonin deficiencies in women. *Maturitas* 2002 Apr 15;41 Suppl 1:S85-104

[663] Kelly GS. Larch arabinogalactan: clinical relevance of a novel immune-enhancing polysaccharide. *Altern Med Rev* 1999 Apr;4(2):96-103

[664] Hein G, Franke S Are advanced glycation end-product-modified proteins of pathogenetic importance in fibromyalgia? *Rheumatology* (Oxford) 2002 Oct;41(10):1163-7

[665] Bierhaus A, Chevion S, Chevion M, Hofmann M, Quehenberger P, Illmer T, Luther T, Berentshtein E, Tritschler H, Muller M, Wahl P, Ziegler R, Nawroth PP. Advanced glycation end product-induced activation of NF kappaB is suppressed by alpha-lipoic acid in cultured endothelial cells. *Diabetes* 1997 Sep;46(9):1481-90

[666] Suzuki YJ, Aggarwal BB, Packer L. Alpha-lipoic acid is a potent inhibitor of NF-kappa B activation in human T cells. *Biochem Biophys Res Commun* 1992 Dec 30;189(3):1709-15

[667] Zhang WJ, Frei B. Alpha-lipoic acid inhibits TNF-alpha-induced NF kappaB activation and adhesion molecule expression in human aortic endothelial cells. *FASEB J* 2001 Nov;15(13):2423-32

[668] Lee HA, Hughes DA. Alpha-lipoic acid modulates NF kappaB activity in human monocytic cells by direct interaction with DNA. *Exp Gerontol* 2002 Jan-Mar;37(2-3):401-10

[669] Nagamatsu M, Nickander K, et al. Lipoic acid improves nerve blood flow, reduces oxidative stress, and improves distal nerve conduction in experimental diabetic neuropathy. *Diabetes Care* 18:1160, 1995.

[670] Ziegler D, and Gries F. Alpha-lipoic acid in the treatment of Diabetic Peripheral and Cardiac Autonomic Neuropathy. *Diabetes* 46(2):S62-S66, 1997.

[671] Christie, R.B. The medical uses of proteolytic enzymes, in Topics in Enzyme and Fermentation Biotechnology, Vol. 4, Wiseman, A., Ed., Ellis Horwood Ltd., Chichester, 1980, 25

[672] Taussig SJ, Batkin S. Bromelain, the enzyme complex of pineapple (Ananas comosus) and its clinical application. An update. *J Ethnopharmacol* 1988 Feb-Mar;22(2):191-203

[673] Wadsworth TL, McDonald TL, Koop DR. *Biochem Pharmacol* Effects of Ginkgo biloba extract (EGb 761) and quercetin on lipopolysaccharide-induced signaling pathways involved in the release of tumor necrosis factor-alpha. 2001 Oct 1;62(7):963-74

[674] Surh YJ, Chun KS, Cha HH, Han SS, Keum YS, Park KK, Lee SS. Molecular mechanisms underlying chemopreventive activities of anti-inflammatory phytochemicals: down-regulation of COX-2 and iNOS through suppression of NF-kappa B activation. *Mutat Res* 2001 Sep 1;480-481:243-68

[675] Chuang SE, Yeh PY, Lu YS, Lai GM, Liao CM, Gao M, Cheng AL. Basal levels and patterns of anticancer drug-induced activation of nuclear factor-kappaB (NF kappaB), and its attenuation by tamoxifen, dexamethasone, and curcumin in carcinoma cells. *Biochem Pharmacol* 2002 May 1;63(9):1709-16

[676] W.Y. John Chen, Ph.D; Giovanni Abetangelo, MD, Ph.D: Functions of hyaluronan in wound repair. *WOUND REP REG* 1999; 7:79-89

[677] Hakkinen K, Pakarinen A, Hannonen P, Hakkinen A, Airaksinen O, Valkeinen H, Alen M. Effects of strength training on muscle strength, cross-sectional area, maximal electromyographic activity, and serum hormones in

pre-menopausal women with fibromyalgia. *J Rheumatol* 2002 Jun;29(6):1287-95

[678] Kang K, Pariza MW. trans-10,cis-12-Conjugated linoleic acid reduces leptin secretion from 3T3-L1 adipocytes. *Biochem Biophys Res Commun* 2001 Sep 21;287(2):377-82

[679] Rahman SM, Wang Y, Yotsumoto H, Cha J, Han S, Inoue S, Yanagita T. Effects of conjugated linoleic acid on serum leptin concentration, body-fat accumulation, and beta-oxidation of fatty acid in OLETF rats. *Nutrition* 2001 May;17(5):385-90

[680] Akahoshi A, Goto Y, Murao K, Miyazaki T, Yamasaki M, Nonaka M, Yamada K, Sugano M. Conjugated linoleic acid reduces body fats and cytokine levels of mice. *Biosci Biotechnol Biochem* 2002 Apr;66(4):916-20

[681] Douyon L, Schteingart DE. Effect of obesity and starvation on thyroid hormone, growth hormone, and cortisol secretion. *Endocrinol Metab Clin North Am* 2002 Mar;31(1):173-89

[682] van der Poll T, Romijn JA, Wiersinga WM, Sauerwein HP. Tumor necrosis factor: a putative mediator of the sick euthyroid syndrome in man. *J Clin Endocrinol Metab* 1990 Dec;71(6):1567-72

[683] Boelen A, Maas MA, Lowik CW, Platvoet MC, Wiersinga WM. Induced illness in interleukin-6 (IL-6) knock-out mice: a causal role of IL-6 in the development of the low 3,5,3'-triiodothyronine syndrome. *Endocrinology* 1996 Dec;137(12):5250-4

[684] Chopra IJ, Solomon DH, Hepner GW, Morgenstein AA. Misleadingly low free thyroxine index and usefulness of reverse triiodothyronine measurement in nonthyroidal illnesses. *Ann Intern Med* 1979 Jun;90(6):905-12

[685] Michalaki M, Vagenakis AG, Makri M, Kalfarentzos F, Kyriazopoulou V. Dissociation of the early decline in serum T(3) concentration and serum IL-6 rise and TNFalpha in nonthyroidal illness syndrome induced by abdominal surgery. *J Clin Endocrinol Metab* 2001 Sep;86(9):4198-205

[686] Friberg L, Drvota V, Bjelak AH, Eggertsen G, Ahnve S. Association between increased levels of reverse triiodothyronine and mortality after acute myocardial infarction. *Am J Med* 2001 Dec 15;111(9):699-703

[687] Pavlou HN, Kliridis PA, Panagiotopoulos AA, Goritsas CP, Vassilakos PJ. Euthyroid sick syndrome in acute ischemic syndromes. *Angiology* 2002 Nov-Dec;53(6):699-707

[688] Schulte C, Reinhardt W, Beelen D, Mann K, Schaefer U. Low T3-syndrome and nutritional status as prognostic factors in patients undergoing bone marrow transplantation. *Bone Marrow Transplant* 1998 Dec;22(12):1171-8

[689] Herrmann F, Hambsch K, Sorger D, Hantzschel H, Muller P, Nagel I. Low T3 syndrome and chronic inflammatory rheumatism *Z Gesamte Inn Med* 1989 Sep 1;44(17):513-8

[690] Goichot B, Schlienger JL, Grunenberger F, Pradignac A, Sapin R. Thyroid hormone status and nutrient intake in the free-living elderly. Interest of reverse triiodothyronine assessment. Eur J Endocrinol 1994 Mar;130(3):244-52

[691] Kranjcec D, Pinter A, Birtic T, Cabrijan T, Halle J, Tomicic D, Halle Z, Pintaric H, Radacic M, Novak N. Metabolic syndrome X—high risk factor for acute myocardial infarction and its complications. *Coll Antropol* 2002 Jun;26(1):23-9

[692] Quentmeier H, Dirks WG, Fleckenstein D, Zaborski M, Drexler HG. Tumor necrosis factor-alpha-induced proliferation requires synthesis of granulocyte-macrophage colony-stimulating factor. *Exp Hematol* 2000 Sep;28(9):1008-15

[693] Karin M, Lin A. NF kappaB at the crossroads of life and death. *Nat Immunol* 2002 Mar;3(3):221-7

[694] Yamamoto Y, Gaynor R B. Role of the NF kappaB pathway in the pathogenesis of human disease states. *Curr Mol Med* 2001 Jul;1(3):287-96

[695] Kasof GM, Lu JJ, Liu D, Speer B, Mongan KN, Gomes BC, Lorenzi MV. Tumor necrosis factor-alpha induces the expression of DR6, a member of the TNF receptor family, through activation of NF kappaB. *Oncogene* 2001 Nov 29;20(55):7965-75

[696] Chen S, Fribley A, Wang CY. Potentiation of tumor necrosis factor-mediated apoptosis of oral squamous cell carcinoma cells by adenovirus-mediated gene transfer of NF kappaB inhibitor. *J Dent Res* 2002 Feb;81(2):98-102

[697] Staudt LM. Gene expression profiling of lymphoid malignancies. *Annu Rev Med* 2002;53:303-18

[698] Delhalle S, Deregowski V, Benoit V, Merville MP, Bours V. NF kappaB-dependent MnSOD expression protects adenocarcinoma cells from TNF-alpha-induced apoptosis. *Oncogene* 2002 May 30;21(24):3917-24

[699] Javelaud D, Poupon MF, Wietzerbin J, Besancon F. Inhibition of constitutive NF-kappa B activity suppresses tumorigenicity of Ewing sarcoma EW7 cells. *Int J Cancer* 2002 Mar 10;98(2):193-8

[700] Sanlioglu S, Luleci G, Thomas KW. Simultaneous inhibition of Rac1 and IKK pathways sensitizes lung cancer cells to TNFalpha-mediated apoptosis. *Cancer Gene Ther* 2001 Nov;8(11):897-905

[701] Javelaud D, Poupon MF, Wietzerbin J, Besancon F. Inhibition of constitutive NF-kappa B activity suppresses tumorigenicity of Ewing sarcoma EW7 cells. *Int J Cancer* 2002 Mar 10;98(2):193-8

[702] Takada M, Koizumi T, Toyama H, Suzuki Y, Kuroda Y. Differential expression of RAGE in human pancreatic carcinoma cells. *Hepatogastroenterology* 2001 Nov-Dec;48(42):1577-8

[703] Beppu M, Ikebe T, Shirasuna K. The inhibitory effects of immunosuppressive factors, dexamethasone and interleukin-4, on NF kappaB-mediated protease production by oral cancer. *Biochim Biophys Acta* 2002 Jan 2;1586(1):11-22

[704] Jones DR, Broad RM, Comeau LD, Parsons SJ, Mayo MW. Inhibition of nuclear factor kappaB chemosensitizes non-small cell lung cancer through cytochrome c release and caspase activation. *J Thorac Cardiovasc Surg* 2002 Feb;123(2):310-7

[705] Sugita S, Kohno T, Yamamoto K, Imaizumi Y, Nakajima H, Ishimaru T, Matsuyama T. Induction of macrophage-inflammatory protein-3alpha gene expression by TNF-dependent NF kappaB activation. *J Immunol* 2002 Jun 1;168(11):5621-8

[706] Tharappel JC, Lee EY, Robertson LW, Spear BT, Glauert HP. Regulation of cell proliferation, apoptosis, and transcription factor activities during the promotion of liver carcinogenesis by polychlorinated biphenyls.

Toxicol Appl Pharmacol 2002 Mar 15;179(3):172-84
[707] Szabo G, Catalano D, Bellerose G, Mandrekar P. Interferon alpha and alcohol augment nuclear regulatory factor-kappaB activation in HepG2 cells, and interferon alpha increases pro-inflammatory cytokine production. *Alcohol Clin Exp Res* 2001 Aug;25(8):1188-97
[708] Wright G, Singh IS, Hasday JD, Farrance IK, Hall G, Cross AS, Rogers TB. Endotoxin stress-response in cardiomyocytes: NF kappaB activation and tumor necrosis factor-alpha expression. *Am J Physiol Heart Circ Physiol* 2002 Mar;282(3):H872-9
[709] Ginis I, Jaiswal R, Klimanis D, Liu J, Greenspon J, Hallenbeck JM. TNF-alpha-induced tolerance to ischemic injury involves differential control of NF kappaB transactivation: the role of NF kappaB association with p300 adaptor. *J Cereb Blood Flow Metab* 2002 Feb;22(2):142-52
[710] Bouloumie A, Marumo T, Lafontan M, Busse R. Leptin induces oxidative stress in human endothelial cells. *FASEB J* 1999 Jul;13(10):1231-8
[711] Viita H, Sen CK, Roy S, Siljamaki T, Nikkari T, Yla-Herttuala S. High expression of human 15-lipoxygenase induces NF kappaB-mediated expression of vascular cell adhesion molecule 1, intercellular adhesion molecule 1, and T-cell adhesion on human endothelial cells. *Antioxid Redox Signal* 1999 Spring;1(1):83-96
[712] Napoleone E, Di Santo A, Bastone A, Peri G, Mantovani A, de Gaetano G, Donati MB, Lorenzet R. Long pentraxin PTX3 upregulates tissue factor expression in human endothelial cells: a novel link between vascular inflammation and clotting activation. *Arterioscler Thromb Vasc Biol* 2002 May 1;22(5):782-7
[713] Ialenti A, Ianaro A, Maffia P, Carnuccio R, D'Acquisto F, Maiello FM, Di Rosa M. Role of nuclear factor-kappaB in a rat model of vascular injury. *Naunyn Schmiedebergs Arch Pharmacol* 2001 Oct;364(4):343-50
[714] Mattson MP, Culmsee C, Yu Z, Camandola S. Roles of nuclear factor kappaB in neuronal survival and plasticity. *J Neurochem* 2000 Feb;74(2):443-56
[715] Del Rio MJ, Velez-Pardo C. Monoamine neurotoxins-induced apoptosis in lymphocytes by a common oxidative stress mechanism: involvement of hydrogen peroxide (H(2)O(2)), caspase-3, and nuclear factor kappa-B (NF kappaB), p53, c-Jun transcription factors. *Biochem Pharmacol* 2002 Feb 15;63(4):677-88
[716] Paganelli R, Di Iorio A, Patricelli L, Ripani F, Sparvieri E, Faricelli R, Iarlori C, Porreca E, Di Gioacchino M, Abate G. Pro-inflammatory cytokines in sera of elderly patients with dementia: levels in vascular injury are higher than those of mild-moderate Alzheimer's disease patients. *Exp Gerontol* 2002 Jan-Mar;37(2-3):257-63
[717] Perry RT, Collins JS, Wiener H, Acton R, Go RC. The role of TNF and its receptors in Alzheimer's disease. *Neurobiol Aging* 2001 Nov-Dec;22(6):873-83
[718] Grammas P, Ovase R. Inflammatory factors are elevated in brain microvessels in Alzheimer's disease. *Neurobiol Aging* 2001 Nov-Dec;22(6):837-42
[719] McGeer PL, McGeer EG. Polymorphisms in inflammatory genes and the risk of Alzheimer disease. *Arch Neurol* 2001 Nov;58(11):1790-2
[720] Bruunsgaard H, Andersen-Ranberg K, Jeune B, Pedersen AN, Skinhoj P, Pedersen BK. A high plasma concentration of TNF-alpha is associated with dementia in centenarians. *J Gerontol A Biol Sci Med Sci* 1999 Jul;54(7):M357-64
[721] Knight DS, Mahajan DK, Qiao X. Dietary fat up-regulates the apolipoprotein E mRNA level in the Zucker lean rat brain. *Neuroreport* 2001 Oct 8;12(14):3111-5
[722] Calderon-Garciduenas L, Azzarelli B, Acuna H, Garcia R, Gambling TM, Osnaya N, Monroy S, DEL Tizapantzi MR, Carson JL, Villarreal-Calderon A, Rewcastle B. Air pollution and brain damage. *Toxicol Pathol* 2002 May-Jun;30(3):373-89
[723] Campbell A, Yang EY, Tsai-Turton M, Bondy SC. Pro-inflammatory effects of aluminum in human glioblastoma cells. *Brain Res* 2002 Apr 12;933(1):60-5
[724] Carpenter DO. Effects of metals on the nervous system of humans and animals. *Int J Occup Med Environ Health* 2001;14(3):209-18
[725] Busso N, So A, Chobaz-Peclat V, Morard C, Martinez-Soria E, Talabot-Ayer D, Gabay C. Leptin signaling deficiency impairs humoral and cellular immune responses and attenuates experimental arthritis. *J Immunol* 2002 Jan 15;168(2):875-82
[726] Nguyen VT, Benveniste EN. Critical role of tumor necrosis factor-alpha and NF-kappa B in interferon-gamma -induced CD40 expression in microglia/macrophages. *J Biol Chem* 2002 Apr 19;277(16):13796-803
[727] Brennan FM, Hayes AL, Ciesielski CJ, Green P, Foxwell BM, Feldmann M. Evidence that rheumatoid arthritis synovial T cells are similar to cytokine-activated T cells: involvement of phosphatidylinositol 3-kinase and nuclear factor kappaB pathways in tumor necrosis factor alpha production in rheumatoid arthritis. *Arthritis Rheum* 2002 Jan;46(1):31-41
[728] Kwok BH, Koh B, Ndubuisi MI, Elofsson M, Crews CM. The anti-inflammatory natural product parthenolide from the medicinal herb Feverfew directly binds to and inhibits IkappaB kinase. *Chem Biol* 2001 Aug;8(8):759-66
[729] Reuter U, Chiarugi A, Bolay H, Moskowitz MA. Nuclear factor-kappaB as a molecular target for migraine therapy. *Ann Neurol* 2002 Apr;51(4):507-16
[730] Kang BY, Chung SW, Kim TS. Inhibition of interleukin-12 production in lipopolysaccharide-activated mouse macrophages by parthenolide, a predominant sesquiterpene lactone in Tanacetum parthenium: involvement of nuclear factor-kappaB. *Immunol Lett* 2001 Jul 2;77(3):159-63
[731] Kang SN, Kim SH, Chung SW, Lee MH, Kim HJ, Kim TS. Enhancement of 1 alpha,25-dihydroxyvitamin D(3)-induced differentiation of human leukaemia HL-60 cells into monocytes by parthenolide via inhibition of NF-kappa B activity. *Br J Pharmacol* 2002 Mar;135(5):1235-44
[732] Patel NM, Nozaki S, Shortle NH, Bhat-Nakshatri P, Newton TR, Rice S, Gelfanov V, Boswell SH, Goulet RJ Jr, Sledge GW Jr, Nakshatri H.Paclitaxel sensitivity of breast cancer cells with constitutively active NF kappaB is enhanced by IkappaBalpha super-repressor and parthenolide. *Oncogene* 2000 Aug 24;19(36):4159-69
[733] Li-Weber M, Giaisi M, Baumann S, Treiber MK, Krammer PH. The anti-inflammatory sesquiterpene lactone parthenolide suppresses CD95-mediated activation-induced-cell-death in T-cells. *Cell Death Differ* 2002 Nov;9(11):1256-65

[734] Mogensen TH, Paludan SR. Virus-cell interactions: impact on cytokine production, immune evasion and tumor growth. *Eur Cytokine Netw* 2001 Jul-Sep;12(3):382-90

[735] Hiscott J, Kwon H, Genin P. Hostile takeovers: viral appropriation of the NF kappaB pathway. *J Clin Invest* 2001 Jan;107(2):143-51

[736] Tai DI, Tsai SL, Chang YH, Huang SN, Chen TC, Chang KS, Liaw YF. Constitutive activation of nuclear factor kappaB in hepatocellular carcinoma. *Cancer* 2000 Dec 1;89(11):2274-81

[737] Tai DI, Tsai SL, Chen YM, Chuang YL, Peng CY, Sheen IS, Yeh CT, Chang KS, Huang SN, Kuo GC, Liaw YF. Activation of nuclear factor kappaB in hepatitis C virus infection: implications for pathogenesis and hepatocarcinogenesis. *Hepatology* 2000 Mar;31(3):656-64

[738] Liu X, Zou S, Qiu F. NF-kappa B expression in cholangiocarcinoma transfected with hepatitis C virus core gene. [Article in Chinese] *Zhonghua Zhong Liu Za Zhi* 2002 Jan;24(1):20-3

[739] Huo TI, Wang XW, Forgues M, Wu CG, Spillare EA, Giannini C, Brechot C, Harris CC. Hepatitis B virus X mutants derived from human hepatocellular carcinoma retain the ability to abrogate p53-induced apoptosis. *Oncogene* 2001 Jun 21;20(28):3620-8

[740] Diao J, Garces R, Richardson CD. X protein of hepatitis B virus modulates cytokine and growth factor related signal transduction pathways during the course of viral infections and hepatocarcinogenesis. *Cytokine Growth Factor Rev* 2001 Jun-Sep;12(2-3):189-205

[741] Vockerodt M, Tesch H, Kube D. Epstein-Barr virus latent membrane protein-1 activates CD25 expression in lymphoma cells involving the NF kappaB pathway. *Genes Immun* 2001 Dec;2(8):433-41

[742] Portis T, Harding JC, Ratner L. The contribution of NF-kappa B activity to spontaneous proliferation and resistance to apoptosis in human T-cell leukemia virus type I Tax-induced tumors. *Blood* 2001 Aug 15;98(4):1200-8

[743] Mahieux R, Pise-Masison C, Gessain A, Brady JN, Olivier R, Perret E, Misteli T, Nicot C. Arsenic trioxide induces apoptosis in human T-cell leukemia virus type I- and type II-infected cells by a caspase-3-dependent mechanism involving Bcl-2 cleavage. *Blood* 2001 Dec 15;98(13):3762-9

[744] Vancurova I, Wu R, Miskolci V, Sun S. Increased p50/p50 NF kappaB activation in human papillomavirus type 6- or type II-induced laryngeal papilloma tissue. *J Virol* 2002 Feb;76(3):1533-6

[745] Shepard LW, Yang M, Xie P, Browning DD, Voyno-Yasenetskaya T, Kozasa T, Ye RD. Constitutive activation of NF-kappa B and secretion of interleukin-8 induced by the G protein-coupled receptor of Kaposi's sarcoma-associated herpesvirus involve G alpha(13) and RhoA. *J Biol Chem* 2001 Dec 7;276(49):45979-87

[746] Esposito E, Rotilio D, Di Matteo V, Di Giulio C, Cacchio M, Algeri S. A review of specific dietary antioxidants and the effects on biochemical mechanisms related to neurodegenerative processes. *Neurobiol Aging* 2002 Sep-Oct;23(5):719

[747] Cadenas S, Cadenas AM. Fighting the stranger-antioxidant protection against endotoxin toxicity. *Toxicology* 2002 Oct 30;180(1):45-63

[748] Carcamo JM, Pedraza A, Borquez-Ojeda O, Golde DW. Vitamin C suppresses TNF alpha-induced NF kappa B activation by inhibiting I kappa B alpha phosphorylation. *Biochemistry* 2002 Oct 29;41(43):12995-3002

[749] Fletcher RH, Fairchild KM Vitamins for chronic disease prevention in adults:clinical applications. *JAMA* June 19, 2002;287:3217-3219

[750] Mundy GR. Directions of drug discovery in osteoporosis. *Annu Rev Med* 2002;53:337-54

[751] Wolf AS. The overweight and underweight girl: from findings to prevention *Zentralbl Gynakol* 2002 Mar;124(3):146-52

[752] Espallargues M, Sampietro-Colom L, Estrada MD, Sola M, del Rio L, Setoain J, Granados A. Identifying bone-mass-related risk factors for fracture to guide bone densitometry measurements: a systematic review of the literature. *Osteoporos Int* 2001;12(10):811-22

[753] Barker ME, Blumsohn A. Is weight loss in obese premenopausal women associated with a decline in bone mass? *J Bone Miner Res* 2002 Apr;17(4):746-9

[754] Morley JE. Anorexia, body composition, and ageing. *Curr Opin Clin Nutr Metab Care* 2001 Jan;4(1):9-13

[755] Laharrague P, Truel N, Fontanilles AM, Corberand JX, Penicaud L, Casteilla L. Regulation by cytokines of leptin expression in human bone marrow adipocytes. *Horm Metab Res* 2000 Oct;32(10):381-5

[756] Holloway WR, Collier FM, Aitken CJ, Myers DE, Hodge JM, Malakellis M, Gough TJ, Collier GR, Nicholson GC. Leptin inhibits osteoclast generation. *J Bone Miner Res* 2002 Feb;17(2):200-9

[757] Amling M, Schilling AF, Haberland M, Rueger JM. Leptin: factor in the central nervous system regulation of bone mass. Development of a new understanding of bone remodeling, skeletal reconstruction, skeletal preservation and skeletal repair. *Orthopade* 2001 Jul;30(7):418-24

[758] Karsenty G. Leptin controls bone formation through a hypothalamic relay. *Recent Prog Horm Res* 2001;56:401-15

[759] Watkins BA, Li Y, Seifert MF. Nutraceutical fatty acids as biochemical and molecular modulators of skeletal biology. *J Am Coll Nutr* 2001 Oct;20(5 Suppl):410S-416S; discussion 417S-420S

[760] Romas E, Gillespie MT, Martin TJ. Involvement of receptor activator of NF kappaB ligand and tumor necrosis factor-alpha in bone destruction in rheumatoid arthritis. *Bone* 2002 Feb;30(2):340-6

[761] Kim MS, Chae HJ, Shin TY, Kim HM, Kim HR. Estrogen regulates cytokine release in human mast cells. *Immunopharmacol Immunotoxicol* 2001 Nov;23(4):495-504

[762] Roggia C, Gao Y, Cenci S, Weitzmann MN, Toraldo G, Isaia G, Pacifici R. Up-regulation of TNF-producing T cells in the bone marrow: a key mechanism by which estrogen deficiency induces bone loss in vivo. *Proc Natl Acad Sci U S A* 2001 Nov 20;98(24):13960-5

[763] Ota N, Hunt SC, Nakajima T, Suzuki T, Hosoi T, Orimo H, Shirai Y, Emi M. Linkage of human tumor necrosis factor-alpha to human osteoporosis by sib pair analysis. *Genes Immun* 2000;1(4):260-4

[764] Habtezion A, Silverberg MS, Parkes R, Mikolainis S, Steinhart AH. Risk factors for low bone density in Crohn's disease. *Inflamm Bowel Dis* 2002 Mar;8(2):87-

92

[765] Hansen CM, Hansen D, Holm PK, Binderup L. Vitamin D compounds exert anti-apoptotic effects in human osteosarcoma cells in vitro. *J Steroid Biochem Mol Biol* 2001 Apr;77(1):1-11

[766] Farmer PK, He X, Schmitz ML, Rubin J, Nanes MS. Inhibitory effect of NF kappaB on 1,25-dihydroxyvitamin D(3) and retinoid X receptor function. Am *J Physiol Endocrinol Metab* 2000 Jul;279(1):E213-20

[767] Norazlina M, Ima-Nirwana S, Abul Gapor MT, Abdul Kadir Khalid B. Tocotrienols are needed for normal bone calcification in growing female rats. *Asia Pac J Clin Nutr* 2002;11(3):194-9

[768] Rude RK, Gruber HE, Wei LY, Frausto A, Mills BG. Magnesium Deficiency: Effect on Bone and Mineral Metabolism in the Mouse. *Calcif Tissue Int* 2002 Oct 10;

[769] Tucker KL, Hannan MT, Kiel DP. The acid-base hypothesis: diet and bone in the Framingham Osteoporosis Study. *Eur J Nutr* 2001 Oct;40(5):231-7

[770] Hsing AW, Chua S Jr, Gao YT, Gentzschein E, Chang L, Deng J, Stanczyk FZ. Prostate cancer risk and serum levels of insulin and leptin: a population-based study. *J Natl Cancer Inst* 2001 May 16;93(10):783-9

[771] Stattin P, Soderberg S, Hallmans G, Bylund A, Kaaks R, Stenman UH, Bergh A, Olsson T. Leptin is associated with increased prostate cancer risk: a nested case-referent study. *J Clin Endocrinol Metab* 2001 Mar;86(3):1341-5

[772] Chang S, Hursting SD, Contois JH, Strom SS, Yamamura Y, Babaian RJ, Troncoso P, Scardino PS, Wheeler TM, Amos CI, Spitz MR. Leptin and prostate cancer. *Prostate* 2001 Jan 1;46(1):62-7

[773] Gurumurthy S, Vasudevan KM, Rangnekar VM. Regulation of apoptosis in prostate cancer. *Cancer Metastasis Rev* 2001;20(3-4):225-43

[774] Chen CD, Sawyers CL. NF-kappa B activates prostate-specific antigen expression and is upregulated in androgen-independent prostate cancer. *Mol Cell Biol* 2002 Apr;22(8):2862-70

[775] Gasparian AV, Yao YJ, Kowalczyk D, Lyakh LA, Karseladze A, Slaga TJ, Budunova IV. The role of IKK in constitutive activation of NF kappaB transcription factor in prostate carcinoma cells. *J Cell Sci* 2002 Jan 1;115(Pt 1):141-51

[776] Maliner-Stratton MS, Klein RD, Udayakumar TS, Nagle RB, Bowden GT. Interleukin-1beta-induced promatrilysin expression is mediated by NF kappaB-regulated synthesis of interleukin-6 in the prostate carcinoma cell line, LNCaP. *Neoplasia* 2001 Nov-Dec;3(6):509-20

[777] Catz SD, Johnson JL. Transcriptional regulation of bcl-2 by nuclear factor kappa B and its significance in prostate cancer. *Oncogene* 2001 Nov 1;20(50):7342-51

[778] Kimura K, Markowski M, Bowen C, Gelmann EP. Androgen blocks apoptosis of hormone-dependent prostate cancer cells. *Cancer Res* 2001 Jul 15;61(14):5611-8

[779] Lindholm PF, Bub J, Kaul S, Shidham VB, Kajdacsy-Balla A. The role of constitutive NF kappaB activity in PC-3 human prostate cancer cell invasive behavior. *Clin Exp Metastasis* 2000;18(6):471-9

[780] Huang S, Pettaway CA, Uehara H, Bucana CD, Fidler IJ. Blockade of NF kappaB activity in human prostate cancer cells is associated with suppression of angiogenesis, invasion, and metastasis. *Oncogene* 2001 Jul 12;20(31):4188-97

[781] Muenchen HJ, Lin DL, Walsh MA, Keller ET, Pienta KJ. Tumor necrosis factor-alpha-induced apoptosis in prostate cancer cells through inhibition of nuclear factor-kappaB by an IkappaBalpha "super-repressor". *Clin Cancer Res* 2000 May;6(5):1969-77

[782] Uzzo RG, Leavis P, Hatch W, Gabai VL, Dulin N, Zvartau N, Kolenko VM. Zinc Inhibits Nuclear Factor-kappaB Activation and Sensitizes Prostate Cancer Cells to Cytotoxic Agents. *Clin Cancer Res* 2002 Nov;8(11):3579-83

[783] Verhoeven, D.T.H., Verhagen, H., Goldbohm, R.A., van den Brandt, P.A., and van Poppel, G. 1997 A review of mechanisms underlying anticarcinogenicity by brassica vegetables. *Chem. Bio. Interactions.* 103:79-129.

[784] Cohen JH, Kristal AR, Stanford JL. Fruit and vegetable intakes and prostate cancer risk. *J Natl Cancer Inst* 2000 Jan 5;92(1):61-8

[785] Chinni SR, Sarkar FH. Akt Inactivation Is a Key Event in Indole-3-carbinol-based Apoptosis in PC-3 Cells. *Clin Cancer Res* 2002 Apr;8(4):1228-36

[786] Chinni SR, Li Y, Upadhyay S, Koppolu PK, Sarkar FH. Indole-3-carbinol (I3C) induced cell growth inhibition, G1 cell cycle arrest and apoptosis in prostate cancer cells. *Oncogene* 2001 May 24;20(23):2927-36

[787] Mukhopadhyay A, Bueso-Ramos C, Chatterjee D, Pantazis P, Aggarwal BB. Curcumin downregulates cell survival mechanisms in human prostate cancer cell lines. *Oncogene* 2001 Nov 15;20(52):7597-609

[788] Hour TC, Chen J, Huang CY, Guan JY, Lu SH, Pu YS. Curcumin enhances cytotoxicity of chemotherapeutic agents in prostate cancer cells by inducing p21(WAF1/CIP1) and C/EBPbeta expressions and suppressing NF kappaB activation. *Prostate* 2002 May 15;51(3):211-8

[789] Dhanalakshmi S, Singh RP, Agarwal C, Agarwal R. Silibinin inhibits constitutive and TNFalpha-induced activation of NF kappaB and sensitizes human prostate carcinoma DU145 cells to TNFalpha-induced apoptosis. *Oncogene* 2002 Mar 7;21(11):1759-67

[790] Tozawa K, Okamoto T, Hayashi Y, Sasaki S, Kawai N, Kohri K. N-acetyl-L-cysteine enhances chemotherapeutic effect on prostate cancer cells. *Urol Res* 2002 Mar;30(1):53-8

[791] O'brien SN, Welter BH, Price TM. Presence of leptin in breast cell lines and breast tumors. *Biochem Biophys Res Commun* 1999 Jun 16;259(3):695-8

[792] Tessitore L, Vizio B, Jenkins O, De Stefano I, Ritossa C, Argiles JM, Benedetto C, Mussa A. Leptin expression in colorectal and breast cancer patients. *Int J Mol Med* 2000 Apr;5(4):421-6

[793] Petridou E, Papadiamantis Y, Markopoulos C, Spanos E, Dessypris N, Trichopoulos D. Leptin and insulin growth factor I in relation to breast cancer (Greece). *Cancer Causes Control* 2000 May;11(5):383-8

[794] Dieudonne MN, Machinal-Quelin F, Serazin-Leroy V, Leneveu MC, Pecquery R, Giudicelli Y. Leptin mediates a proliferative response in human MCF7 breast cancer cells. *Biochem Biophys Res Commun* 2002 Apr 26;293(1):622-8

[795] Laud K, Gourdou I, Pessemesse L, Peyrat JP,

Djiane J. Identification of leptin receptors in human breast cancer: functional activity in the T47-D breast cancer cell line. *Mol Cell Endocrinol* 2002 Feb 25;188(1-2):219-26

[796] Okumura M, Yamamoto M, Sakuma H, Kojima T, Maruyama T, Jamali M, Cooper D, Yasuda K. Leptin and high glucose stimulate cell proliferation in MCF-7 human breast cancer cells: reciprocal involvement of PKC-alpha and PPAR expression. *Biochim Biophys Acta* 2002 Oct 21;1592(2):107

[797] Bhat-Nakshatri P, Sweeney CJ, Nakshatri H. Identification of signal transduction pathways involved in constitutive NF kappaB activation in breast cancer cells. *Oncogene* 2002 Mar 27;21(13):2066-78

[798] Toillon RA, Descamps S, Adriaenssens E, Ricort JM, Bernard D, Boilly B, Le Bourhis X. Normal breast epithelial cells induce apoptosis of breast cancer cells via Fas signaling. *Exp Cell Res* 2002 Apr 15;275(1):31-43

[799] Marttunen MB, Andersson S, Hietanen P, Karonen SL, Koistinen HA, Koivisto VA, Tiitinen A, Ylikorkala O. Antiestrogenic tamoxifen and toremifene increase serum leptin levels in postmenopausal breast cancer patients. Maturitas 2000 May 29;35(2):175-9

[800] Ozet A, Arpaci F, Yilmaz MI, Ayta H, Ozturk B, Komurcu S, Yavuz AA, Tezcan Y,Acikel C. Effects of tamoxifen on the serum leptin level in patients with breast cancer. *Jpn J Clin Oncol* 2001 Sep;31(9):424-7

[801] Goodwin PJ, Ennis M, Pritchard KI, Trudeau ME, Koo J, Madarnas Y, Hartwick W, Hoffman B, Hood N. Fasting insulin and outcome in early-stage breast cancer: results of a prospective cohort study. *J Clin Oncol* 2002 Jan 1;29(1):42-51.

[802] Nishino M, Hayakawa K, Nakamura Y, Morimoto T, Mukaihara S. Effects of tamoxifen on hepatic fat content and the development of hepatic steatosis in patients with breast cancer: high frequency of involvement and rapid reversal after completion of tamoxifen therapy. *AJR Am J Roentgenol* 2003 Jan;180(1):129-34

[803] Wang H, Isaksson E, Von Schoultz B, Cline JM, Sahlin L. The effect of long-term treatment with steroid hormones or tamoxifen on oestrogen receptors (alpha and beta) in the endometrium of ovariectomized cynomolgus macaques. *J Endocrinol* 2002 Dec;175(3):673-81

[804] The ATAC Trialists' Group. Arimidex, tamoxifen alone or in combination. Anastrozole alone or in combination with tamoxifen versus tamoxifen alone for adjuvant treatment of postmenopausal women with early breast cancer: first results of the ATAC randomised trial. *Lancet 2002* Jun 22;359(9324):2131-9

[805] Baum M. Has tamoxifen had its day? *Breast Cancer Res* 2002;4(6):213-7

[806] Gadd SL, Hobbs G, Miller MR. Acetaminophen-induced proliferation of estrogen-responsive breast cancer cells is associated with increases in c-myc RNA expression and NF kappaB activity. *Toxicol Sci* 2002 Apr;66(2):233-43

[807] Schwenke DC. Does lack of tocopherols and tocotrienols put women at increased risk of breast cancer? *J Nutr Biochem* 2002 Jan;13(1):2-20

[808] Sylvester PW, Nachnani A, Shah S, Briski KP. Role of GTP-binding proteins in reversing the antiproliferative effects of tocotrienols in preneoplastic mammary epithelial cells. *Asia Pac J Clin Nutr* 2002 Oct;11 Suppl 7:S452-S459

[809] Nesaretnam K, Dorasamy S, Darbre PD. Tocotrienols inhibit growth of ZR-75-1 breast cancer cells. *Int J Food Sci Nutr* 2000;51 Suppl:S95-103

[810] McIntyre BS, Briski KP, Gapor A, Sylvester PW. Antiproliferative and apoptotic effects of tocopherols and tocotrienols on preneoplastic and neoplastic mouse mammary epithelial cells. *Proc Soc Exp Biol Med* 2000 Sep;224(4):292-301

[811] Yu W, Simmons-Menchaca M, Gapor A, Sanders BG, Kline K. Induction of apoptosis in human breast cancer cells by tocopherols and tocotrienols. *Nutr Cancer* 1999;33(1):26-32

[812] Nesaretnam K, Stephen R, Dils R, Darbre P. Tocotrienols inhibit the growth of human breast cancer cells irrespective of estrogen receptor status. *Lipids* 1998 May;33(5):461-9

[813] Guthrie N, Gapor A, Chambers AF, Carroll KK. Inhibition of proliferation of estrogen receptor-negative MDA-MB-435 and -positive MCF-7 human breast cancer cells by palm oil tocotrienols and tamoxifen, alone and in combination. *J Nutr* 1997 Mar;127(3):544S-548S

[814] Theriault A, Chao JT, Gapor A.Tocotrienol is the most effective vitamin E for reducing endothelial expression of adhesion molecules and adhesion to monocytes. *Atherosclerosis* 2002 Jan;160(1):21-30

[815] Ip C, Chin SF, Scimeca JA, Pariza MW. Mammary cancer prevention by conjugated dienoic derivative of linoleic acid. *Cancer Res* 1991 Nov 15;51(22):6118-24

[816] Choi Y, Park Y, Storkson JM, Pariza MW, Ntambi JM. Inhibition of stearoyl-CoA desaturase activity by the cis-9,trans-11 isomer and the trans-10,cis-12 isomer of conjugated linoleic acid in MDA-MB-231 and MCF-7 human breast cancer cells. *Biochem Biophys Res Commun* 2002 Jun 21;294(4):785-90

[817] Devery R, Miller A, Stanton C. Conjugated linoleic acid and oxidative behaviour in cancer cells. *Biochem Soc Trans* 2001 May;29(Pt 2):341-4

[818] Hubbard NE, Lim D, Summers L, Erickson KL. Reduction of murine mammary tumor metastasis by conjugated linoleic acid. *Cancer Lett* 2000 Mar 13;150(1):93-100

[819] O'Shea M, Devery R, Lawless F, Murphy J, Stanton C. Milk fat conjugated linoleic acid (CLA) inhibits growth of human mammary MCF-7 cancer cells. *Anticancer Res* 2000 Sep- Oct;20(5B):3591-601

[820] Park Y, Allen KG, Shultz TD. Modulation of MCF-7 breast cancer cell signal transduction by linoleic acid and conjugated linoleic acid in culture. *Anticancer Res* 2000 Mar-Apr;20(2A):669-76

[821] Aro A, Mannisto S, Salminen I, Ovaskainen ML, Kataja V, Uusitupa M. Inverse association between dietary and serum conjugated linoleic acid and risk of breast cancer in postmenopausal women. *Nutr Cancer* 2000;38(2):151-7

[822] Majumder B, Wahle KW, Moir S, Schofield A, Choe SN, Farquharson A, Grant I, Heys SD. Conjugated linoleic acids (CLAs) regulate the expression of key apoptotic genes in human breast cancer cells. *FASEB J* 2002 Sep;16(11):1447-9

[823] Suganuma M, Sueoka E, Sueoka N, Okabe S, Fujiki H. Mechanisms of cancer prevention by tea polyphe-

nols based on inhibition of TNF-alpha expression. *Biofactors* 2000;13(1-4):67-72

[824] Pianetti S, Guo S, Kavanagh KT, Sonenshein GE. Green tea polyphenol epigallocatechin-3 gallate inhibits Her-2/neu signaling, proliferation, and transformed phenotype of breast cancer cells. *Cancer Res* 2002 Feb 1;62(3):652-5

[825] Vergote D, Cren-Olive C, Chopin V, Toillon RA, Rolando C, Hondermarck H, Le Bourhis X. (-)-Epigallocatechin (EGC) of green tea induces apoptosis of human breast cancer cells but not of their normal counterparts. *Breast Cancer Res Treat* 2002 Dec;76(3):195-201

[826] Brownson DM, Azios NG, Fuqua BK, Dharmawardhane SF, Mabry TJ. Flavonoid effects relevant to cancer. *J Nutr* 2002 Nov;132(11 Suppl):3482S-3489S

[827] Banerjee S, Bueso-Ramos C, Aggarwal BB. Suppression of 7,12-dimethylbenz(a)anthracene-induced mammary carcinogenesis in rats by resveratrol: role of nuclear factor-kappaB, cyclooxygenase 2, and matrix metalloprotease 9. *Cancer Res* 2002 Sep 1;62(17):4945-54

[828] Bhat KP, Lantvit D, Christov K, Mehta RG, Moon RC, Pezzuto JM. Estrogenic and antiestrogenic properties of resveratrol in mammary tumor models. *Cancer Res* 2001 Oct 15;61(20):7456-63

[829] Serrero G, Lu R. Effect of resveratrol on the expression of autocrine growth modulators in human breast cancer cells. *Antioxid Redox Signal* 2001 Dec;3(6):969-79

[830] Bove K, Lincoln DW, Tsan MF. Effect of resveratrol on growth of 4T1 breast cancer cells in vitro and in vivo. *Biochem Biophys Res Commun* 2002 Mar 8;291(4):1001-5

[831] Waffo-Teguo P, Hawthorne ME, Cuendet M, Merillon JM, Kinghorn AD, Pezzuto JM, Mehta RG. Potential cancer-chemopreventive activities of wine stilbenoids and flavans extracted from grape (Vitis vinifera) cell cultures. *Nutr Cancer* 2001;40(2):173-9

[832] Choi JA, Kim JY, Lee JY, Kang CM, Kwon HJ, Yoo YD, Kim TW, Lee YS, Lee SJ. Induction of cell cycle arrest and apoptosis in human breast cancer cells by quercetin. *Int J Oncol* 2001 Oct;19(4):837-44

[833] Han D, Tachibana H, Yamada K. Inhibition of environmental estrogen-induced proliferation of human breast carcinoma MCF-7 cells by flavonoids. *In Vitro Cell Dev Biol Anim* 2001 May;37(5):275-82

[834] Scambia G, Ranelletti FO, Benedetti Panici P, et al. Quercetin inhibits the growth of a multidrug-resistant estrogen-receptor-negative MCF-7 human breast-cancer cell line expressing type II estrogen-binding sites. *Cancer Chemother Pharmacol* (Germany) 28:255-258; 1991.

[835] Piantelli M, Tatone D, Castrilli G, Savini F, Maggiano N, Larocca LM, Ranelletti FO, Natali PG. Quercetin and tamoxifen sensitize human melanoma cells to hyperthermia. *Melanoma Res* 2001 Oct;11(5):469-76

[836] Michnoviez JJ, Bradlow HL. Altered estrogen metabolism and excretion in humans following consumption of indole-3-carbinol. *Nutr Cancer*. 1991; 16(1): 59-66.

[837] Michnoviez JJ., Bradlow HL. Induction of estradiol metabolism by dietary indole-3-carbinol in humans. *J Natl Cancer Inst*. 1990; 82(11):947-949.

[838] Michnoviez JJ, Bradlow HL. Altered estrogen metabolism and excretion in humans following consumption of indole-3-carbinol. *Nutr Cancer*. 1991; 16(1): 59-66.

[839] Cover CM, Hsieh SJ, Tran SH, Hallden G, Kim GS, Bjeldanes LF and Firestone GL. Indole-3-Carbinol inhibits the expression of cyclin-dependent kinase-6 and induces a G1 cell cycle arrest of human breast cancer cells independent of estrogen receptor signaling. *J Biol Chem*. 1998; 273:3838-3847.

[840] Cover CM, Hsieh SJ, Cram EJ, Hong C, Riby JE, Bjeldanes LF, and Firestone GL. Indole-3-carbinol and tamoxifen cooperate to arrest the cell cycle of MCF-7 human breast cancer cells. *Cancer Research* 1999; 59:1244-1251.

[841] Fujiki H, Suganuma M, Okabe S, Kurusu M, Imai K, Nakachi K. Involvement of TNF-alpha changes in human cancer development, prevention and palliative care. *Mech Ageing Dev* 2002 Nov;123(12):1655-63

INDEX

cancer
  acetaminophen, 366
  andropause, 281
  body rhythm, 14
  breast cancer, 267-268, 288, 298, 307, 363-368
  cachexia, 241, 245
  curcumin, 360
  cyclosporine, 19
  Epstein Barr Virus, 350
  estrogen, 293, 364-365
  GM-CSF, 340, 342
  green tea, 367
  growth hormone risk, 265, 267
  IL-6, 358-359
  indole-3-caribinol, 360, 367
  insulin resistance, 365
  leptin, 32, 49, 138, 357, 363
  liver, 345, 349
  N-Acetyl-Cysteine, 361
  NF-kappaB, 339, 342, 357-360
  pancreatic, 245, 343
  parthenolide, 349
  prostate, 357-361
  quercetin, 367
  silymarin, 361
  Tamoxifen, 364-367
  TNFa, 56, 63-64, 339-340, 342-343, 350-351, 357, 363
  tocotrienols, 366
  trans-resveratrol, 367
  viral, 349-350
  zinc deficiency, 358
candida, 63-66, 79, 112
carbohydrate
  breakfast, 150
  dinner, 260
  fluid retention, 162
  ghrelin, 190
  hyperglycemia, 260
  insulin resistance, 150, 155-156, 228
  leptin rhythm, 41
  liver metabolism, 149
  male sexual dysfunction, 284
  serotonin, 180
  snacking, 155, 260

  snacking - raising cholesterol, 130
  too low an amount, 156, 158, 231
  total body reserves, 128
carnosine, 181-182, 323
cellulite, 238-239, 246
cholesterol, 7, 11, 20, 54, 130, 132, 136, 139
choline, 199
chromium, 336
cirrhosis, 62
cocaine and amphetamine regulating transcript (CART), 67-68, 71, 106
corticotrophin-releasing hormone (CRH), 321
cortisol, 41, 167-168, 218, 220-221, 224-226, 228-229, 232-233, 238, 240, 244-245, 259-260, 267, 271, 273-274, 281, 283, 320, 322, 334
cravings
  alcohol, 59-61
  caffeine, 174
  dopamine, 185
  ghrelin, 187
  histamine, 181
  hyperglycemia, 145
  hypoglycemia, 150
  leptin causing, 5, 25, 41, 53, 253
  low calcium causing, 182
  neuropeptide Y, 177-178
  physical fitness, 185, 253-254
  serotonin, 180, 186
  stress, 180-181
  stress eating, 61, 168-169
  sugar cravings, 150
  sunshine reduces, 183
curcumin, 327, 360

D

DHA, 203, 323
DHEA, 282
diabetes, 3, 12, 48-49, 125, 128-129, 132, 135, 138, 281, 293
diet drugs, dangers of, 68, 192
digestive system, 146, 151, 156, 169, 189, 201, 216

G

H

I

Mastering Leptin
ONLINE RESOURCES

- Tips for success
- Nutritional supplements
- Free e-newsletter from Byron J. Richards
- Latest findings on leptin and weight loss
- Take the Leptin Quiz
- Watch free videos online
- Leptin Diet approved recipes

Visit:

www.WellnessResources.com/leptin
or call: 800-717-9355 for more information.